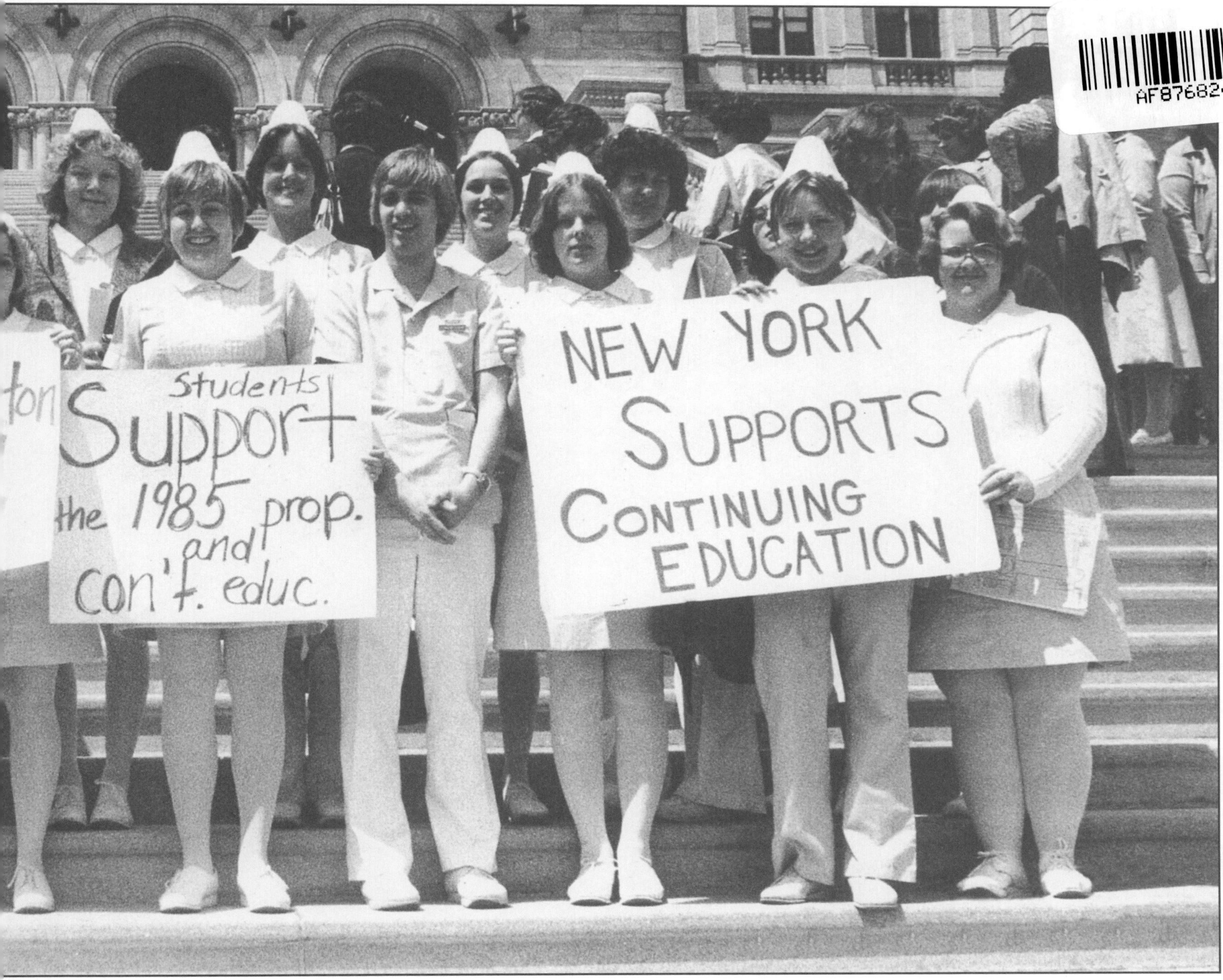
ton
Students
Support
the 1985 prop.
and
con't. educ.
NEW YORK
SUPPORTS
CONTINUING
EDUCATION

THE NEW YORK STATE NURSES ASSOCIATION

EXCELSIOR

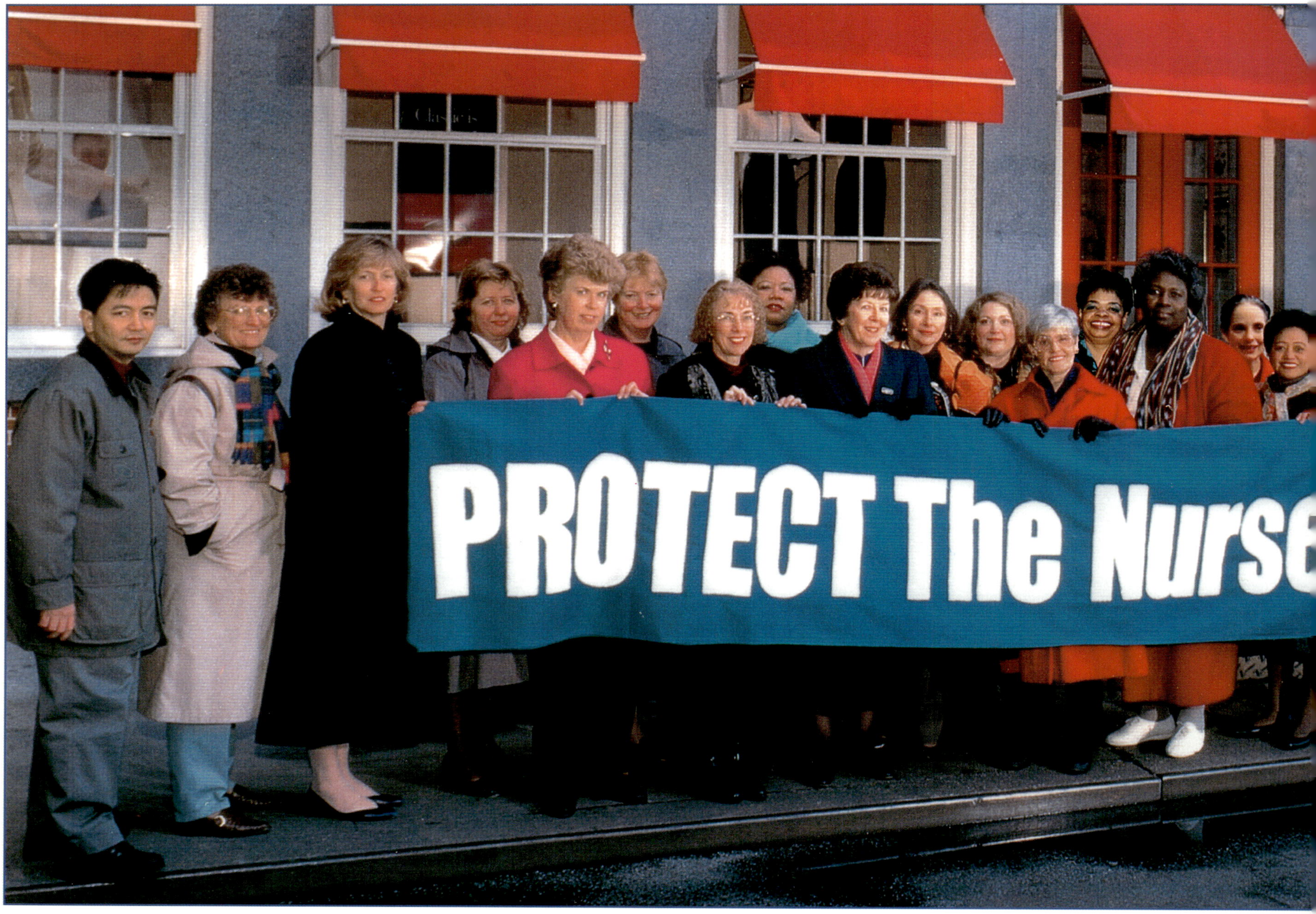
PROTECT The Nurse

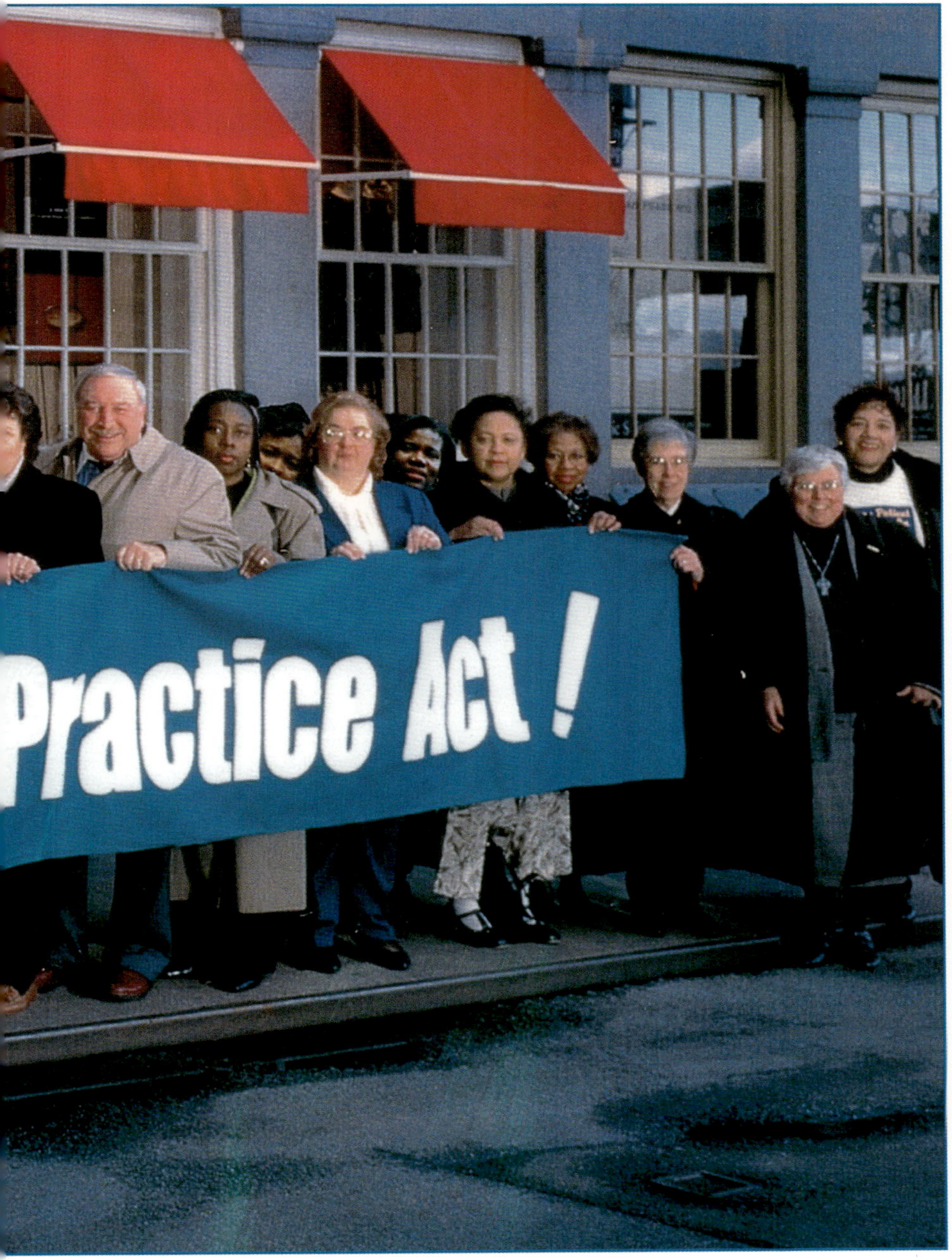

Honoring Our Past ~ Building Our Future

A History of The New York State Nurses Association

By

Julie M. Pavri

Dedicated to New York nurses — past, present, and future.

PREVIOUS PAGE: In 1997 the association celebrated the twenty-fifth anniversary of the 1972 Nurse Practice Act revision. NYSNA leaders gathered to demonstrate their ongoing commitment to protection of the act. *Photograph by Ansell Horn.*

CONTENTS

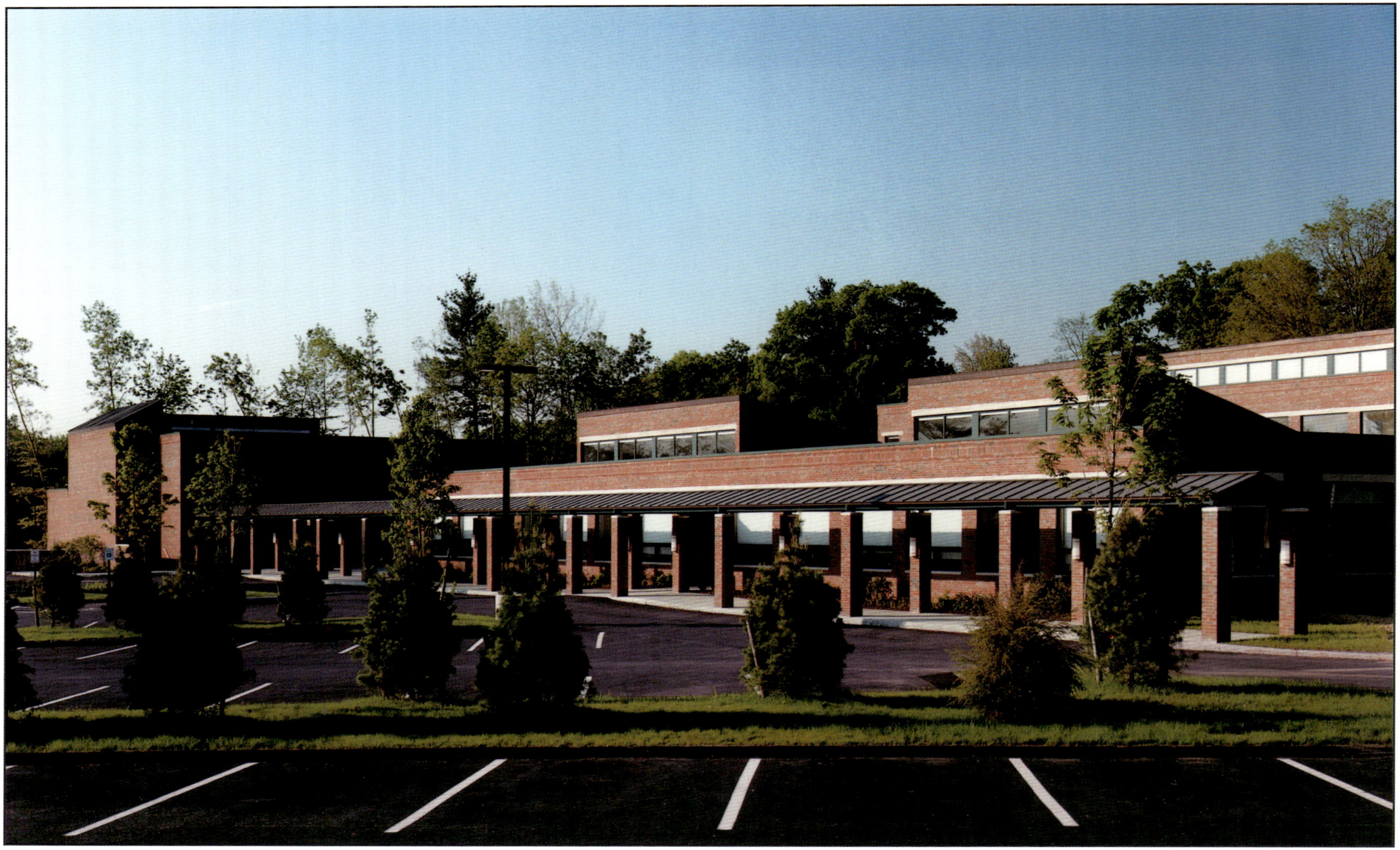

NYSNA's new headquarters opened in June 1995.
Photograph by Randall Perry.

FOREWORD

Documenting the rich history of the New York State Nurses Association to celebrate the 100th anniversary of this extraordinary association has been a labor of love. Guided by the thoughtful recommendations of nurse historians and the board of directors, we have sought to place the historical markers of NYSNA within the professional and social contexts of their times. To the extent that we have succeeded, *all* professional nurses in New York will be helped to understand and take pride in the unbroken chain of achievements that has been a product of the visionary, tenacious, resolute, and caring leaders and members of NYSNA.

Fundamentally, the association is about its members' contributions to the advancement of the profession of nursing, the welfare of all nurses, and the policies that shape the provision of health care to the people of New York. The courage and conviction of nurses everywhere is nowhere more vividly demonstrated than in New York. Since 1901, the leaders of our association have worked with tireless energy and commitment to empower nurses through securing (and then protecting) appropriate legislation, most especially a Nurse Practice Act that enables, recognizes, and promotes the independent practice of autonomous professional nursing.

NYSNA has led the nation with uncompromising dedication to the highest possible standards of practice, education, and professionalism, often at great cost and in spite of enormous opposition from without and within the profession. This book seeks to describe the passion for nursing and for NYSNA that is the heart and soul of so many of the members, leaders, and staff of the association.

FACING PAGE: Throughout NYSNA's history, members have faithfully attended and participated in ANA conventions. The directors of visiting nurse associations in Yonkers, Mt. Vernon, and New Rochelle attended ANA's convention in Atlantic City. *Photograph by Fred Hass & Son.*

For much of its history, NYSNA was built solely upon the drive of its member leaders. Their personal sacrifices and contributions could not be overstated in *volumes* of histories. Our collective consciousness as an organization flows from their definition of the work of a professional association. In later years, these leaders were joined by expert staff, many of whom have dedicated large parts of their careers to supporting and carrying out the directions of countless boards, committees, task forces, and Voting Bodies. To each of them, and to successive generations of the members of NYSNA, this book is given with unending appreciation.

MARTHA L. ORR MN, RN, CAE
Executive Director

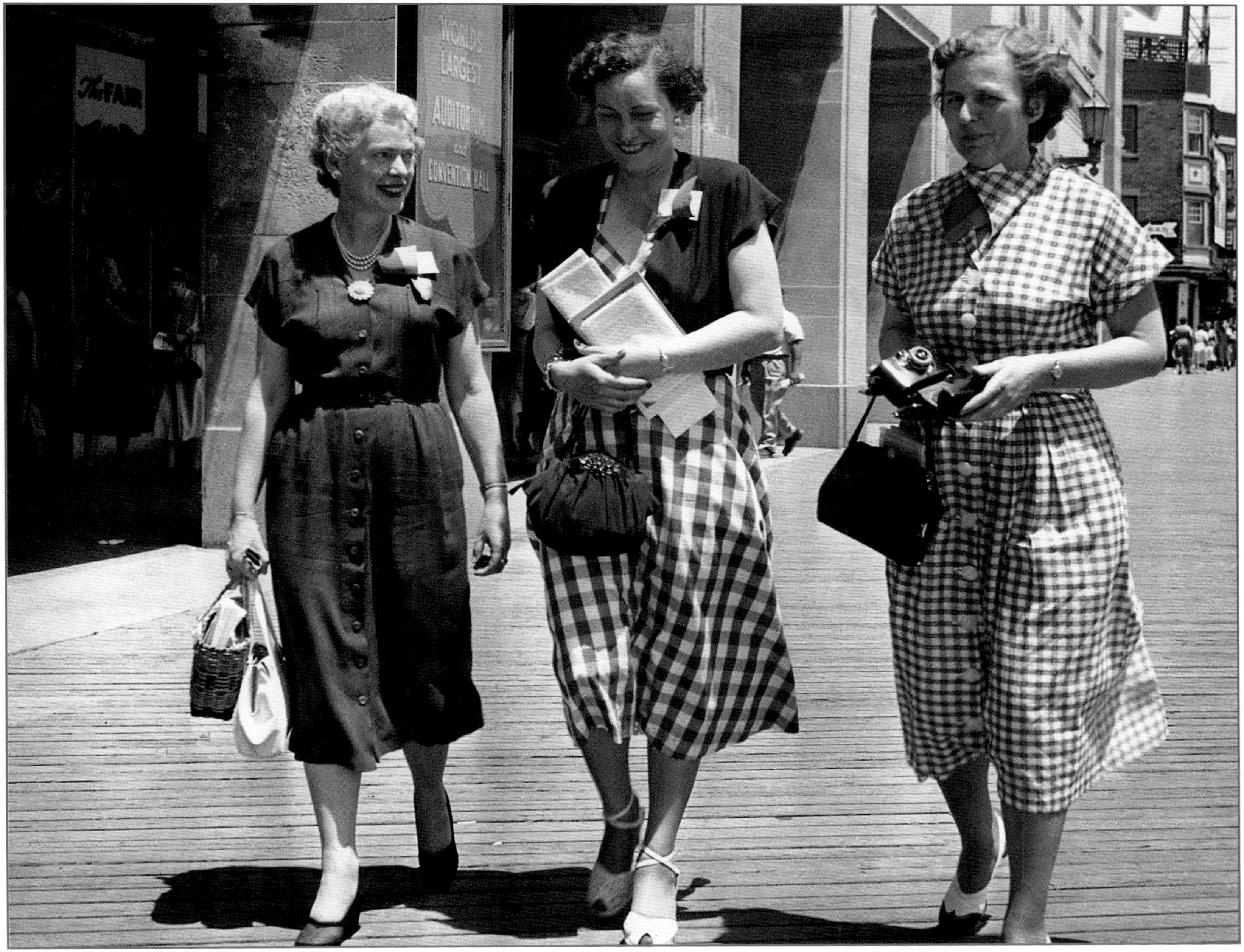
The FAIR
WORLD'S LARGEST AUDITORIUM and CONVENTION HALL

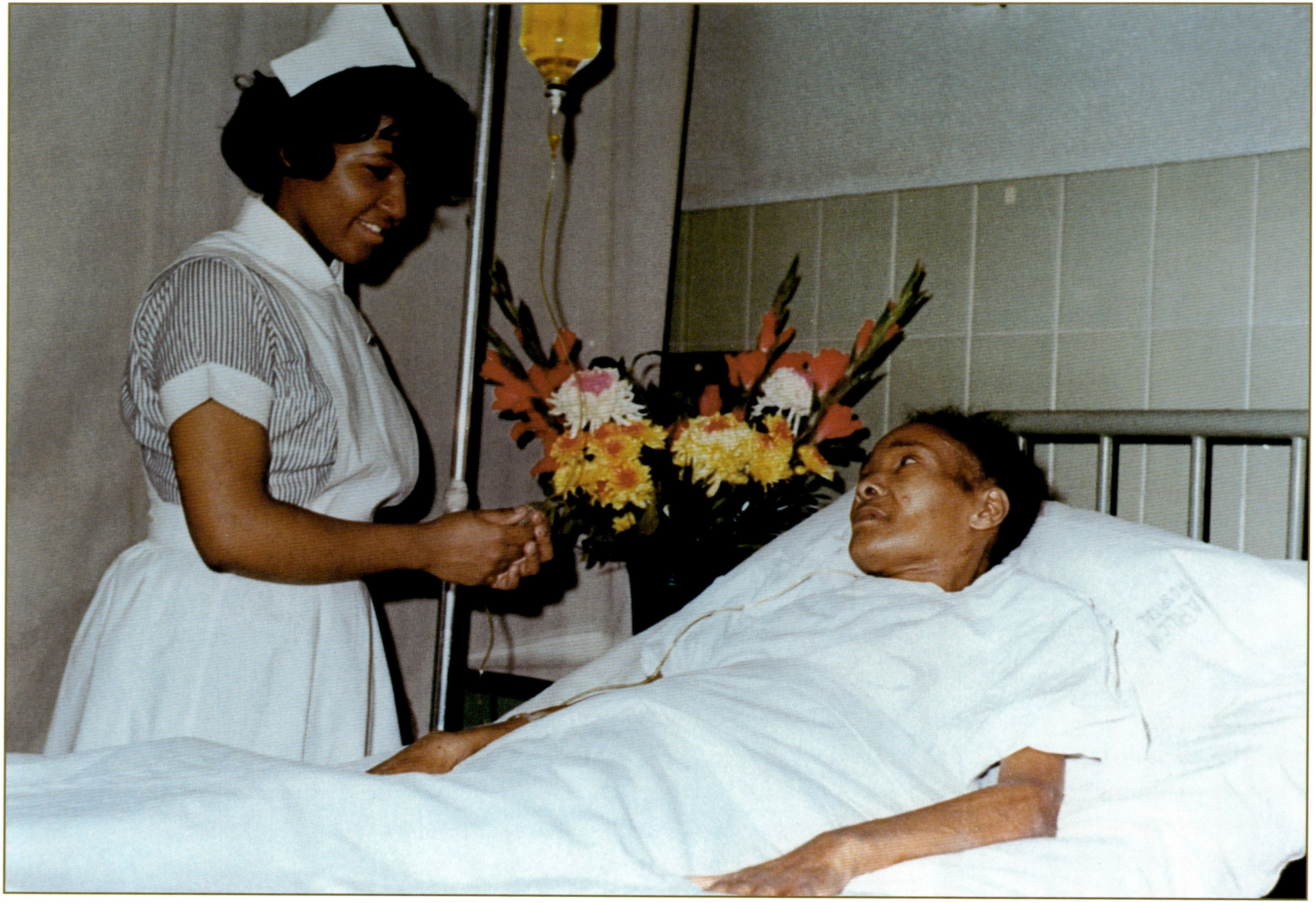

ACKNOWLEDGMENTS

This history could not have been completed without the help of many colleagues, and the support of my family. Special thanks go to Dr. Nettie Birnbach, Martha Orr, Dr. Cindy Gurney, and Dr. Cathryne Welch for their thoughtful review of the manuscript and helpful suggestions. Despite their many other obligations, NYSNA staff members Martha Orr, Tina Gerardi, Wendy Burbank, Karen Ballard, Nancey Agard, Gail DeMarco, Barbara Garrett, Ellen Ellis, and Warren Hawkes generously assisted in the research process by reviewing original documents, and Anne Schott provided invaluable assistance in photograph selection and reproduction. NYSNA library staff, and Linda Sickler at the Foundation of NYSNA cheerfully provided needed information, often at a moment's notice. Thanks go to all who provided photographs, especially Phil Maples at Rochester General Hospital, Mary Tomaselli of the Bellevue School of Nursing Alumnae Association, Mildred M. Norman of the Alumni Association of Harlem Hospital School of Nursing, Steve Hooper, Julie Colon, and the Westchester Medical Center. All photographs not otherwise credited were obtained from the NYSNA Archives at the Foundation of NYSNA. For their daily support, thanks go to my husband and my daughters. Kate gently prodded and encouraged me throughout this project, while AK provided long distance support. ■

FACING PAGE: Administering and managing intravenous therapy became a routine component of nursing care after NYSNA sought an opinion from New York's attorney general. *Courtesy Alumni Association of Harlem Hospital Center School of Nursing.*

CHAPTER ONE

Nursing in 1900

AS THE NINETEENTH CENTURY ROLLED INTO THE TWENTIETH, A TIME OF revolutionary change in every sphere of life and learning, the vast majority of practicing nurses lacked any formal training, even though modern training schools had been graduating nurses for more than twenty-five years. Although hospital use was growing rapidly, most people avoided them if at all possible, and nursing care was provided primarily in the home. By far the majority of nurses worked in homes as private duty nurses, with some employed as superintendents or head nurses in hospitals, and a few nurses in large cities provided nursing and social services to the poor in the emerging field of visiting nursing.

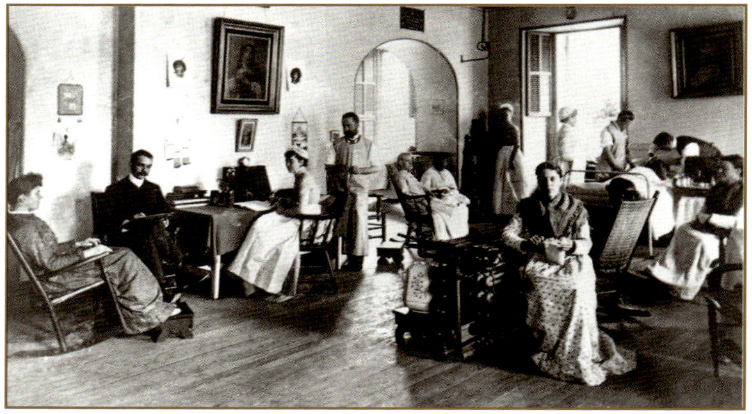

LEFT: Private hospital rooms were much more home-like than the large wards. *Courtesy Bellevue Alumnae Association.*

Nurses cared for surgical patients and those with chronic illness and contagious diseases. Typhoid fever and pneumonia were especially prevalent and required lengthy periods of convalescence. Techniques of sterilization, disinfection, and isolation were critical elements of patient care, as were massage, the prevention and treatment of decubiti, mouth care, and nutrition. Instructions for preparing various skin care ointments, mouth washes, and enemas, as well as recipes for various sickroom nourishments were frequently included in the nursing journals of the day.

The private duty nurse was engaged by the patient's family to provide around-the-clock care in the home. She was responsible not only to the physician, but to the family as well. She was expected to attend to the patient day and night, sleeping for short periods only if the patient was resting comfortably. A daily walk—at the convenience of the family—was her only "time off." The average salary in large cities was $25 per week or $4 a day. The rate for "special cases" — male patients, obstetrical patients, or patients with contagious diseases — was $5 per day. If she was a hard worker, and had established a coterie of loyal families and physicians, the private duty nurse could expect to work nine to ten months each year.

The nurse had to manage her earnings carefully to provide for living expenses when she was not employed. Both hospital and private duty nurses were admonished to set aside money for the future when they were no longer able to withstand the hard work and long hours.[1] Between assignments, private duty nurses stayed with family or secured lodging at a boardinghouse. Nurses' clubs and residences, often established by training school alumnae associations, were gaining popularity as places for rest, relaxation, and socialization, and as more desirable temporary living quarters.

RIGHT: Most graduate nurses at the turn of the century, such as Esther Wahlquist shown here, worked in homes as private duty nurses. *Courtesy Foundation of NYSNA Archives.*

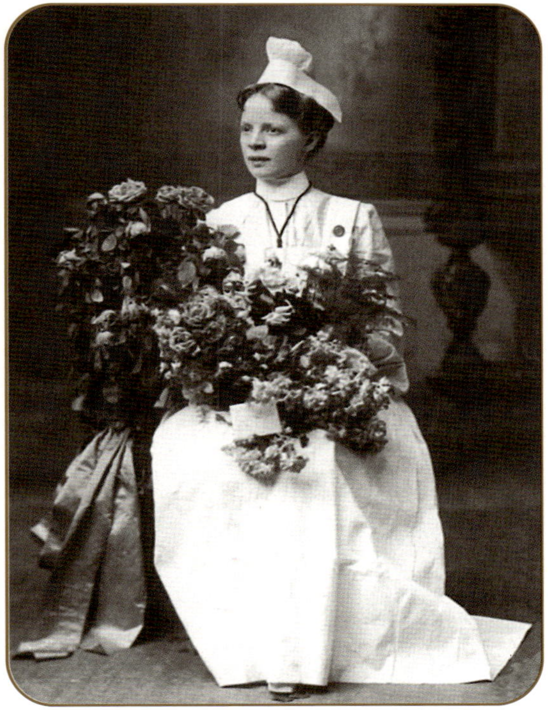

Whether in home or hospital, absolute loyalty and obedience to the physician were expected, and the nurse was solely responsible for carrying out all of the physician's orders. This included the administration of medications and various treatments. Special baths were ordered, as were applications of leeches and poultices, "cupping," dressing changes, and bandaging. The nurse was also responsible for maintaining the comfort of the patient, preparing and serving food, and maintaining the sickroom environment. Although maid service was sometimes available, nurses spent many hours mopping, washing windows, scrubbing, washing and folding clothing and linen, rolling bandages, bringing in coal, and filling and cleaning oil or kerosene lamps. Surgery was performed in both home and hospital. The nurse prepared the room, the patient, and all instruments and supplies, assisted the physician during the procedure, and often administered the anesthetic.

Despite long hours, back-breaking work, and poor pay, nursing was one of the few "respectable" professions for women, and would-be nurses flocked to training schools. The emerging profession offered stimulating, rewarding work, and a rare opportunity for independence.[2]

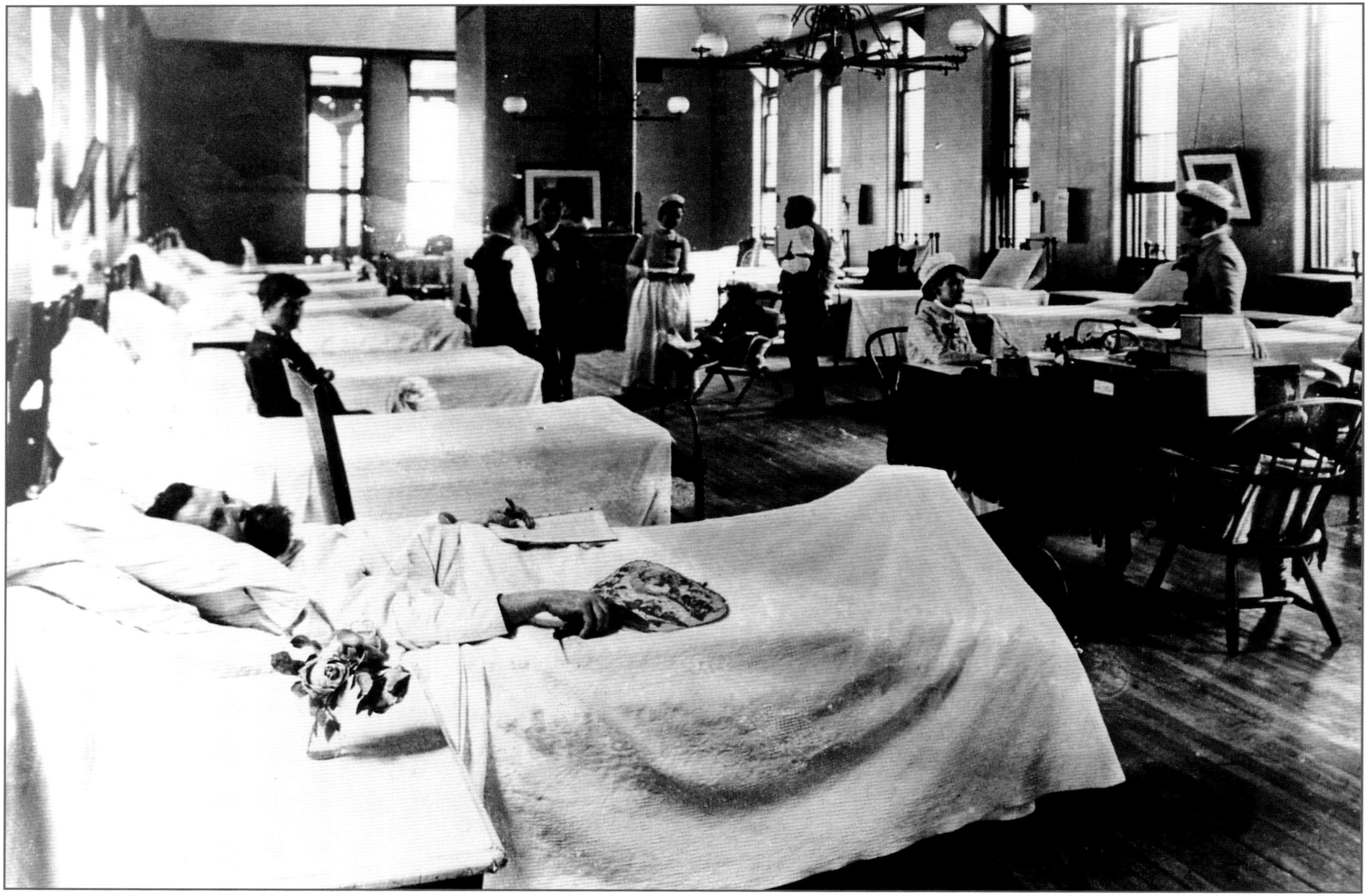

ABOVE: At the turn of the century, hospitalized patients were cared for in large wards like this one at Bellevue Hospital.
Courtesy Bellevue Alumnae Association.

AN INSTITUTION THAT WILL ENDURE 1901~1910

At the turn of the century, the United States was in the midst of sweeping economic, social, and political reforms. Soaring immigration and the shift from an agrarian to an industrial society sent rural Americans streaming to the cities, creating overcrowded living conditions, poor sanitation, poverty, and high rates of disease. The newly arrived lived in crowded, squalid tenements and were cut off from their former network of support and health care. The popular "literature of protest" exposed a variety of social ills to the public and contributed to a proliferation of humanitarian activities. As the gap between the wealthy and the poor widened, well-to-do reformers formed charitable organizations, funded settlement houses, and advocated for legislative changes both in the spirit of altruism and to protect the spread of disease into their own neighborhoods.[3] Hospitals proliferated at the rate of two or three a week, with 40 percent of the hospitals in New York in 1910 having been established after 1900.[4] Most of the newly established hospitals were small, private institutions, many specializing in mental illness, nervous disorders, women's and children's diseases, or contagious illnesses.

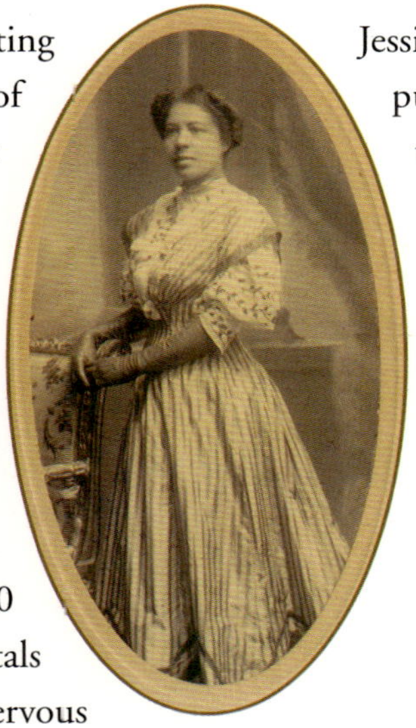

Jessie Sleet, the first black public health nurse in the United States, was a charter member of NYSNA and one of its incorporators. *Courtesy the family of Jessie Sleet Scales.*

The formal training of nurses in the United States had begun in 1873, when three schools of nursing based on the model of Florence Nightingale were established, one at New York's Bellevue Hospital. In England, the Nightingale schools were endowed.

However, in the United States, financing was secured by agreements with the hospitals whereby nursing services were provided in exchange for clinical experience for the pupil nurses.[5] These two-year apprentice programs markedly improved the care provided by these hospitals. As hospitals realized the economic advantages, the number of training schools skyrocketed from 432 in 1900 to 1,129 a mere ten years later. In New York alone, there were 84 training schools for nurses in 1903, and 123 registered schools by 1911.[6]

In 1900 New York was at the very center of the evolving profession of nursing. The state was home to Bellevue Hospital's training school, as well as several other large and prestigious schools for nurses. The *Trained Nurse and Hospital Review,* one of the first nursing journals, was published in Buffalo, and Rochester was home to the new *American Journal of Nursing* (AJN). A visiting nurse association was established in Brooklyn in 1888, and in 1893 Lillian Wald launched public health nursing when she established the famous Henry Street Settlement in a slum neighborhood on New York's lower east side. On the western edge of the state, nurses in Buffalo formed one of the country's first visiting nurse associations, opened a nurse's registry in 1896, and organized the Trained Nurses Association of Buffalo in 1895. Across the state, nurses formed alumnae associations to provide mutual support and advance the profession.

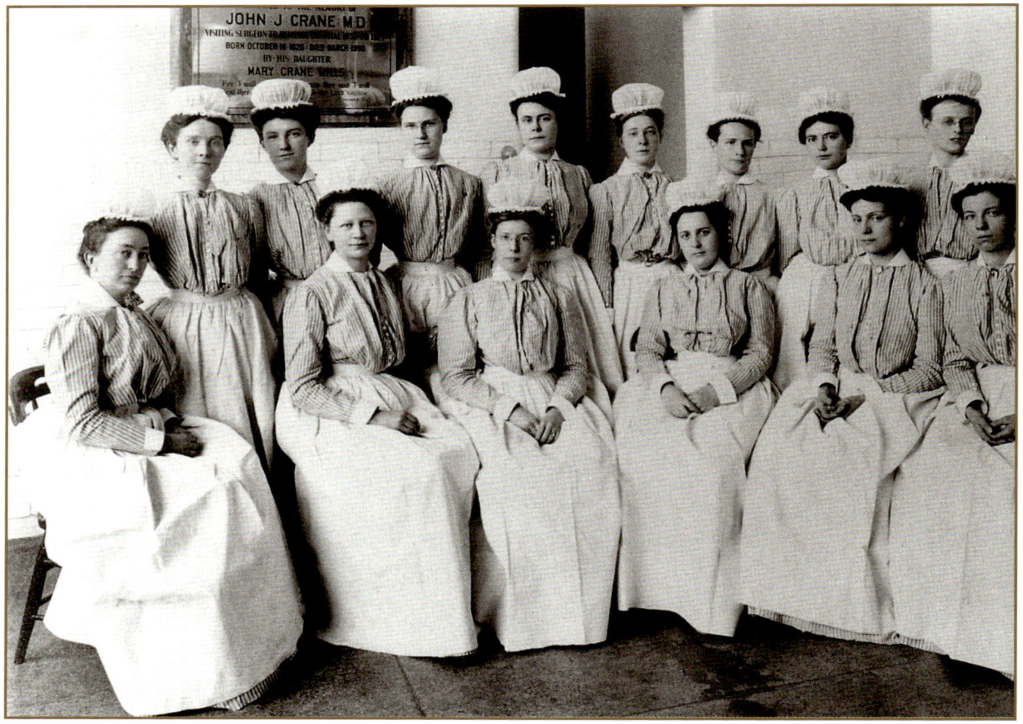

ABOVE: Many Bellevue School of Nursing graduates, perhaps some from this 1903 class, were active in NYSNA, and many went on to assume positions of state and national leadership. *Courtesy Bellevue Alumnae Association.*

Hospital superintendents, nurses who were often in charge of both the training school and the hospital nursing service, had administrative, supervisory, and teaching responsibilities. There was little coordination or communication among the superintendents, and there were no standard entrance requirements, length of program, or curricula for these early schools. A nurse could be trained in a large, well-established school in a general hospital, in a small specialty hospital, or even through a correspondence course. Many small schools lacked equipment and failed to provide a variety of clinical experiences, while correspondence schools provided no hospital experience at all. "Private individuals and hospitals operated schools of nursing for personal profit; the pupils did work which saved the management the wages of servants; and, when they were turned out of the hospital, they had little nursing education, but they did have a big diploma . . . Commercial promoters of schools of nursing found that a liberal distribution of pins and badges could serve as substitute for a burdensome curriculum."[7]

This was an era when the frontier individualism of American society was giving way to cooperative effort, and several occupational groups were forming associations. The settlement house, labor, and suffrage movements had also begun to demonstrate the value of uniting and organizing to achieve goals. Superintendents of the larger schools, concerned about the disparities in the quality of training programs, met in 1893 to form a society to raise educational standards. This American Society of Superintendents of Training Schools for Nurses became the National League of Nursing Education (NLNE), and later the National League for Nursing (NLN). Nurses who formed this first national nursing organization identified the need for nursing to control its own educational standards and promoted unification as a means to this end.[8]

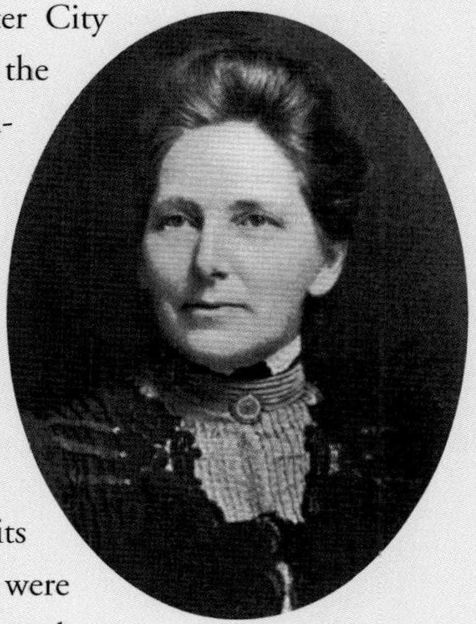

Sophia French Palmer came to Rochester in 1896 as the Superintendent of the Rochester City Hospital. She was a founder of the American Society of Superintendents of Training Schools for Nurses, and was an organizer of the Nurses' Associated Alumnae. She was a guiding force behind the establishment of the *American Journal of Nursing,* and served as editor for its first twenty years. For its first twelve years, journal offices were located in Palmer's Rochester home. *Courtesy Baker-Cederberg Museum and Archives.*

While the Superintendents' Society was grappling with educational issues, the Nurses' Associated Alumnae of the United States and Canada (later the American Nurses Association) was established in 1896 to tackle a broader range of problems. Trained nursing had gained widespread acceptance, but untrained nurses continued to dominate the workforce, and the public was unaware of the distinction between the two groups. In 1900 New York had twenty-five hundred trained nurses and fifteen thousand untrained nurses.[9] The large number of practicing untrained nurses was seen as a threat both to the public's health and to the welfare of graduate nurses. To address these concerns, the Nurses' Associated Alumnae's first task was to secure legislation that would provide a legal credentialing mechanism for nursing practice. However, since professional regulation was the right of individual states, registration and licensure would have to be achieved state by state.

ORGANIZATION FOR REGISTRATION: Although a state organization for trained nurses had been suggested as early as 1889, it was ten years before nursing leaders became alarmed enough about the need for state legislation to take definite steps. In 1899 two Rochester nurses, Sophia Palmer and Eva Allerton, presented papers on "State Registration for Nurses" at a meeting of the New York State Federation of Women's Clubs. Palmer stated that "The greatest need in the nursing profession today is a law that shall place training schools for nurses under the supervision of the University of the State of New York. Such a law would require every training school to bring its standard up to a given point . . . would require every woman who wished to practise nursing to obtain a diploma from a training school recognised by the University, to pass a regents' examination, and to register her license to practise . . . It is of vital importance that examining boards shall be selected from among nurses."[10] The assembly adopted a resolution endorsing the inclusion of nursing education as one of the professions supervised by the regents and the formation of a board of nurse examiners chosen by a state society of nurses. A few days later, a representative of the regents met with Palmer, Allerton, and the president of the Nurses' Associated Alumnae, Isabel Hampton Robb. About the same time, Sylveen Nye offered her suggestions to Buffalo physician Charles Butler, and Palmer talked with a Rochester physician. Both men wrote to the Board of Regents in support of the concept of registration for nurses.[11]

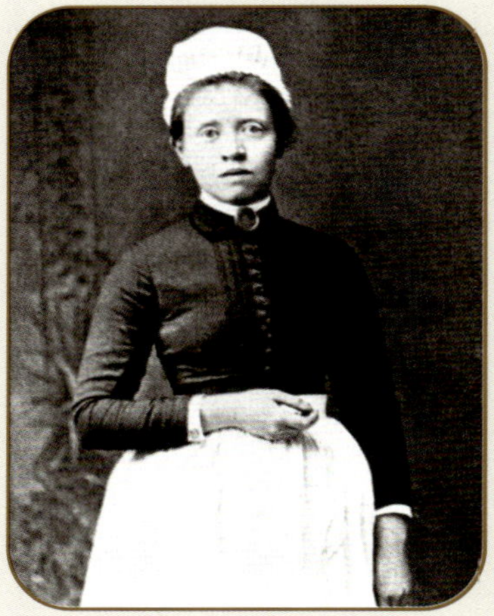

Annie Damer was instrumental in the founding of NYSNA, and was an exceedingly active leader of nursing organizations. She served as president of NYSNA (1904–1906), the Buffalo Nurses' Association (1900–1901), the Nurses' Associated Alumnae (1901–1902 and 1905–1909), and the Board of Nurse Examiners. She was also a pioneer in public health and tuberculosis nursing. *Courtesy the American Nurses Association.*

Although little information is available on activities in subsequent weeks, no doubt discussions among nurses, state officials, and influential citizens continued. In March 1900 Allerton, Sophia Palmer, and her sister Ida Palmer formed the Monroe County Graduate Nurses' Association to "bring all of the nurses of this county into closer professional and social relationship, and to have a local society organized which should be in proper form to take active steps when State meetings should be agitated."[12]

When the Nurses' Associated Alumnae gathered in New York for its third annual convention in 1900, Isabel Hampton Robb used her president's address as an "opportunity to hold a general review of our forces" — to look at the past and the present in order to plan for the future. For Robb, that future included state associations working for state registration of nurses. ". . . we trust steps may very soon be taken to formulate State associations, beginning in all probability, with the State of New York . . . It is only fitting that this State should take the initiative. Its educational institutions are controlled by the University of the State of New York . . . Again, as New York is the home of the mother of training schools in this country, it is but fitting that this State should first receive the crowning glory of the work she so bravely undertook."[13]

Following the meeting, a small group met at the Presbyterian Training School to discuss the steps necessary to form a state society. Sophia Palmer, reporting on the meeting in the first issue of the *American Journal of Nursing,* laid out the rationale for the formation of a state organization. "The diploma now held by a nurse from Smith's Corners or Split Rock Hospital, with four beds, seven nurses, and six-months' hospital training, has as much legal value as that of a graduate of Bellevue, Philadelphia, or Johns Hopkins, who has spent two or three years in hard work to obtain it. 'Practical' nurses, trained attendants, trained nursery maids, discharged pupils, and probationers all don the 'stripes,' compete with, and claim the name and rank of those who justly are the only ones entitled to bear them . . . Do we desire to make it so that those who bear the name of nurse shall be so not in name only, but in deed and truth? If so, a State Association is necessary which can work for State registration and a uniform system of education."[14] A committee was formed to arrange for a statewide meeting.

Sylveen Nye thoroughly discussed the proposed goals of a state association in the *Trained Nurse and Hospital Review.* She emphasized, "We want it to be an institution that will endure as long as the profession and the State . . . We should progress slowly and endeavor to work wisely and judiciously. Give every step careful consideration and opportunity for discussion."[15] Over the next few months, committee members Lavinia Dock and Annie Damer attended meetings of nursing groups around the state in an attempt to bring the issue of state organization to every trained nurse and hospital. It must have been a frustrating task, for there existed no lists or directories of either. Finally, a call went out to all New York State nurses to gather in Albany on April 16 and 17, 1901, to form a New York State Nurses Association (NYSNA). The call stated that the purpose of such an association would be to secure legislation to advance the profession.[16]

Fifty-six nurses from New York City, Brooklyn, Staten Island, Albany, Poughkeepsie, Rochester, Buffalo, Saratoga, Jamestown, Utica, Ogdensburg, Middletown, and Gloversville assembled at City Hall in Albany on the appointed date. Sylveen Nye, Chairman of the State Committee on Organizing a Convention, opened the meeting and addressed the group. "We have met here to form a New York State Nurses' Association, the object of which shall be to raise the standard of the nursing profession; to make better nurses; to help those of us already in the work to be broader, more intelligent, more useful; to help us to grow . . . We believe the proper means of attaining this desired purpose is by suitable legislation: not a legislation by a few for a few, but legislation that will affect all nurses and hospitals beneficially, that will bring about better teaching, better conditions for all nurses, better nursing for all classes of people, and legal recognition of our profession."[17] Discussion then opened on how the organization should be formed. Many advocated for individual membership while some argued for a membership of local societies. Others, including Damer and Palmer, suggested a membership system that would provide for

SYLVEEN V. NYE

1860 – 1936

Sylveen V. Nye, NYSNA's first president, was "a strong, capable, and earnest woman."[1] Born in Schuyler County to a distinguished New York family, she became superintendent of the Lexington Heights Hospital in Buffalo, and was instrumental in founding the Buffalo Nurses' Association in 1895.

Nye was an early proponent of state organization and legislation to regulate the profession. She advocated for a broadly representative membership, and strongly believed that NYSNA should be open to all trained nurses, regardless of the quality or size of their training program, positions that put her at odds with other leaders. Animosity increased when Nye called for legislation which protected the title "nurse," and provided for physician representation on the Board of Nurse Examiners. "Instantly there stood forth two opposing standard-bearers, and a duel typically illustrative of all subsequent struggles began . . . Her belief . . . was that, in organisation and legislation, as well as in the sick-room, nurses should be subordinate to medical associates."[2]

At her death in 1936, she was remembered as forthright, clear thinking, and courageous, and her defense of the simple title "nurse" was viewed as prophetic, ". . . she held that by adopting one of the other titles which must necessarily be misleading in its significance, we were creating difficulties for the future."[3]

both individual and group membership.[18] The day ended with the appointment of a committee to draft a constitution for consideration the following day.

The second day's meeting opened with the passage of a motion, *"Resolved,* That we do form a State Society." There followed the adoption of a constitution providing for the name, object, and officers. The difficult and contentious issue of membership was deferred, and following the election of officers, the meeting was adjourned. Thus was born the first state nurses' association in the country, the New York State Nurses Association, its adopted constitutional object "the advancement of the educational standard of nursing; the furtherance of the efficient care of the sick; the maintenance of the honor and character of the nursing profession; also the furtherance of cordial relations between the New York State nurses and the nurses of other States and countries."[19]

The second meeting of the association was to be held in Buffalo the following fall. However, the September 1901 meeting of the International Council of Nurses in conjunction with the Pan American Exposition in Buffalo involved so many nurses in meetings and hostessing responsibilities, the officers deemed it wiser to postpone the meeting. A letter from President Nye explained the postponement. "After Pan-American and all its attendant work and worry are over we shall all be in a better condition to give the subject the calm and judicious attention that is necessary."[20] The "State movement" was of enormous interest to the nurses assembled in Buffalo, and a resolution was unanimously adopted. "It is the duty of the nursing profession of every country to work for suitable legislative enactments regulating the education of nurses, and protecting the interests of the public, by securing State examinations and public registration with the proper penalties for enforcing same."[21] The movement was discussed at an informal meeting of the New York State Nurses Association with foreign delegates and representatives of the newly established state associations in Illinois and Virginia. "The discussions brought out the fact that all countries and States represented were working along the same lines, and that all have about the same difficulties to overcome."[22]

> "The thinkers and workers in the nursing profession all over the world are considering the questions of registration ...The difficulty lies in the question of responsibility. Who should bear it?"
>
> —*Katherine DeWitt*[1]

CONTROVERSIAL ISSUES: The association's second meeting, held in January 1902 in New York City, was contentious and frustrating. Focusing on the issue of membership structure and eligibility, the meeting demonstrated the difficulties of organizing such a geographically large and diverse state, and highlighted the strong personalities of leaders Palmer, Nye, and Dock. Two vexing procedural issues emerged. The first had to do with the status of visitors at the meeting. Twenty-two of the fifty-six members enrolled at the previous meeting were present, "while on the other side of the house was a much larger body of nurses who had come into the meeting, many of them prominent, well-known women in the profession."[23] A motion to give this group of non-member visitors the opportunity to join and fully participate was followed by animated discussion. Members objected that it was "irregular and inexpedient" to admit additional members until eligibility requirements for membership were established, and the motion was defeated. However, the following morning the motion was re-introduced and finally passed. Sixty-two nurses were then enrolled as new members.[24]

The second procedural issue involved the Bylaws Committee, composed of the officers and five appointed members. Half of this group resided in the greater New York City area and half in western New York. At a brief meeting of the committee immediately following the April 1901 organizational meeting, it was decided that the eastern group would meet and submit suggestions to the president to be presented to the western group. At the January meeting, committee chairman Anna Davids presented the proposals of the eastern group to the assembly. This was immediately followed by President Nye's introduction of her own proposals. Unbeknown to committee members, she had failed to pass on the suggestions of the eastern group to the other members of the western group, instead formulating her own recommendations. The result was confusion and tension, and "was most demoralizing in its influence upon the audience."[25]

Debate over these procedural issues and bylaws provisions was extensive. The membership eligiblity debate, a "prolonged and bitter struggle," addressed the educational standard that would be required for membership in the association.[26] The critical question was, would graduates from schools of a twenty-four-bed obstetrical hospital, for example, be admitted to membership on the same basis as graduates of a well-established large hospital school or a state hospital for the insane? Bylaws finally were adopted which accepted nurse graduates from all general hospitals offering at least a two-year training program, and from any state hospital for the insane offering at least a two-year training program and giving a course equal to that of New York State hospitals.[27]

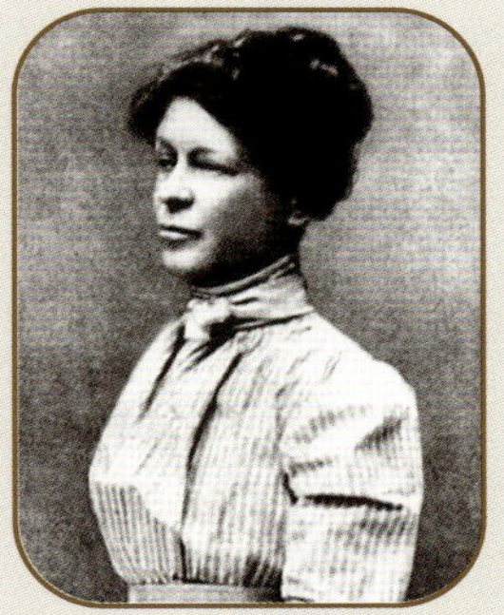

Lavinia Dock was a visiting nurse at the famous Henry St. Settlement, a social reformer, author of the first definitive history of nursing, and an ardent suffragist. As a columnist for the *American Journal of Nursing,* Dock influenced the profession both nationally and internationally. She researched the organizational structure of many groups and advised the first nursing associations on organizational matters. She was a charter member of NYSNA, and a vigorous supporter of registration legislation. *Courtesy Lavinia L. Dock, "What We May Expect From the Law,"* AMERICAN JOURNAL OF NURSING, *vol. 50, no. 10, 599–600.*

"The meeting of many nurses from many schools is stimulating to the individual, and rouses the cooperative spirit and the desire to do something besides 'talk shop' at the society meetings."

—Ida Palmer[2]

The second membership issue was that of structure. Here the question was, would members be admitted as individuals or as members of local organizations, such as alumnae associations? Individual membership was viewed as too unwieldy by many, yet membership restricted to alumnae associations would bar from membership nurses who graduated from out-of-state schools.

Palmer strongly promoted county and city associations as a solution. Ultimately, a compromise was reached, providing for both individual and organizational membership. However, twenty-five or more individual members from one county would be asked to organize into a local association. The membership provisions of the bylaws were adopted by a vote of 54 to 19 only an hour before adjournment, and then only after firm parliamentary maneuvering and direction from Lavinia Dock. Other bylaws were adopted in the final hour, and committees on nominations and incorporation were appointed before adjournment.[28]

Work on the bylaws continued at the association's first annual meeting in Albany on April 15, 1902. Procedures for admission of both organizations and individuals were established, providing for a Credentials Committee to review membership applications and make recommendations to the delegates. Other adopted bylaws established a committee structure, and set dues at $1 per year for individuals and $1 per year per every 10 members for organizations. The *American Journal of Nursing* was selected as "the recognized voice of the association," with all meeting reports to be submitted for publication. Finally, new officers and trustees were elected, and chairmen were chosen for committees on bylaws, legislation, press and publication, finance, and credentials. The first elected trustees were an impressive trio of national nursing leaders: Anna Maxwell, beloved founder and superintendent of the prestigious school of nursing at New York City's Presbyterian Hospital; national and international leader, Lavinia Dock; and the powerful Sophia Palmer.[29]

In contrast to the tone of the previous meeting, it was reported the April meeting was "a notably well-conducted and harmonious gathering."[30] A notice in the *Americn Journal of Nursing,* however, indicates that at least one group felt disenfranchised. A resolution adopted by the Buffalo Nurses' Association was printed which expressed its dissatisfaction with the constitution and bylaws. "The said New York State Nurses' Association admits to membership only graduates of general hospitals and hospitals for the insane, and we believe that such action is not Christian-like and is unwise, and we believe that nurses from all schools connected with reputable hospitals should be recognized . . . and we believe that a few women have no moral or legal right to discriminate against the recognition of such nurses . . . *Resolved,* That it is the sense of this association not to affiliate with the New York State Nurses' Association in its present form . . ."[31] Palmer's editorial comment was scathing, "So the Buffalo Nurses' Association, not being able to dictate arbitrarily to the nurses of New York State, have decided to 'take their dolls and go home.' There is a pettishness in the action that we are sorry to see, but as the question of eligibility was decided by a body of women including delegates who represented a constituency of more than nine hundred nurses, it is certainly according to the principle of American liberty that the 'majority' should rule."[32]

"Personally, I believe the State association will be a much broader and stronger organization if all distinction of school is eliminated."

— Beatrice Van Homrigh[3]

In 1902 NYSNA's incorporation committee filed papers and met all legal obligations before the association's first annual meeting. The signatures of Jessie Sleet, Sophia Palmer, Anna Maxwell, Lavinia Dock, Mary Thornton, Mary Emma Cameron, Mary Bohling, and Mary Miner appear on the incorporation papers. Legally incorporated, funded through dues, its structure established, and its formidable leadership in place, the newly formed association was ready to direct its energies into legislatively securing registration for nurses. The Publication Committee formulated a letter to be sent to two thousand New York nurses, preparing them for the upcoming legislative thrust, and stating that legislation "can prevent a probationer or pupil dismissed for unfitness from donning a uniform and calling herself a trained nurse, thus imposing upon the public and endangering the lives of sick people . . . Such women must be known for what they really are, untaught and untrained women, and in this way they will be prevented from competing with the fully trained nurse who has given two or three years to the study of her profession. Then, little by little, and year by year, the law can require the training-schools to give better and more complete training. It can fix a 'minimum' standard of teaching. This will be what we all agree upon as the least that any woman ought to know in order to call herself a trained nurse . . ."[33] The letter encouraged nurses to discuss the issue with friends, colleagues, physicians, and most importantly, legislators.

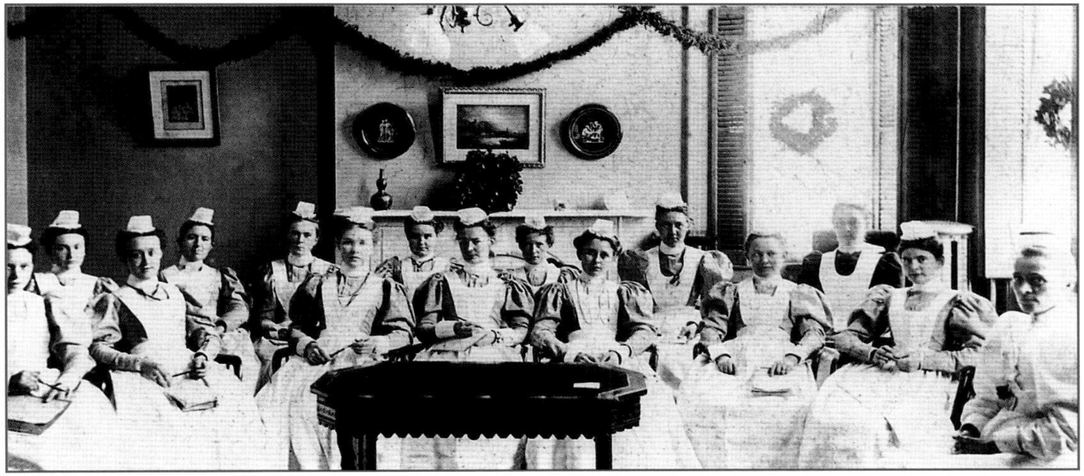

The October 1902 quarterly meeting of NYSNA was held in this room of the Rochester City Hospital's Nurses Home. After dinner, members joined in dancing a lively "two-step." *Courtesy Baker-Cederberg Museum and Archives.*

LEGISLATION FOR REGISTRATION: Eva Allerton, superintendent of Rochester's Homeopathic Hospital and Training School, was appointed the chairman of NYSNA's first Committee on Legislation. Allerton had a thorough knowledge of the functions of the University of the State of New York and its Board of Regents. "A woman of the utmost ability and remarkable magnetism,"[34] Allerton met with prominent Rochester residents Rev. Thomas Hendricks, member of the Board of Regents, and State Senator William W. Armstrong. The Senator suggested a simple bill modeled after existing laws regulating physicians, and indicated his willingness to introduce and carry through legislation. He noted that a decision also needed to be made regarding the title which would be protected under the law. At NYSNA's 1902 midsummer meeting, delegates voted to begin developing widespread support, and to ask Senator Armstrong to present a bill. No decision on the title was made, but a notice appeared in the *American Journal of Nursing* asking members to forward opinions to NYSNA's secretary.[35]

Rochester, site of the next regular meeting of the association in October 1902, had become the center of the New York registration movement. Nearly all of its trained nurses were NYSNA members, and the city was home to Palmer, Allerton, Hendricks, and Armstrong.[36] The importance of the meeting was not underestimated. "The nurses of today are making history, and the result of their work will influence the status of nurses during the century."[37]

The first speaker of the day was the great suffragette Susan B. Anthony. Palmer reported that ". . . although now in exceedingly frail health, Miss Anthony's interest in the discussions was so great that she remained in her seat on the platform through both the morning and afternoon sessions . . . she referred to the great power of women's organizations, and she emphasized the point that if the thirty thousand graduate nurses in this country had the right to vote they would obtain what they desire much more easily. She closed her address with an earnest appeal to the nurses to remember the power and the influence of their work, and to improve it to the utmost." Miss Anthony received a standing ovation.[38]

Following encouraging remarks by a member of the State Board of Medical Examiners and Regent Hendricks, the assembly turned its attention to a reading of the proposed bill by Miss Damer. All thirty-nine delegates present, together with more than a hundred visitors, were encouraged to participate fully in the discussion, which focused on the title under which nurses would be registered.

> "Valuable as educational fitness may be, it has been recognized that unscrupulousness, or a low standing of integrity can quickly overturn what years of education and intelligence cannot replace."
>
> *—Jane Elizabeth Hitchcock*[4]

Three titles were debated by three strong personalities in an animated discussion. Eva Allerton represented the Committee on Legislation's preference for "Trained Nurse," believing the term was familiar and already understood by the public. The most impassioned speaker, former President Sylveen Nye " . . . believed the title should be simply 'Nurse;' that a woman should have the right to use that title or she should not have it; that there should be no qualifying or half-way measures." Sophia Palmer advocated for the term "Registered Nurse." Following a spirited debate between Palmer and Nye, a member moved to defer the decision until the opinions of other state nurses' associations could be solicited. Damer responded that "all of the State associations were equally undecided in the choice of the title, and they were looking to the New York State Nurses Association to make a decision at this meeting."[39] The membership defeated the motion, and Damer immediately moved that the title "Registered Nurse" be incorporated into the bill. The strong Rochester delegation carried the motion, the only opponents being the "out-of-towners." The large group of non-voting visitors was polled, and unanimously supported the vote. The remaining sections of the bill were adopted without debate, and there was "great applause and enthusiasm."[40] The Buffalo nurses, the "out-of-towners," however, were not celebratory. "Miss Nye declared that . . . Buffalo was strongly opposed to the action and would stand out for what it considers is the right." This "very small but determined minority" strongly condemned the proceedings, believing the proposed bill would not recognize graduates of special and smaller hospitals.[41]

The proposed bill called for registration of New York State residents over the age of 23, of "good moral character," holding a diploma from a training school for nurses connected with a general hospital or a hospital for the insane with a course of at least two years. The training school was required to be registered by the regents as maintaining standards to be determined by the regents. Only nurses possessing these qualifications and obtaining registration would be permitted to use the title "Registered Nurse." The bill provided for a Board of Examiners selected from nominations submitted by the association. In consultation with the Board of Examiners, the regents would make rules for examinations and set appropriate fees. At the discretion of the regents and with unanimous approval of the Board of Examiners, a waiver of the examination would be granted to individuals who graduated before the passage of the law. Any violation of the act would be a misdemeanor.

Nurses were encouraged to attend the next scheduled meeting in New York City in January 1903. ". . . the movement for registration is a movement of the nurses of the present day to better the conditions of the nurses of the future. Who can afford not to march with the spirit of the times?" The meeting hall was filled to overflowing to hear physicians and others speak in support of the proposed legislation. Every member was asked to work to influence public opinion, especially members of the legislature's Committee on Public Health.[42]

Despite the secretary's report that "there were no criticisms of the bill made either by members present or by the visitors, and no amendment proposed," opposition to the bill was growing, and it was coming from within as well as from outside the association. A number of small private hospitals and sanatoria, dependent on student labor and fearful their nursing schools would not meet state standards, were "commercially opposed to the bill," and there was growing opposition among physicians who wanted to exert greater control over the nursing profession. Immediately prior to Senate hearings on the bill, the association was informed that a physician-prepared bill, which called for registration of nurses with three years of hospital experience but no formal training, and which included physicians on the Board of Examiners, would be introduced.[43]

A faction within the association also proved troublesome. Sylveen Nye and her followers (according to Palmer, "the *minority* of the New York State Nurses Association, the 'rule or ruin' element that almost every large organization has to contend with") proved to be a formidable force. Nye's brother, State Assemblyman Olin Nye, represented her position that NYSNA's proposals would restrict many nurses from registration eligibility. On February 16 he introduced his own bill that put control of registration with the secretary of state, and granted licensure to anyone providing a sworn statement that the individual was entitled to registration. No diploma was required, and the bill called for no educational standards.[44] Six days later, on February 23, Senator Armstrong introduced NYSNA's bill in the Senate, and Martin Davis, also from Rochester, introduced it in the Assembly the following day.[45]

Hearings were held on the bill in March. Opposition speakers, primarily physicians from Albany and Buffalo, focused on the bill's "discrimination" toward untrained nurses, who "were equally well-qualified for their work," and the plea for physician representation on the Board of Nurse Examiners. Opponents also charged that the association was too powerful, and not representative of the state's nurses. Speakers in support of the bill included physicians, members of hospital boards, and nurses, including an impressive delegation of supportive nurses and training school superintendents

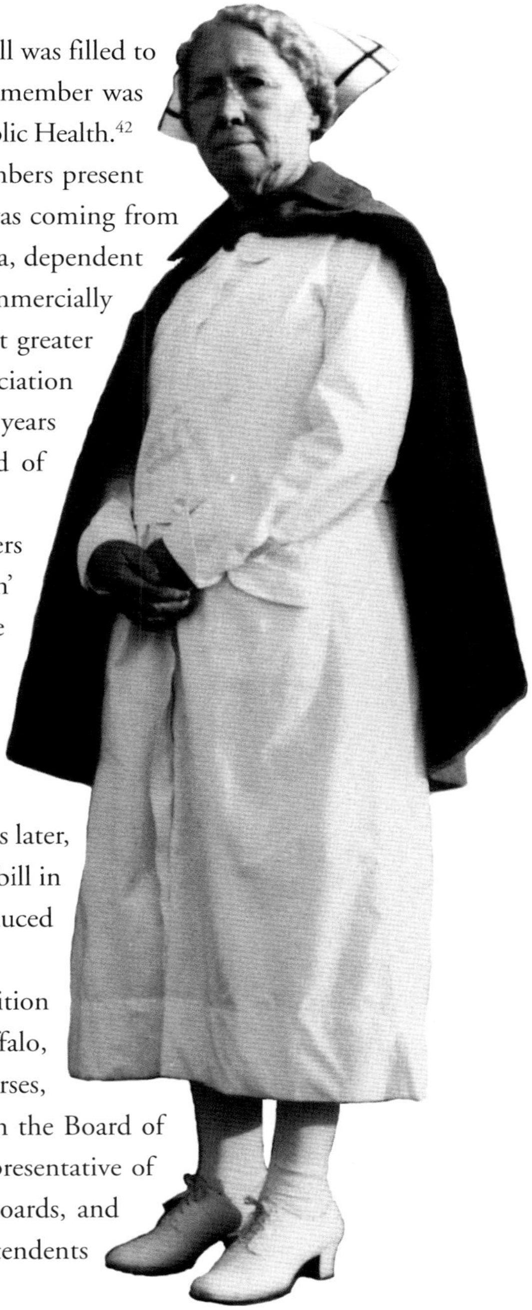

RIGHT: Ida Jane Anderson, a 1902 graduate of the Genesee Hospital School of Nursing in Rochester, was the first nurse to receive an RN license in New York State. *Courtesy ViaHealth Genesee Hospital.*

from New York City's largest hospitals. Supporters emphasized the "injustice" of a Board of Nurse Examiners which included physicians, and defended the strength of NYSNA in both the size of its membership and its geographical representativeness. It was also pointed out that the bill would not prohibit untrained nurses from practicing, only from using the title "registered nurse."[46]

"It has been a year of great anxiety for all of us who realize what this bill means to us, namely, making the art of nursing a profession."

—Nancy E. Cadmus[5]

Following the hearings, the association met with legal counsel and representatives of the medical societies to address objections. The association stood firmly behind the proposed composition of the Board of Examiners, but agreed to broaden the waiver provisions for untrained nurses.[47] The bill was quickly passed in the Senate. The opposition Nye bill was successfully amended to conform to the Senate bill and easily passed in the Assembly April 20, 1903.[48] The following day, New York nurses assembled in Albany for NYSNA's second annual meeting, and triumphantly celebrated its first legislative victory.

Although not the first state registration bill to be passed, New York's law is widely considered to be the most progressive and influential of the early legislation. The New York law was the most restrictive in that the waiver provisions were administered rigorously, and the qualifying examination was not easy. More than any other state's legislation, the New York law most closely fulfilled the dreams of the early leaders for a law that provided for the development of educational standards, protected the public from unsafe nursing care, and placed the regulation of the profession firmly in the hands of nurses. Nurses across the country followed the early work of the New York Board of Nurse Examiners. New York "had become the 'central source of registration wisdom' and nurses in other states measured their gains against the Empire State's achievements."[49]

A LAW DOES NOT ENFORCE ITSELF: Legislation enacted, the association's efforts turned to implementation and protection of the law. By 1904 the five members of the Board of Nurse Examiners were selected by the regents from a list of ten nominations submitted by NYSNA. L. Bissell Sanford, Annie Damer, Dorothy McDonald, Sophia Palmer, and Jane Elizabeth Hitchcock comprised the first Board of Nurse Examiners. Early reports at NYSNA conventions detail the board's precedent-setting decisions, including the establishment of a training school curriculum and preliminary requirements, application procedures, waiver requirements, and examination content. Palmer described the board's work during the first year as "exceedingly difficult . . . the board was called upon to define, for the first time in nursing history, what should constitute a general training."[50] It is evident that the early boards relied heavily on the input and expertise of the state association. A Committee on Education was formed by NYSNA in 1905 specifically to make recommendations to the State Board on a uniform curriculum, and a "bureau of information" was established to collect data on curricula utilized by the state's training schools.[51]

NYSNA's Committee on Legislation remained vigilant, utilizing various legislative information services to stay apprised of legislative activity. "With the passage of a bill the real work commences. A law does not enforce itself, continued pressure must be constantly felt from someone. A pernicious amendment allowed to pass because no one is on hand to object may undo the work of years."[52] It wasn't long before just such amendments began to be introduced. In 1905 a bill was introduced which provided for the registration of an applicant who had been "rejected by the examiners as being unable to comply with any of the requirements of the law." The following year a bill was introduced to repeal the existing law and create a Commission on Nursing, composed of physicians, to regulate the practice of nursing, and a second bill was introduced to replace nurses with physicians on the examining board. Committee on Legislation chairman Jane Delano worked to successfully defeat all three bills. "The result of our work has given us the greatest satisfaction and has been most encouraging, all alumnae associations and county societies working in harmony and with the determination that no outsiders should tamper with our present law . . ."[53]

A Firm Foundation: By its second annual meeting, the membership of the association had grown from 56 to 1,509, "a fair proportion of the twenty-five hundred trained nurses of the State."[54] The new law necessitated bylaws changes, including provisions for the nomination of candidates for the State Board of Nurse Examiners and for making registration a requirement of association membership.[55] By 1907 dues for individual members were increased to $2 and the October annual meeting had been established. As the financial base of the organization became more secure, NYSNA began a rich tradition of providing support for national and international nursing endeavors of a professional, educational, and charitable nature.[56]

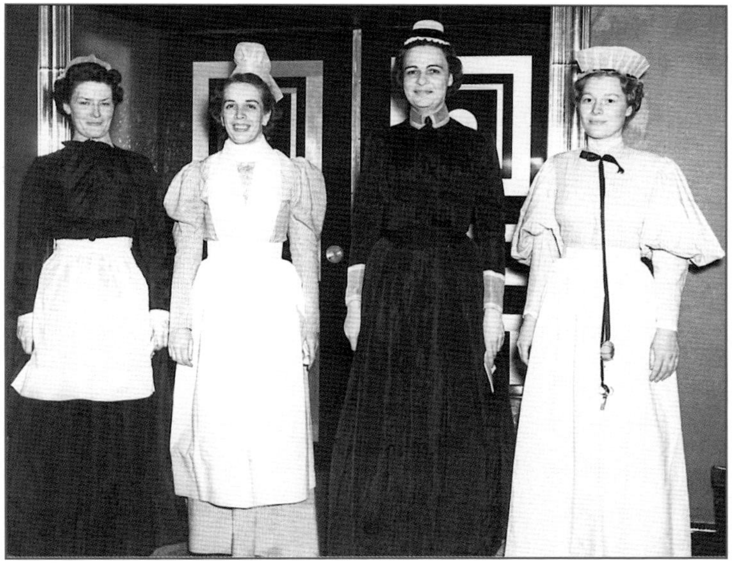

above: Nurses at NYSNA's fortieth anniversary convention donned vintage uniforms to portray early NYSNA leaders; from left to right are Annie Damer, Eva Allerton, Sophia Palmer, and Sylveen Nye. They demonstrate the typically voluminous uniforms, often with leg o' mutton sleeves. During this period, it was considered highly unethical for nurses (with the exception of visiting nurses) to wear their uniforms outside of the home or hospital. *Courtesy District 14 Collection, Foundation of NYSNA Archives; Knickerboker Photographers.*

In 1904 the association officially voted to affiliate with the Nurses' Associated Alumnae, and for the first time included papers on clinical topics in its meeting program. These papers addressed timely clinical topics, from tuberculosis in 1904 to pharmacy, public health problems, obstetrics, surgery, contagious diseases, and "nervous work" in subsequent years. Professional issues were also raised. Ethical questions such as "Should a Nurse Take a Case from Which Another Nurse Has Been Dismissed Without Just Cause," were popular discussion topics. Nurses' registries and clubhouses, and the developing field of visiting nursing were frequently addressed. A 1907 paper on "A Physician's Advice on Caring for People of Moderate Means" advocated "the introduction of trained assistants, in the hospital and out." Annie Damer led a spirited discussion on the reported accusation of "nurses of the spirit of the trades-unions in sitting at home idle, waiting for a call, yet refusing to go where there is need for their services at reduced rates." Damer asked, "'Where can you find more of a trades-union spirit than in the New York Medical Society?' She added that the whole burden of caring for these people at reduced rates falls on the shoulders of the private duty nurse who is criticised on the one hand for not saving money for the future and on the other hand for not giving her services more often. She suggested that hospitals should do their share . . ."[57]

In its first decade, the New York State Nurses Association established a firm foundation for the development of organized nursing in New York State. It built a sound organizational structure and established a forum for nurses to debate professional issues and enhance clinical knowledge. Most dramatically, though none of its women members could vote, it demonstrated it was a formidable political and legislative force by initiating and defending legislation to protect the public and advance the profession.

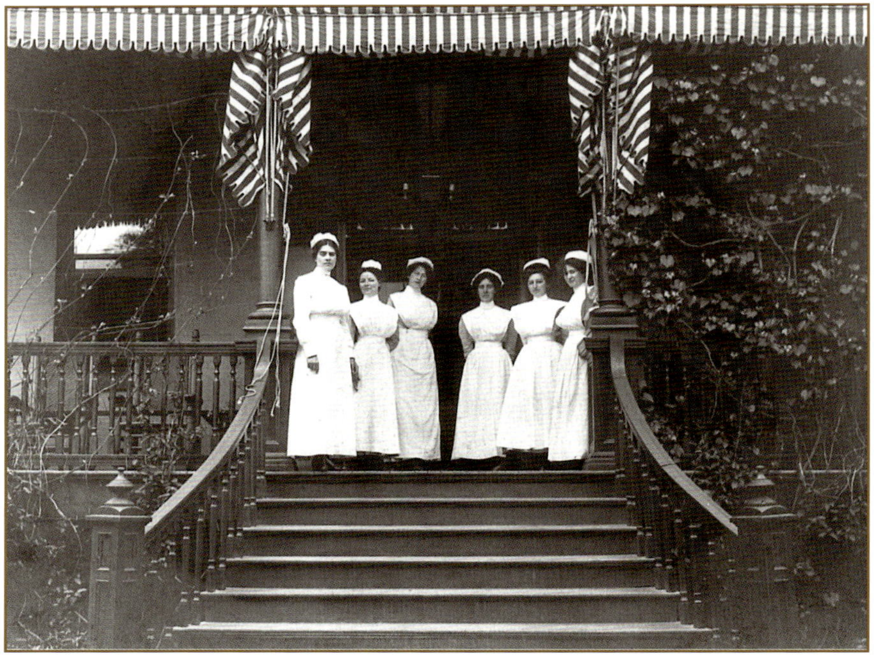

ABOVE: Hospital nursing staff, such as shown here from the Westchester Medical Center at the turn of the century, were primarily responsible for teaching and supervising students. *Courtesy Westchester Medical Center.*

CHAPTER NOTES

TEXT

1. The private duty nurse's vitality diminished after age 40, and physicians and families preferred to hire younger nurses. Consequently, the private duty nurse rarely practiced beyond age 50. Neither the hospital nurse nor the private duty nurse had employer-provided or governmental pension plans. (Philip A. Kalisch and Beatrice J. Kalisch, *The Advance of American Nursing,* 3rd ed. [Philadelphia: J. B. Lippincott, 1995], 148–49.)

2. Margaret L. Rogers, "Private Nursing," *American Journal of Nursing* 2 (November 1901): 83; and Kalisch and Kalisch, *Advance of American Nursing,* 133–52.

3. Samuel Eliot Morrison, Henry Steele Commager and William E. Leuchtenburg, *A Concise History of the American Republic* (New York: Oxford University Press, 1977), 504–6.

4. "Hospital Service in the United States," *Journal of the American Medical Association* 82 (12 January 1924): 120.

5. Jo Ann Ashley, *Hospitals, Paternalism, and the Role of the Nurse* (New York: Teachers College Press, 1976), 9.

6. Sophia F. Palmer, "Editorial Comment," *American Journal of Nursing* 5 (February 1905): 281; and Annie W. Goodrich, "Report of the Inspector of Training Schools of New York State," *American Journal of Nursing* 11 (January 1911): 305.

7. Victor Robinson, *White Caps: The Story of Nursing* (New York: J. B. Lippincott, 1946), 265.

8. Nettie Birnbach, "Credentialing-Chaos to Accountability," in *Prologue to Professionalism: A History of Nursing,* ed. M. Louise Fitzpatrick (Bowie, Md.: Brady Communications, 1983), 107.

9. "Official Reports of Societies," *American Journal of Nursing* 3 (April 1903): 558. Nationwide, the 1900 United States census listed 12,000 trained nurses and 109,000 untrained nurses and midwives. (Ellen D. Baer, *Editor's Notes* [New York: National League for Nursing, 1990], 24.)

10. Lavinia L. Dock, *A History of Nursing* 3 (New York: G.P. Putnam's Sons, 1912), 144. The University of the State of New York was created in 1784. Supervised by a Board of Regents, the organization was authorized to establish secondary schools and colleges in the state. Until legislation was enacted, however, the regents had no control over training schools for nurses. (David M. Ellis et al., *A History of New York State* [Ithaca, N.Y.: Cornell University Press, 1967], 199.)

11. Dock, *History of Nursing,* 144–45.

12. "American Delegates and Societies," *American Journal of Nursing* 1 (September 1901): 909.

13. Isabel Hampton Robb, "Address of the President," *American Journal of Nursing* 1 (November 1900): 102.

14. "Practical nurses" refers to individuals employed as nurses who were not graduates of a training school. They received their education and training through "practice." Committee members were Lavinia Dock and Isabel Merritt from New York, Sylveen Nye, and Annie Damer from Buffalo, and Eva Allerton from Rochester. (Sophia F. Palmer, "Editor's Miscellany," *American Journal of Nursing* 1 [October 1900]: 60.)

15. Sylveen V. Nye, "The Proposed New York State Nurses' Association," *The Trained Nurse and Hospital Review* 25 (December 1900): 400.

16. The letter was dated February 26, 1901. Nye had also written a letter in January, making it clear that, in an effort to reach every trained nurse in New York State, meeting notices would be sent to every known hospital and nursing organization in the state, and that a notice of the meeting would be printed in the *American Journal of Nursing* (AJN). The information was also included in an editorial of the other major nursing publication of that time, *The Trained Nurse and Hospital Review.* (Sophia F. Palmer, "Editor's Miscellany," *American Journal of Nursing* 1 [April 1901]: 525.)

17. "Official Reports of Societies," *American Journal of Nursing* 1 (May 1901): 594.

18. The Nurses' Associated Alumnae was comprised of nurses who were members solely through their alumnae associations, and membership was restricted to alumnae associations of schools of nursing connected with general hospitals of not less than one hundred beds, and which provided not less than two full years of training in the hospital. See Lyndia Flanagan, *One Strong Voice* (Kansas City: American Nurses' Association, 1976), 44.

19. The elected officers were: Sylveen V. Nye, President; Isabel Merritt, Vice-President; Annie R.

Young, Second Vice-President; Elizabeth Sandford, Secretary; and Mary E. Thornton, Treasurer. *Report of the New York State Nurses' Association 1901–06* (New York: Irving Press, 1907), 3–7 is the official published report for the meeting. A more comprehensive report is that given in the "Official Reports of Societies," cited in note 17.

20. "Official Reports of Societies," *American Journal of Nursing* 1 (September 1901): 933.

21. Nettie Birnbach, "The Development of Organized Nursing and the Pan-American Exposition at Buffalo in 1901: Doing Historical Research," in *Nursing Research: A Qualitative Perspective,* 2nd ed., ed. Patricia L. Munhall and Carolyn O. Boyd (New York: NLN Press, 1993), 385.

22. "Official Reports of Societies," *American Journal of Nursing* 2 (October 1901): 51.

23. Sophia F. Palmer, "Editorial Comment," *American Journal of Nursing* 2 (January 1902): 487.

24. Ibid., 487–88.

25. Palmer also noted that during the discussion it was apparent that the officers had not met since their election in January, and that the president had failed to engage an official stenographer for the January meeting, "the unfortunate result being much trouble for the secretary, and leaving the sensational newspaper reports as the only public records of the proceedings." Nye's explanation of lack of time owing to unusual business pressures, complicated with serious illness in her family, was accepted "in a cordial spirit." (Ibid.)

26. Ibid.

27. "Official Reports of Societies," *American Journal of Nursing* 2 (September 1902): 1023. For individuals who graduated before January 1, 1897, the program must have been at least one year. The bylaws made no provision for the size of the hospital or the training program, and "general" meant "where general diseases are nursed."

28. Palmer, "Editorial Comment," January 1902, 489.

29. "Official Report of Societies," *American Journal of Nursing* 2 (May 1902): 622–23. Trustees were later changed to directors, then to an Executive Committee before being again changed to directors.

30. "State Meetings," *American Journal of Nursing* 2 (May 1902): 646.

31. "Official Reports of Societies," *American Journal of Nursing* 2 (June 1902): 699–700. The Buffalo Nurses' Association was accepted as an organizational member of NYSNA in 1911.

32. Sophia F. Palmer, "Editorial Comment," *American Journal of Nursing* 2 (June 1902): 730.

33. "Official Reports of Societies," September 1902, 1023–24.

34. Dock, *History of Nursing,* 148. In Robinson's *White Caps,* 303, Allerton is described as ". . . of Mayflower descent, and herself a pilgrim when she led the nurses of New York to the new land of state registration."

35. "Official Reports of Societies," *American Journal of Nursing* 3 (October 1902): 54. Suggested titles were Graduate Nurse, Trained Nurse, Certified Nurse, Registered Nurse, and Registered Graduate Nurse. (*Report 1901–06,* 10–11.)

36. "Trained Nurses in Convention," *Rochester Democrat and Chronicle,* 19 October, 1902.

37. Palmer, "Editorial Comment," May 1902, 562.

38. Sophia F. Palmer, "Editorial Comment," *American Journal of Nursing* 3 (November 1902): 158. Anthony later participated in the discussion on title, and expressed the optimistic opinion that "the day is coming when trained nurses will be required to possess a college education before being admitted to training, saying that the older generation of women had not had the opportunities for college education which the younger generation now have." ("Official Reports of Societies," *American Journal of Nursing* 3 [December 1902]: 216. See also "Nurses Had a Lively Debate," *Rochester Democrat and Chronicle,* 22 October 1902.)

39. "Official Reports," December 1902, 218.

40. Ibid.

41. "Nurses Had Lively Debate." The article lists the "out-of-towners" and the city from which they came. Most were from Buffalo. The article also includes a full text of the Buffalo Nurses' Association resolution adopted following the April meeting.

42. Sophia F. Palmer, "Editorial Comment," *American Journal of Nursing* 3 (January 1903): 332; and Sophia F. Palmer, "Editorial Comment," *American Journal of Nursing* 3 (February 1903): 411–12.

43. "Official Reports," April 1903, 556. The bill was never introduced, and was later viewed as a "bluff." However, many physicians wanted representation of the medical community on the Examining Board. Most popular was a proposal for three physician examiners, one from each medical society — allopathic, homeopathic, and eclectic — thus embroiling nursing in the medical politics of the day. The six-thousand-member Medical Society of the State of New York, however, unanimously endorsed the legislation. Dr. Van Fleet, chair of the Medical Society's Legislative Committee, provided invaluable assistance. "During the Albany Campaign without his presence, advice, and assistance the leaders would many times, in their inexperience, have been brought to confusion . . ." However, another member of the committee, Dr. Root of Albany, seemed to be leading the opposition to the bill during the hearings. (Sophia F. Palmer, "Editorial Comment," *American Journal of Nursing* 3 [April 1903]: 590–91.)

44. Sophia F. Palmer, "Editorial Comment," *American Journal of Nursing* 3 (March 1903): 503.

45. Nye and the Buffalo Nurses' Association deplored requirements that would restrict many nurses from registration and from NYSNA membership. NYSNA believed these restrictions were necessary to elevate the standards of the profession. Pressured by the secretary of the Board of Regents, the Committee on Legislation agreed to several changes in the bill. The age requirement was changed from 23 to 21, the size of the Board of Examiners was increased from three to five, and the time of waiver was extended from two to three years. (Veronica M. Driscoll, *Legitimizing the Profession of Nursing: The Distinct Mission of The New York State Nurses Association* [Guilderland, N.Y.: Foundation of NYSNA, 1976], 15.)

46. "Official Reports," April 1903, 557–62.

47. Graduates of good moral character from approved schools, those training at the time the law was passed, and nurses with three years' experience in a general hospital could apply within three years for waiver of the examination. The examination could also be waived for any nurse of good moral character who had practiced nursing for at least three years and passed a practical examination. (*Report 1901–06,* 20.)

48. "Official Reports of Societies," *American Journal of Nursing* 3 (May 1903): 727. Palmer gives credit to the influence exerted by the Committee on Legislation, who were all present in Albany: Eva Allerton, Nancy Cadmus and Annie Damer, as well as other influential nurses Anna Maxwell, Mary Thornton, and Sophia Palmer herself. (Sophia F. Palmer, "Editorial Comment," *American Journal of Nursing* 3 [May 1903]: 671.) The governor signed the bill on April 27. See also Driscoll, *Legitimizing the Profession,* 17–18.

49. Nancy Tomes, "The Silent Battle-Nurse Registration in New York State, 1903 to 1920," in *Nursing History — New Perspectives, New Possibilities,* ed. Ellen C. Lagemann (New York: Teachers College Press, 1983): 110–20. Tomes notes that graduate nurses could not register under the waiver until their school was registered by the regents, and for nurses without formal training, the nurse examiners insisted on a personal reference from an individual known by a member of the Board of Nurse Examiners.

50. Sophia F. Palmer, "Editorial Comment," *American Journal of Nursing* 4 (May 1904): 663. Palmer was elected the Board of Examiner's first president, and Hitchcock its first secretary.

51. *Report 1901–06,* 56. The committee was short-lived, and was soon dissolved. Nursing education activities were handled by the New York State League of Nursing Education, and it was several decades before a Committee on Education was again appointed.

52. Sophia F. Palmer, "Editorial Comment," *American Journal of Nursing* 5 (April 1905): 416.

53. *Report 1901–06,* 48–50.

54. Palmer, "Editorial Comment," May 1903, 672.

55. *Report 1901–1906,* 20. The relatively low number of applicants for registration was a disappointment to those who worked so hard to achieve registration legislation, and frequent calls went out urging nurses to register. Many who did apply to register expressed profound frustration when their applications were denied because their training school did not meet the state requirements. (Nettie Birnbach, "The Genesis of the Nurse Registration Movement in the United States, 1893–1903" [Ed.D. diss., Teachers College, 1982], 93).

56. In the beginning, the association met quarterly, then semi-annually, and finally annually. Bylaws provided for an annual April meeting until it was changed to October in 1907. Funds were allocated to the Nurses' Associated Alumnae toward purchase of stock in the *American Journal of Nursing,* and toward the endowment fund for the Hospital Economics course at Teachers College, Columbia University. Established in 1899, this was the first course established to teach teachers of nursing. ("Official Reports of Societies," *American Journal of Nursing* 8 [January 1908]: 305.)

57. Sophia F. Palmer, "Editorial Comment," *American Journal of Nursing* 8 (November 1907): 105–6.

FEATURE

SYLVEEN V. NYE

1. Dock, *History of Nursing,* 148.

2. Ibid.

3. "Sylveen V. Nye," *Quarterly News* 9 (January 1937): 19.

EXCERPTS

1. "The Opportunity and Responsibility of the Graduate Nurse of To-Day," *American Journal of Nursing* 2 (November 1901): 6.

2. Ida R. Palmer, "The Necessity of Organizing County Associations," *American Journal of Nursing* 6 (September 1906): 857.

3. "Letters to the Editor," *American Journal of Nursing* 2 (January 1902): 298

4. "State Board of Nurse Examiners Yearly Report," *Report 1901–06,* 34.

5. "Official Reports," May 1903, 727.

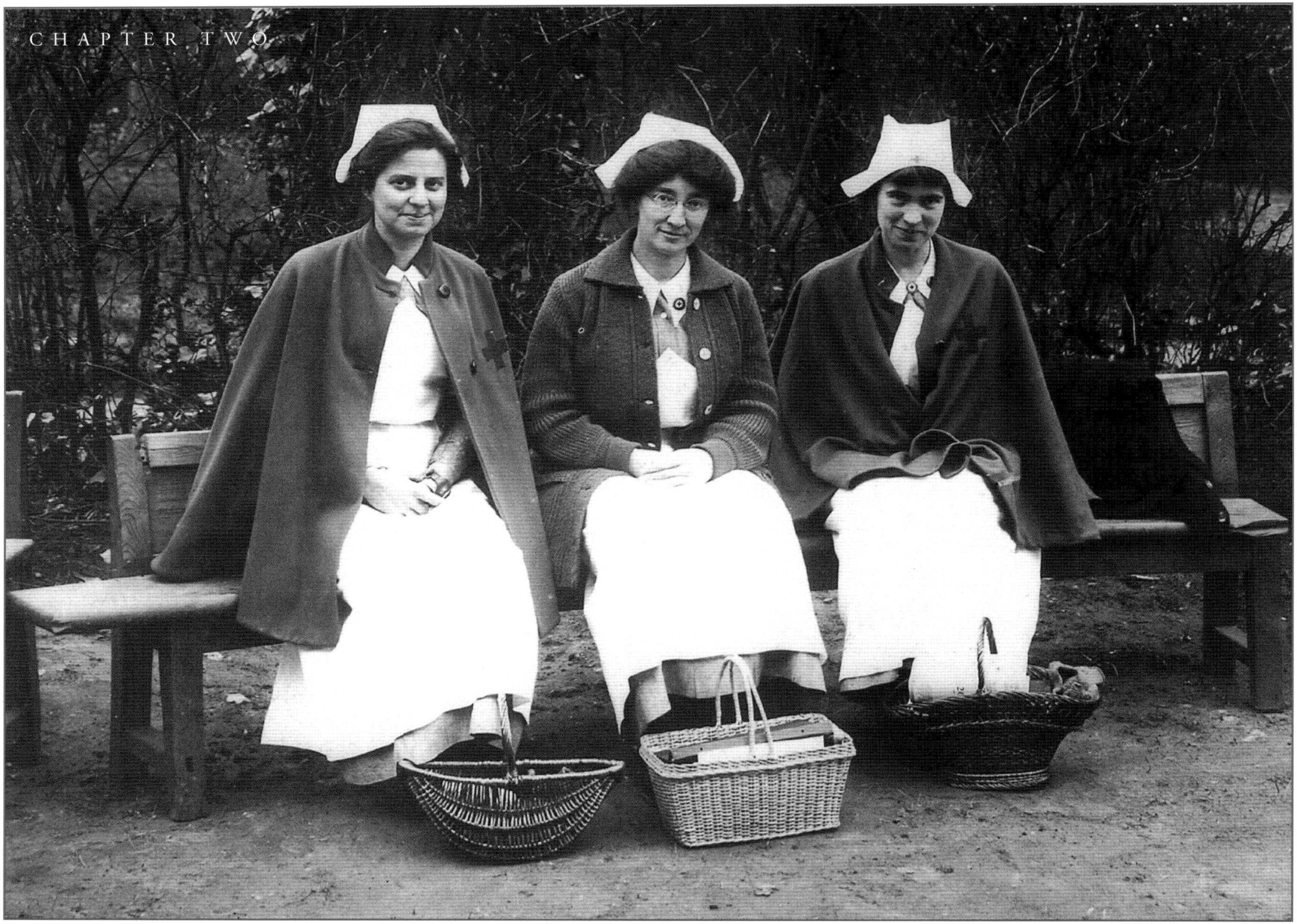

CHAPTER TWO

A PROFESSION WORTH FIGHTING FOR 1911–1920

In its first decade NYSNA achieved national stature by securing registration legislation. However, many of the conditions that precipitated the 1903 legislation persisted, and even worsened. Statistics showed only one in ten practicing nurses was hospital trained, and because the law was not compulsory, the association's goal of protecting the public from untrained practitioners remained a dream. Hospital use was rising, and confronted with more and more patients, hospitals needed more and more students to provide the necessary nursing care. More correspondence schools and "short-courses" were established, with one New York school boasting three thousand graduates in one year.[1] The desire for more nurses was so great, even hospitals with the most prestigious schools vigorously protested a 1910 Department of Education ruling that required the equivalent of just one year of high school for admission to nurse training schools.

FACING PAGE: Marion McCune Rice at left, of Rochester posed with fellow Red Cross nurses Helen Spaulding, center, and Miss McCracken, at right, in France during World War I. *Courtesy the Rice Collection.*

WHO IS CARING FOR THE SICK? The association held its tenth annual meeting in Albany in October 1911. President Louise Twiss remarked that "we have had a quiet year," and the *American Journal of Nursing* reported harmony and peace in the nursing world.[2] However, papers presented at the meeting roused the nursing community out of its complacency and set the agenda for the association's work for nearly a decade.

Dr. Augustus Downing, first assistant commissioner of the Department of Education, presented a paper enumerating the strengths and weaknesses of the Nurse Practice Act, and the difficulties of its administration. Downing highlighted the lack of compulsory registration as the law's primary weakness. While only registered nurses could use the title "registered nurse" or "RN," anyone — trained or untrained — could practice as a nurse. The law provided no protection of the "innocent public" against the deception of untrained persons practicing as expert nurses, and no protection of the registered nurse against the competition of untrained nurses in the workplace. He laid the blame squarely on the "commercialization" of nurse training schools, and recommended that the law be amended "to strengthen its fundamental principle — education — and to eradicate its weakness by making it possible only for the truly trained nurse to act as nurse." Specifically, he called for protection of the title "nurse" and registration of "trained attendants."[3]

Downing's impassioned plea for education as "prerequisite to intelligent nursing" was followed by an equally impassioned paper by M. Adelaide Nutting, professor of nursing at Teachers College, Columbia University. In a paper entitled "The New Demands in Nursing," Nutting expressed "gravest concern" over recent changes in the profession, notably technical advances "involving highly complicated procedures," the newly placed emphasis on disease prevention, and the expressed concern that nurses were not being adequately prepared. "We can never more be satisfied with our old blind, blundering methods of tinkering up sick bodies and ignoring all those deeper causes and complications . . ." She strongly advocated for an increase in theoretical content and better prepared teachers and superintendents, but knew such change would be difficult. "There is no cause for discouragement if we only keep our purpose clear, and know what we want, and why we want it. We have overcome difficulties before, and we are not going to be intimidated or rebuffed by specious arguments, or open opposition. We have a profession that is worth fighting for, a body of women most of whom I'm sure are loyal and devoted, and traditions that any profession might envy. Nothing will prevent us but our own blindness or apathy, or faithlessness."[4]

Immediately following the Nutting paper, ANA's new interstate secretary, Isabel McIsaacs, addressed the group. It is clear from her remarks that New York had already established a national leadership role. "What the New York nurses do very largely sets the pace for what the nurses do in other states."[5] After hearing the passion, enthusiasm, and encouragement of these speakers, it is no wonder that delegates were inspired to initiate a legislative campaign to improve the law.

Delegates to the 1912 meeting came prepared to formally vote on amending the Nurse Practice Act. In a welcome address to delegates, Sophia Palmer remembered the importance of the July 1902 meeting in formulating New York's first nurse practice act, and reminded delegates of NYSNA's leadership role in a new national movement toward mandatory registration. "We come back to Utica to again take up the discussion of the amendments to our law . . . The movement has commenced, New York is leading it. It has led it before and in every state it

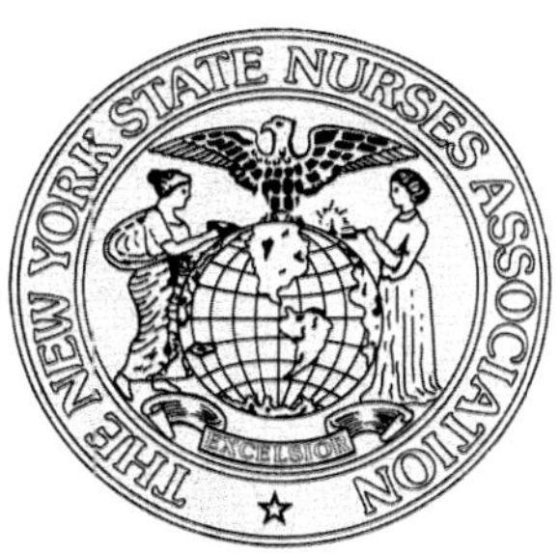

NYSNA's seal, first used in 1912, was designed by Beatrice Stevenson, NYSNA's president from 1913 to 1915. Stevenson served as a Red Cross nurse in the Spanish American War, and as superintendent of nurses at Rikers Island Hospital. The eagle on the seal represents leadership, and the globe represents nurses' field of work. Hygieia, the Goddess of Health, stands on the globe's left, and Florence Nightingale on the right. "Excelsior" expresses the association's ideals for professional advancement to higher standards.

is the subject for discussion and agitation in this year."[6] A paper by Miss Nutting reported on a Teachers College study of nurse training schools that found the majority seriously lacked standards and demonstrated even greater deficiencies than twenty years ago. "We are, therefore, more convinced than ever that a stringent law is absolutely necessary to check that downward flow by making registration compulsory."[7] Delegates empowered the Legislative Committee to prepare amendments to the Nurse Practice Act to restrict the practice of nursing and use of the title "nurse" to graduates of approved and registered schools of nursing.[8]

> "Possibly we need another title for the amending of our bill. It could be 'Registered Real Nurses.'"
>
> — *Annie Rhodes*[1]

In January 1913 the Legislative Committee sent the proposed amendments to association members and superintendents of registered training schools, asking for endorsement by physicians, boards of trustees, and other interested parties. Senator Seeley, chairman of the Public Health Committee, introduced a bill on February 18, 1913, and a letter prepared by Lavinia Dock was sent to each member of the Legislature.

Hearings on the bill were held in March. Legislative Committee chairman Annie Goodrich reported that "None of us who were present at that first hearing will, I am sure, ever forget the day. The Assembly Room two-thirds filled by our opponents, the hour and a half through which we listened to attacks upon our motives, the brief but dignified replies by our women . . ."[9] The correspondence schools, notably the Chautauqua School in Jamestown, and the "short-courses," represented by the National School for Certified Nurses in Albany, vigorously opposed the bill. They contended that their graduates were needed to provide care to the poor and middle class who could not afford the $25 per week charged by registered nurses. Bill supporters retorted that rich and poor alike deserved the highest level of nursing care possible, provided by well-prepared nurses, and pointed out that pupil nurses provided a great deal of care to the poor in public hospitals without compensation.[10]

The Hospital Council of New York City bitterly opposed the bill. In fact, it wanted to loosen the restrictions of the Nurse Practice Act to insure that city hospitals could continue to train nurses in sufficient numbers to meet the demand for service. Sophia Palmer, however, knew there were large numbers of New York City nurses unable to secure work, and concluded "that it is not primarily in the interest of the public that this protest is made, but for the economic advantage of cheap service to the hospital."[11]

The second hearing was expected to be less significant. NYSNA leaders believed the opposition would not even appear, but when President Twiss arrived at Grand Central Station on her way to Albany, "She saw the members of the opposition leave on the Empire express. With her usual quick thought and action, she immediately sent a telegram to warn the chairman and spent the rest of the day getting telegrams sent to the chairman of the Public Health Committee, Senator Seeley." Nurses in Albany and Schenectady were also contacted, and immediately went to work to secure hearing speakers. Meanwhile, telegrams poured in from around the state. During the hearing, when it was stated that the proposed legislation was "the work of a few nurses," Senator Seeley silently passed a stack of telegrams documenting the support of thousands from around the state.[12]

> "The committee labored faithfully to try to plan some satisfactory way to overcome the criticisms of the Medical Society and still maintain the standard of the registered nurse."
>
> — *Mary D. Burrill*[2]

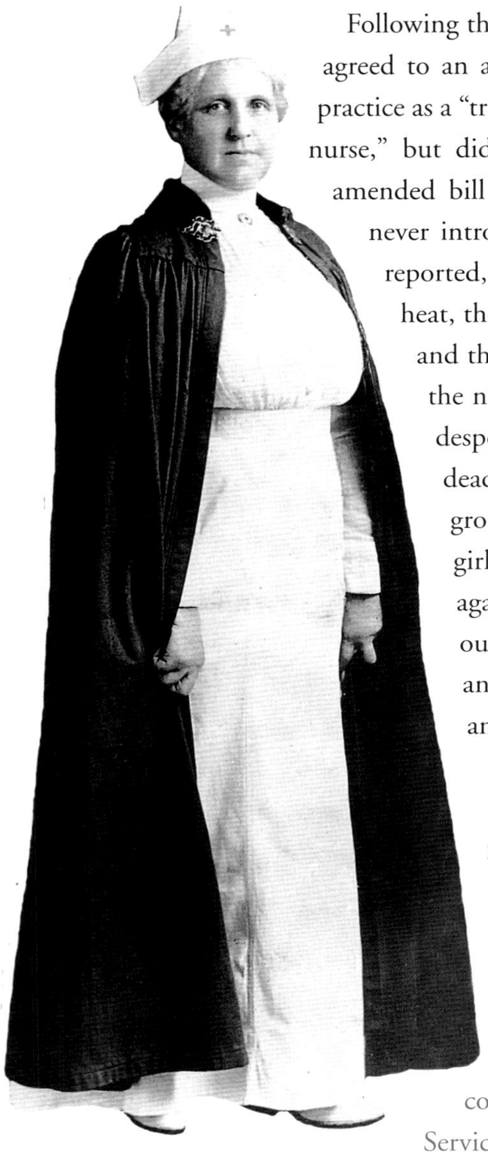

Following the hearings, the association reluctantly agreed to an amendment which defined who may practice as a "trained, certified, graduate or registered nurse," but did not protect the title "nurse." The amended bill was passed by the Senate, but was never introduced into the Assembly. Goodrich reported, "As we went out from the glare, the heat, the flowers, and the gifts to the Speaker and the Leaders, down the Capitol Hill, on the night that the Legislature adjourned, a despondent little group, for *our* Bill was dead, a cheery voice sang out from a group of Assemblymen, 'Never mind, girls, don't feel so badly about it. Come again next year and we will help you out.'"[13] Goodrich blamed the defeat on an inadequate educational campaign and poor organization.

An entirely rewritten bill was introduced in 1914. A proposal to establish several grades of nurses representing various levels of training was gaining support in the medical community, but Palmer declared the grading proposal was "based upon fraud. A woman is either a nurse or not a nurse. If she is not qualified to care for the sick, she should not be called a nurse."[14] Opposition arguments were similar to those voiced the previous year, and the bill was not reported out of committee. Despite another defeat, President Beatrice Stevenson stated, "It is no small thing to have aroused a mighty State like New York on the question, *who* is caring for the sick — it is no small contribution to public health work to have raised the question, *who* is the nurse . . ." Stevenson viewed the legislative struggle, not just as an attempt to pass a bill, but to effect a great reform to improve the care of the sick. She encouraged delegates to persevere. ". . . I am willing to come every year, until we have gained that great reform. That is what we are trying to do. Not just pass a bill."[15]

LEFT: Jane Arminda Delano directed the Bellevue Training School for Nurses from 1902 to 1907. In 1909 she became superintendent of the Army Nurse Corps, president of the ANA, and chairman of the national committee of the Red Cross Nursing Service. She later became director of the Red Cross Nursing Service, recruiting and organizing nurses during World War I. *Courtesy Nurses House Collection, Foundation of NYSNA Archives.*

In 1915, 1916, and 1917, the association endorsed bills prepared and sponsored by the State Education Department. These bills again restricted the use of "trained, graduate, certified and registered nurse." Legislative Committee Chairman Beatrice Stevenson characterized the opposition as "frankly and rankly commercial."[16] Strong opposition continued from the correspondence schools and "short-courses." NYSNA was described as a small coterie of registered nurses, protected by the Board of Regents, who sought to control the practice of nursing. Attacks on the regents were even more venomous, calling them "conspicuously unfit" to regulate nursing, and unsympathetic to the sick poor. The registration exam itself was condemned as "impracticable and absurd."[17]

The bill was referred to as the "Nurses' Monopoly Bill" by many newspapers. The Hospital Conference of New York City and others introduced amendments to eliminate the association's role in the nomination of State Board of Nurse Examiners' candidates, and to add

Annie Wharburton Goodrich
1866 - 1954

Annie Goodrich, graduate of the training school for nurses at New York Postgraduate Hospital, was a beloved and influential nursing leader. She served as Superintendent of Nursing at several New York hospitals, including St. Luke's Hospital and Bellevue Hospital. In 1910 she became the second Inspector of Nurses' Training Schools in New York, and in 1917 became director of nurses at the Henry Street Settlement. She was an active NYSNA member, serving as a trustee and on committees. As president of the American Nurses' Association from 1915 to 1918, Goodrich simplified and reorganized the membership structure.

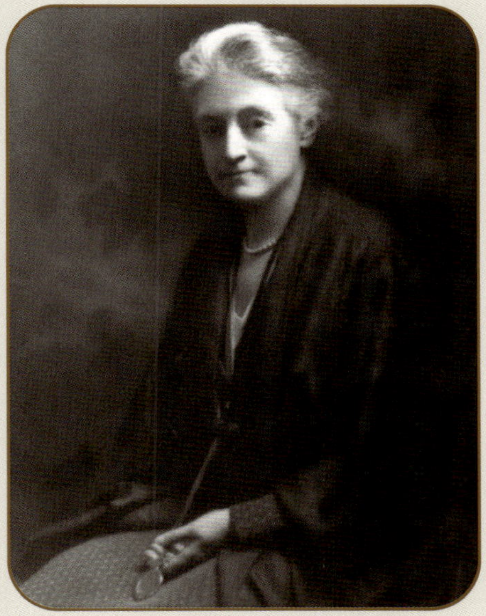

Courtesy Nurses House Collection, Foundation of NYSNA Archives.

Annie Goodrich was a fierce proponent of raising admission and graduation requirements in schools of nursing, and an early supporter of university education for nurses. She strongly supported legislation protecting the title "nurse." "We are asking about the same protection as the pharmacist and the druggist. They do not say 'qualified, certified, trained druggist.' They know better than that. They say one is a pharmacist and one is a druggist and that one shall have five years of preparation, and the other three. As a member of the American Nurses' Association, representing 20,000 trained women in the United States, I protest that I will live and die a nurse."[1] As chairman of NYSNA's Committee on Legislation, she guided the development of a revision of the Nurse Practice Act, and urged the association to continue to introduce legislation until a new bill was finally enacted in 1920.

During World War I, Goodrich was chief inspector nurse of Army hospitals, proposed the Army School of Nursing, and served as its first dean. Despite these heavy demands, she continued as a member of NYSNA's Executive Committee. She frequently presented papers at annual meetings and contributed to discussions, demonstrating her sharp intellect, lively enthusiasm, and inspired leadership. She shared with delegates her view of the future of nursing, where there would be "a coordinated program through which the public may have reasonable assurance of the availability of the required nursing service for the cure and prevention of disease at a minimum cost with assurance to the nurse of economic security."[2] In 1923 Annie Goodrich left New York to become dean of the first experimental university-based independent school of nursing at Yale University.

physicians and hospital representatives to the State Board. Each year the bill was defeated. No doubt deeply discouraged, leaders were nonetheless determined, and the indomitable Beatrice Stevenson encouraged members. "Events may not move as swiftly as we desire but eventually legislative regulation, restriction and standardization of the practice of nursing is inevitable."[18]

"Never before have we worked so harmoniously and untiringly together to accomplish the ultimate ends for which we are organized."

— *Maud Jack*[3]

The association prepared a new bill, introduced in 1919, which added a provision for trained attendants. This decision was not an easy one. A proposal for licensing and registering attendants was rejected by association leaders when Dr. Downing first suggested it in 1911, but since then the world had changed. The serious shortage of nurses experienced during World War I and the 1918 influenza epidemic, and the use of Red Cross trained aides was fresh in everyone's mind. "Since there have been so many women trained as nurses' aids, unless they are controlled by the department many of them are going to pose as nurses . . . I feel that unless we control and can get a bill through, including this class of nurses, that is placing them under the control of the regents, that our difficulties are going to be greater than they have ever been."[19]

At the association's annual meeting in 1919, the Legislative Committee once again had to report defeat. Undaunted, chairman Alice Shepard Gilman submitted detailed recommendations to increase the dissemination of information and raise funds for the 1920 campaign.[20] Facing the same old opposition, the association reluctantly agreed to several major concessions. In response to intense pressure from the State Hospital Commission on Lunacy, NYSNA agreed to delay the preliminary education requirement of one year of high school for entrance into training schools, in effect lowering the entrance requirement and usurping the Board of Regents' authority to determine preliminary requirements. And, as a compromise response to pressure to include physicians on the Board of Nurse Examiners, the association agreed to include physicians and hospital representatives on the Advisory Council to the State Board of Nurse Examiners.[21]

The bill passed the legislature on April 24, and was signed into law by Governor Alfred E. Smith on May 12, the one hundredth anniversary of the birth of Florence Nightingale. After nine years of concerted effort, the association had finally achieved a new law, but it barely resembled the earlier amendments prepared by the association. The law protected the titles "trained, certified, graduate, and registered nurse," rather than "nurse," and a provision restricting unregistered schools from training nurses was eliminated.[22] The law did include a provision for reciprocity, appointment of a paid secretary of the Board of Nurse Examiners, and licensed attendants. Perhaps most significantly, the law included a generous waiver clause "so broad that no injustice can possibly be done to anyone who has made nursing her occupation."[23]

In November 1920 the association publicized the major points of the law in newspapers and in handbills distributed throughout the state, and nurses eligible for licensure through waiver were urged to apply before the January 1921 deadline. On December 16, 1920, the Chautauqua Correspondence School of Nursing served an injunction on NYSNA to cease distribution of the materials. The school charged that the association was "working consistently in opposition to the Chautauqua School," and that the publicity materials contained misleading information. To avoid a court trial, the Chautauqua School offered to accept an amendment to the Nurse Practice Act, removing "graduate nurse" as a protected title.[24] NYSNA refused the offer and a trial ensued during which the association agreed to refrain from disseminating information stating or implying that Chautauqua graduates were not entitled to practice nursing as Chautauqua Nurses. NYSNA leaders believed this to be a mutually satisfactory solution that did not compromise the integrity of the law, and President Alice Gilman viewed the legal struggle as a victory. "The time has come when this Association must take a decisive stand not only in setting professional standards and in placing laws on the statute books but in the enforcement of such laws by fearlessly withstanding the attacks of those who would destroy us. In order to protect a piece of legislation that is of any value we must be prepared to struggle with the forces who are opposed and would commercialize our profession."[25]

NURSES CALLED TO SERVICE: At the 1909 NYSNA convention delegates voted to affiliate with the American Red Cross Nursing Service, and a committee was formed to encourage the establishment of local Red Cross committees and promote enrollment. Qualifications for enrollment included at least two years' training in a hospital that had a daily average of at least fifty patients of both sexes, state registration, and membership in an ANA affiliate organization.[26] Red Cross nurses provided heroic service to disaster victims, and in 1913 the War Department formalized an agreement whereby Red Cross nurses constituted a reserve for the U.S. Army Nurse Corps.[27]

When war broke out in Europe in August 1914, the Red Cross offered units of twelve nurses and three physicians to each country at war. Requests for nurses were sent to many East Coast cities, including New York, Brooklyn, Buffalo, Rochester, and Albany. A month later, the relief ship *Red Cross* carried physicians, supplies, and 120 nurses to serve in eight European countries. Efforts at enrollment were stepped up, and by October over a thousand New York nurses had been enrolled, and forty-eight called to war service.[28]

As the war escalated, the Red Cross began to organize base hospital units in major medical centers. Personnel from the hospital staff, equipment ("from scalpel to laundry plant"), and supplies necessary to set up a five-hundred-bed hospital were readied for mobilization. Each of these base hospital units had a chief nurse whose responsibility it was to secure and organize dietitians, nurses' aides, and fifty nurses.[29] When the United States declared war on Germany in April 1917, a plea went out to each nurse to "give herself to her country in the way she can best be of use . . . Wherever our duty lies, let us be found true women and true nurses, faithful, dependable, working well with others, broad in our sympathies and interests and so doing our part to support our nation's leaders in bringing righteousness and peace once more to this troubled world."[30] The first base hospital units left New York harbor for France in May, 1917.[31]

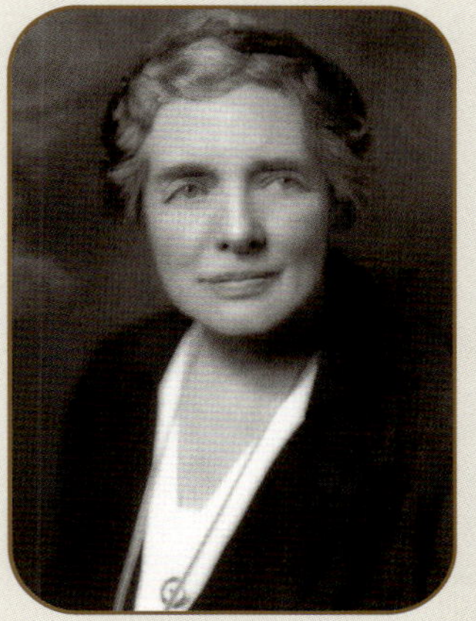

Florence Johnson, Director of the Atlantic Division of the Red Cross Nursing Service, addressed delegates at NYSNA's 1918 convention. Miss Johnson accompanied thousands of nurses to the port of New York when they left for European service during World War I. Her cheerful words and admonitions earned her the title "the nurse on the docks." *Courtesy Nurses House Collection, Foundation of NYSNA Archives.*

At NYSNA's 1917 annual meeting, it was reported that base hospital units had been formed in Albany, Buffalo, Rochester, Syracuse, Brooklyn,

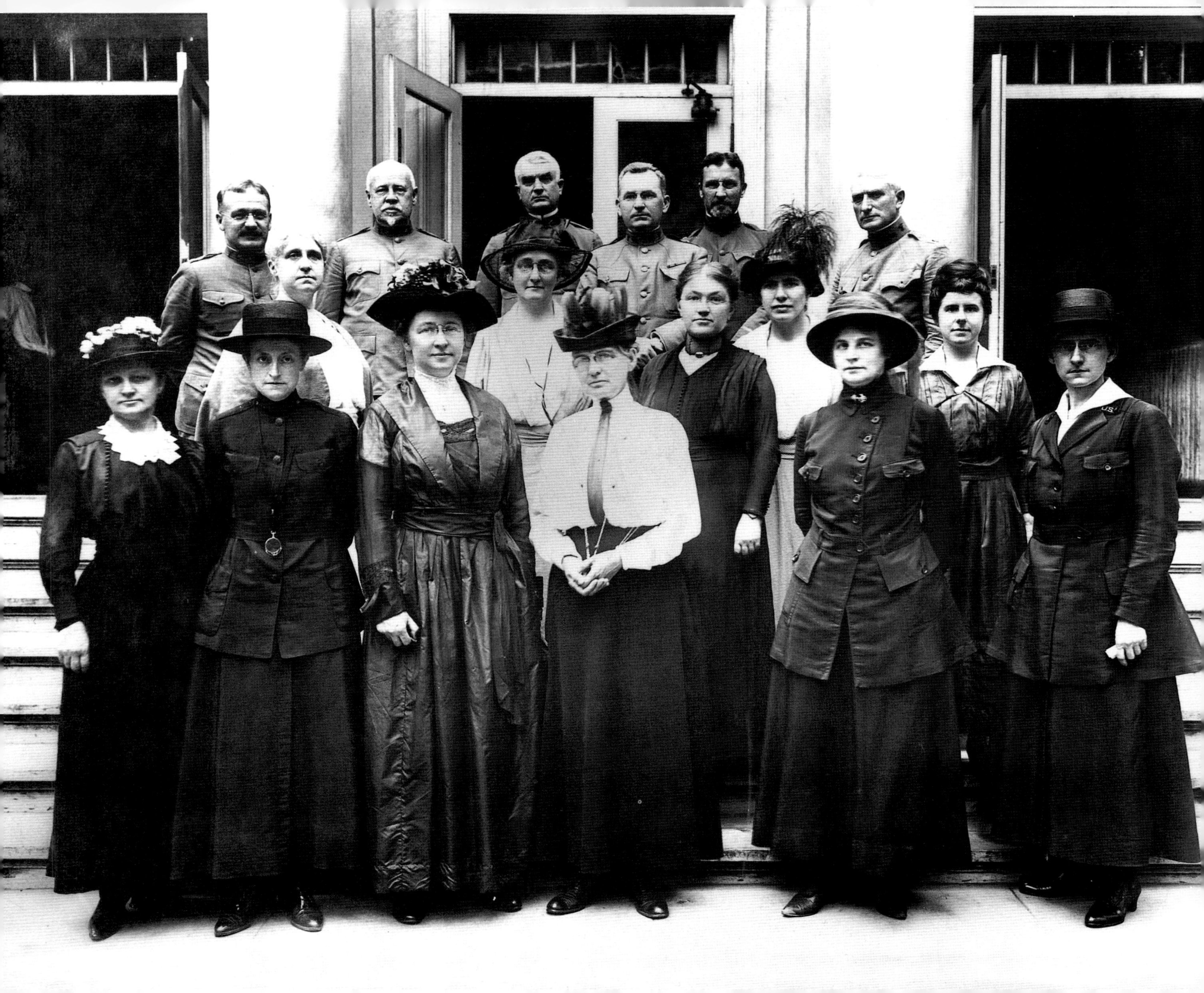

and New York. Two hundred New York Red Cross nurses were serving in "home service," five hundred in foreign service, and nearly a thousand were waiting to be called. "Seventeen hundred seems a large number to take from one State — but many, many more will be needed. We are just entering the war — the call for nurses has just begun and it will increase as the war goes on. To supply this demand is your problem — to meet it will require all your resources — it means a sacrifice even more for those who stay at home than for those who go abroad."[32] NYSNA membership was necessary for Red Cross enrollment, and applications poured in. NYSNA leaders modified membership processing in order to move the enrollment process along smoothly and quickly.[33]

"After this war, there are none of us who will not realize more fully the three words of that learned gentleman who said, 'War is hell,' and I think we who went, and also those who have remained behind, will realize also that those three words mean a great deal."

— *Esmee Everard*[4]

In June 1917 a group of nurses assembled by Adelaide Nutting formed the National Emergency Committee on Nursing to plan for military and civilian nursing needs during the war. In addition to base hospital units, nurses were needed on hospital trains, and in camp, evacuation, and mobile hospitals. Public health nurses were needed in and around military camps where serious health problems developed, and in France to assist with tuberculosis control and the needs of thousands of homeless children. Supervisors and teachers were required to train the increasing numbers of student nurses. The supply of nurses to meet civilian health needs was quickly depleted, and one of the committee's first tasks was to systematically survey the nation's nursing resources. Working with the committee, the American Nurses Association agreed to sponsor a survey conducted by the state nurses' associations. NYSNA's survey was more complete than that of many states, and identified many types of "nurses" and attendants. Survey results revealed large numbers of nurses eligible for Red Cross Service, and heightened the resolve of nursing's leaders to provide an adequate supply of qualified nurses without sacrificing hard-won standards, even though there was pressure to lower admission and graduation requirements in schools of nursing and waive legal requirements.[34]

LEFT: M. Adelaide Nutting, center front, was a frequent speaker at NYSNA annual meetings. During World War I, Nutting helped plan for nursing needs through the Committee on Nursing of the Council of National Defense, shown here. *Courtesy Special Collections, Milbank Memorial Library, Teachers College, Columbia University, New York.*

Hospitals initiated massive recruitment campaigns and new programs developed to increase the supply of nurses. Assuming college educated women could be prepared more quickly to fill needed teaching, administrative, and public health positions, Vassar College initiated an experimental program in the summer of 1918. The program provided a three-month preparatory course, followed by a shortened period of hospital training at affiliated schools. A second program, the Army School of Nursing, was established to increase the nurse supply and to provide a student labor force in military hospitals.[35]

Military nurses serving in Europe cared for soldiers suffering from devastating wounds caused by modern artillery, poison gas, infection, contagious disease, and "shell shock." They worked fourteen to eighteen hours a day for weeks at a time, and some hospitals had only seventy to eighty nurses to care for thousands of patients.[36] While assuming these

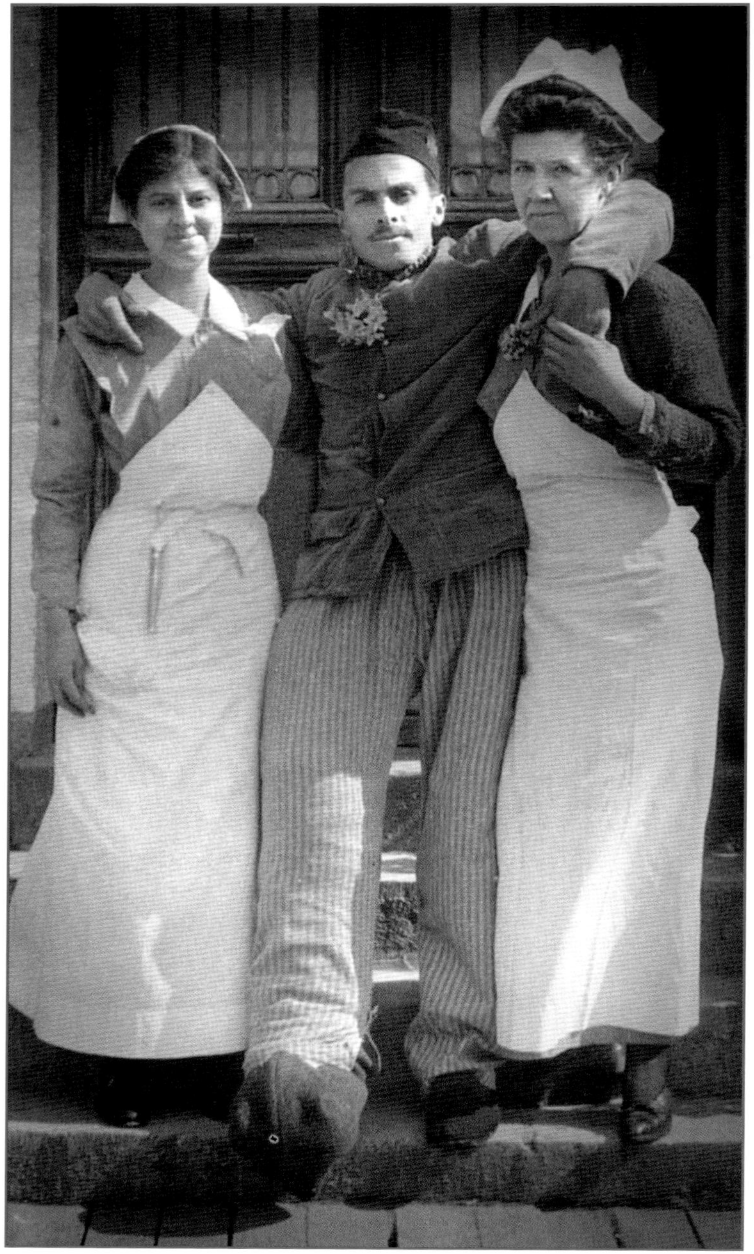

overwhelming responsibilities, nurses were hampered by their lack of military rank, which prohibited them from teaching or directing orderlies or handling administrative problems.[37] Mrs. Helen Hoy Greeley, counsel to the National Committee to Secure Military Rank for Nurses, told delegates to NYSNA's 1918 convention, ". . . it had never occurred to the United States authorities that the position of the nurse should be defined. They have not cared. It has not occurred to them to care whether she was fish, flesh, fowl or good red herring, and nobody has known whether she was an officer, private or hired extra . . . "[38] Delegates were admonished to write their congressional representatives "soon and often," and delegates passed a resolution urging passage of the bill.[39] NYSNA's Executive Committee sent a telegram to the War Department's Chief of Staff, urging "you to use every means in your power to aid in the passage of the bill, now before the Senate, to grant rank to nurses in military service."[40] Although a bill giving military nurses officer status was finally passed in 1920, it did not provide the pay and allowances enjoyed by male officers.[41]

World War I ended with the signing of the Armistice on November 11, 1918. At NYSNA's annual meeting the following month, Annie Goodrich spoke to the delegates. "I could not tell you, of course, what joy is in my heart, and I need not, because I know it is in all our hearts, that we are now come to a meeting without the shadow of a horror over us; that those who have gone and served are coming back, some of them; those who can't come back have served as they desired to serve and have made the supreme contribution and sacrifice to the saving of democracy. Life again seems possible to all of us, therefore we can begin to think in constructive terms."[42] ANA spearheaded a drive to establish the Florence Nightingale School of Nursing at Bordeaux, France as a tribute to the 296 American nurses who lost their lives during war service. NYSNA contributed to this project, which was finally completed in 1931.[43]

LEFT: Red Cross nurses Marion McCune Rice, at left, and Josephine Clay, at right, support French soldier "Leon." *Courtesy the Rice Collection.*

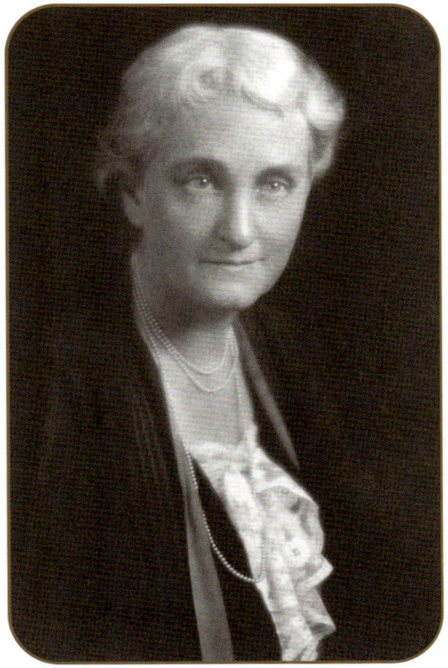

LEFT: Clara Noyes, former superintendent of Bellevue Hospital, was the director of the Red Cross Bureau of Nursing during World War I. She organized base hospitals and assigned nurses, and in 1919 succeeded Jane Delano as director of the Red Cross Nursing Service. Miss Noyes served as President of ANA from 1918 to 1922. *Courtesy Nurses House Collection, Foundation of NYSNA Archives; photograph by Harris and Ewing.*

"IF WE DON'T ALL DIE OF INFLUENZE": In the fall of 1918 a worldwide influenza epidemic further complicated the crisis of war. At home and abroad, wounded and convalescent soldiers and overworked hospital personnel were especially vulnerable to the virulent illness. One base hospital arrived in Europe with so many ill with influenza it was never organized for service.

"The onset of sickness was rapid. A victim felt chilly and weak, suffered pains in his eyes or ears or head or back, complained of dizziness, coughed, clutched his throat because it felt sore, and in a few hours was prostrated. Anyone in close contact with a flu patient could expect to be stricken within the next few hours or days, so quickly did the plague spread." The death toll in New York City reached over eight hundred in a single day. "Hospitals filled up, overflowed, and turned away patients. Doctors urged everyone to stay home. So many staff members at Bellevue Hospital succumbed that a few doctors suggested the place be closed . . . Nurses dragged about their duties, eyes black-ringed with fatigue."[44]

NYSNA's 1918 annual meeting was scheduled for October in Rochester, where "the great and imminent peril to public health" had prompted the closure or limiting of hours of operation of places where groups of people gathered. At Rochester General Hospital, where staff was already depleted by half due to the war, probationary students were assigned to hospital duty, and senior students assumed responsibilities usually assigned to interns.[45] Hospital superintendent Mary Keith, chair of the convention program committee, sent a telegram. "Influenze has reached Rochester. No disengaged nurses in City and other Cities calling for help. Local Health Officer advises postponement of States meeting." Other telegrams and letters were read at NYSNA's Executive Committee meeting. Miss Lightbourne wrote, "Hope convention is postponed. Would be criminal to hold meeting where influenze is raging. I am helping to fight it in Watertown." Amy Hilliard, State Inspector of Training Schools wrote, "I do not know of any nurse in active duty who would be able to attend the convention with a clear conscience." Rochester nurse and associate editor of the *American Journal of Nursing,* Katherine DeWitt, urged postponement. "We all think it would be folly to try to hold the state meeting at the appointed time . . . the epidemic may have subsided in two weeks, but just now it is increasing . . . Cheer up! If we don't all die of influenze, we will have a good state meeting yet."[46] The meeting was postponed until December.

"A great many have been profiteering, while others have given their services free during the epidemic."

— *Miss Cummings*[5]

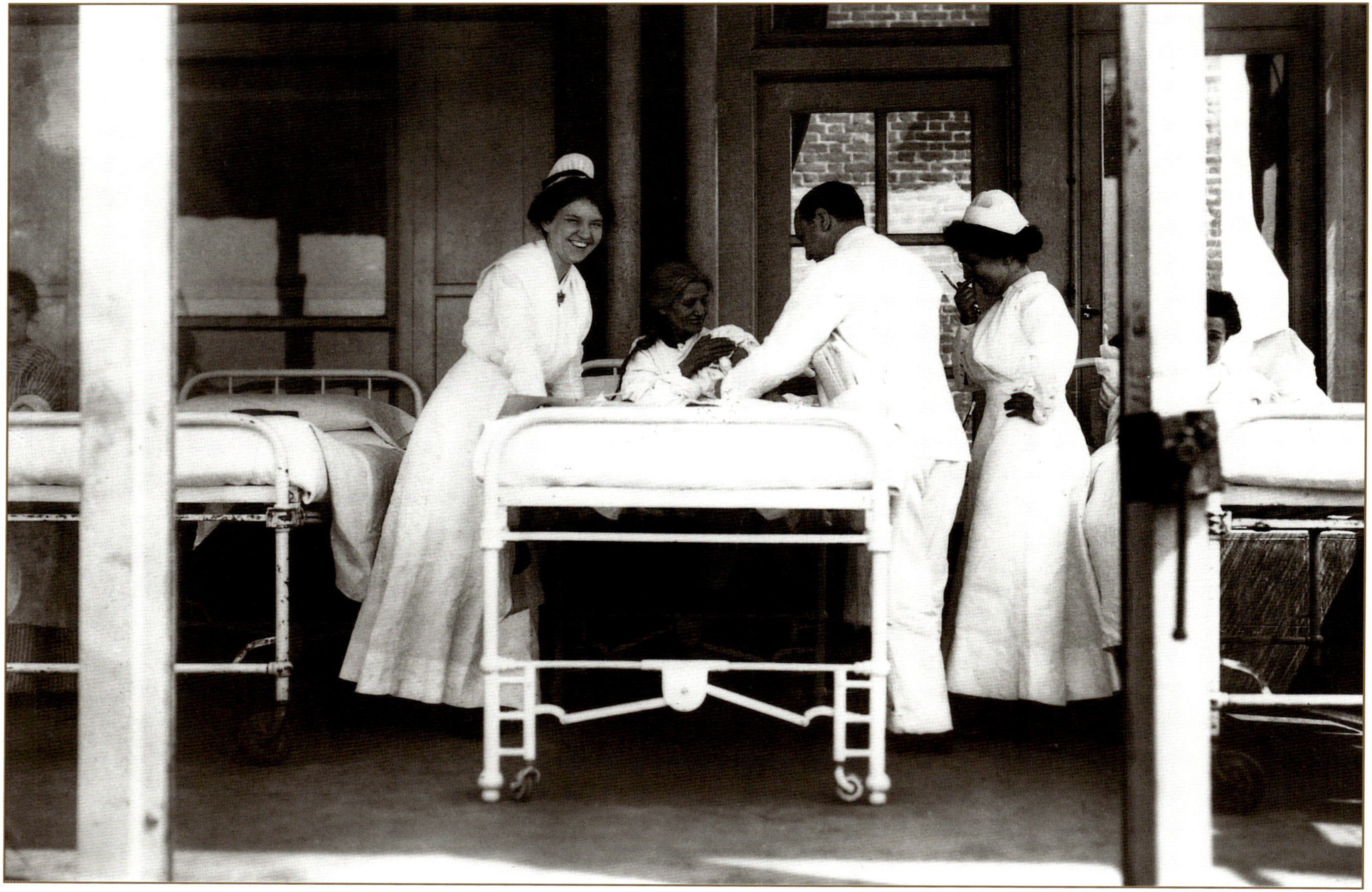

Hospital wards, such as this one at Mount Sinai Hospital, were often moved outdoors.
Courtesy the Archives of the Mount Sinai Medical Center.

Twenty thousand New Yorkers died in the 1918 epidemic, and an alarming number of nurses and nursing students were stricken. Ever the reformer, Sophia Palmer remarked, "When you see the Journal and see the death list this morning I think you will agree with me and some of the rest of us that there was something radically wrong in the life of the nurses of this country, for the long hours and hard work that they did, or that so weakened their resisting powers to a very unnatural degree, because they have gone down as nothing has ever shaken them before."[47]

> "The time would seem to have come when there must be a central directory for registered nurses in the City of New York; one directory where strangers in need of nurses may go or send and be sure of securing a reliable registered nurse."
>
> — *Mary E. Thornton*[6]

Calm after the Crises: At NYSNA's 1919 convention, Annie Goodrich noted the tremendous stress and strain of the past few years. "A speaker recently likened the present situation in the world to the seashore after a great storm . . . The waves have rolled in and there has been tumult on the land; but it is always after the sun is shining and the world is at peace that the waves come in mountain high and that the undercurrents are more than ever dangerous. This is indeed a good picture, I think, of the situation we are facing today."[48]

Nurses and nursing had been in the public eye in recruiting posters, newspapers, and magazines during the war. Large numbers of patriotic young women entered training schools in response to recruitment appeals, yet by 1920 there was a great scarcity of graduate nurses and a serious shortage of applicants to training schools.[49] Other occupations were opening up to women, and nursing leaders advocated for reforms to make nursing more attractive. They called for improved conditions in training schools, an eight-hour day for students, higher educational standards, and altering conditions so that private duty nurses could maintain a home life and "a normal relation to the rest of the world."[50]

While the crises of war, epidemic, and a bitter legislative battle consumed a great deal of NYSNA's resources, NYSNA did achieve successes during these busy years. The existing structure providing for both individual and organizational membership became increasingly burdensome, both at the state and national levels. When Annie Goodrich became ANA president in 1915, she devised a membership plan whereby all nurses became members through their state associations. The establishment of districts throughout each state was encouraged. NYSNA adopted this plan in 1918, and by the following year, ten districts, representing 6,339 nurses, submitted bylaws and were accepted into membership. The acceptance of the four remaining districts in 1920 completed the reorganization.[51] The establishment of the district nurses' associations was a highly significant development. These organizations were instrumental in advancing the mission, programs, and policies of the state association on the regional level.

Annual NYSNA conventions continued to provide a stimulating forum for discussion and opportunities for education. As the field of public health nursing expanded, aspects of this work became popular topics. The newly organized National Organization for Public Health Nursing was discussed at the 1912 meeting, and in 1915 NYSNA's Committee on Public Health became the New York State Organization for Public Health Nursing.[52] Papers on polio were presented in response to epidemics in 1912 and 1916. The Executive Committee approved birth control and health insurance as convention topics in 1917, and venereal disease in 1919. Private duty nursing, registries, and professional ethics were perennially popular topics for discussion.

Mary L. Keith
1865 - 1948

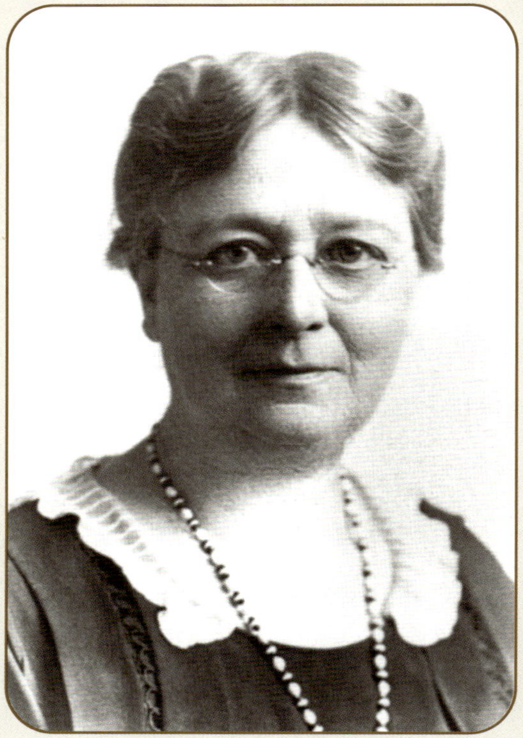

Courtesy Baker-Cederberg Museum and Archives.

Mary Keith graduated from the Boston Training School for Nurses in 1888, and held several positions with Boston hospitals. She replaced Sophia Palmer as superintendent of the Rochester City Hospital in 1901. In that position she established a formal Department of Nursing and oversaw construction of twelve new buildings which doubled the hospital's bed capacity.

Miss Keith was a member of NYSNA and an active participant at annual meetings. She must have been well-loved and respected by her fellow nurses, for her comments usually engendered both laughter and applause. In 1916 she was a speaker on the topic, "The Private Nurse and Twenty-Four Hour Hospital Duty." She believed twenty-four-hour duty was detrimental to both the patient and the nurse, and instead advocated for twelve-hour shifts. Her comments on these issues give a glimpse into the daily routine of private duty nursing in the hospital.

"A nurse on twenty-four duty must necessarily sleep in the patient's room, and her sleep is frequently interrupted, and for what? To rub a back, to give a bed-pan, to open or close a window, fill a hot water bottle or an ice bag, fill a glass with cold water, or get a cup of hot broth, to pull a blanket up or down, or any one of a number of offices which could very well be performed by the general nurse on night duty. Then the day special, refreshed by a night's sleep outside the hospital, takes her duties cheerfully in the morning and is ready to give the bath and serve the meals, make the bed, do the dressing, get a patient outdoors, arrange flowers, read to the patient, amuse her, keep the callers away or entice them in, as the case may be, and do something to help the patient, and the patient is better served."[1]

In 1911 the suffrage movement surged forward with an aggressive national campaign, and suffrage societies were established along the lines of political parties. A delegation from the Woman's Suffrage Party arrived at the 1912 annual meeting and requested time on the program. While it was agreed there was no time available in the crowded convention schedule, Beatrice Stevenson, Katherine DeWitt, and Sophia Palmer declared their positions as "ardent suffragettes." The vote on a motion to send a message of "sympathy in their work" was lost; however, the vote demonstrated a nearly equal division on the issue. The following year, guest speakers presented papers for and against suffrage, and in 1914 delegates granted a suffragette five minutes to address the body. President Stevenson voiced her strong opposition to the association taking a stand, and the voting body took no action on the suffrage question. New York ratified the suffrage amendment in 1917, and in 1920 the amendment became law.[53]

THE END OF AN ERA: In October 1920 convention delegates arrived at the Albany train station and made their way up State Street hill toward the capitol. An electric sign blazed, "Welcome New York State Nurses." In her welcome to delegates, Elizabeth Burgess, secretary of the Board of Nurse Examiners, referred to members' many trips to Albany to lobby legislators in the ongoing struggle to protect and strengthen the Nurse Practice Act. "I am sure . . . that many of you have come with far different feelings than those you had when you made your last trip to Albany. 'Going to Albany,' it meant hard work and not at all an agreeable task to many of you. So we are especially glad to have you this year with the knowledge that that particular piece of work is behind you, and the satisfaction that you have passed another milestone on the road of nurse legislation."[54]

The celebration of legislative success was tempered by the "restlessness of the aftermath of war," and the loss of the beloved Sophia Palmer. Delegates discussed a fitting memorial for the equally beloved Jane Delano, who had died in France the previous year. The following year, delegates commemorated the resignation of the venerable Anna Maxwell from her position at Presbyterian Hospital, and offered a rising vote of thanks to Louise Twiss in recognition of fourteen years of service as an association officer.[55] For the first time, the Nominating Committee's slate included none of the "Old Guard." Instead of Palmer, Maxwell, Goodrich, Twiss, Allerton, and Stevenson, another generation of nurses was assuming leadership. It was the end of an era of nursing in New York State, and the beginning of another.

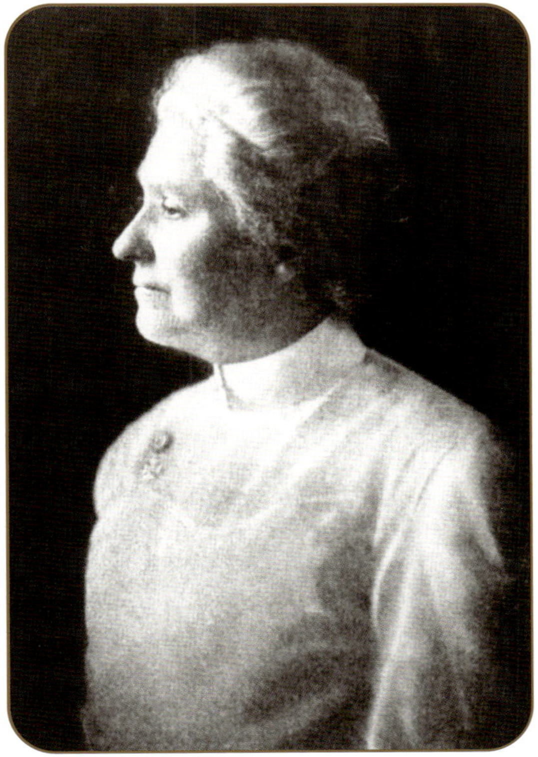

Anna Caroline Maxwell was a prominent nurse educator and administrator. She organized the nursing school at St. Luke's Hospital in New York City, and directed the nursing school at the city's Presbyterian Hospital for nearly thirty years. She was well-known for standardizing many nursing procedures and for building Presbyterian's school on high educational standards. She served on many NYSNA committees, and used her influence to aid in the passage of registration legislation. *Courtesy Nurses House Collection, Foundation of NYSNA Archives.*

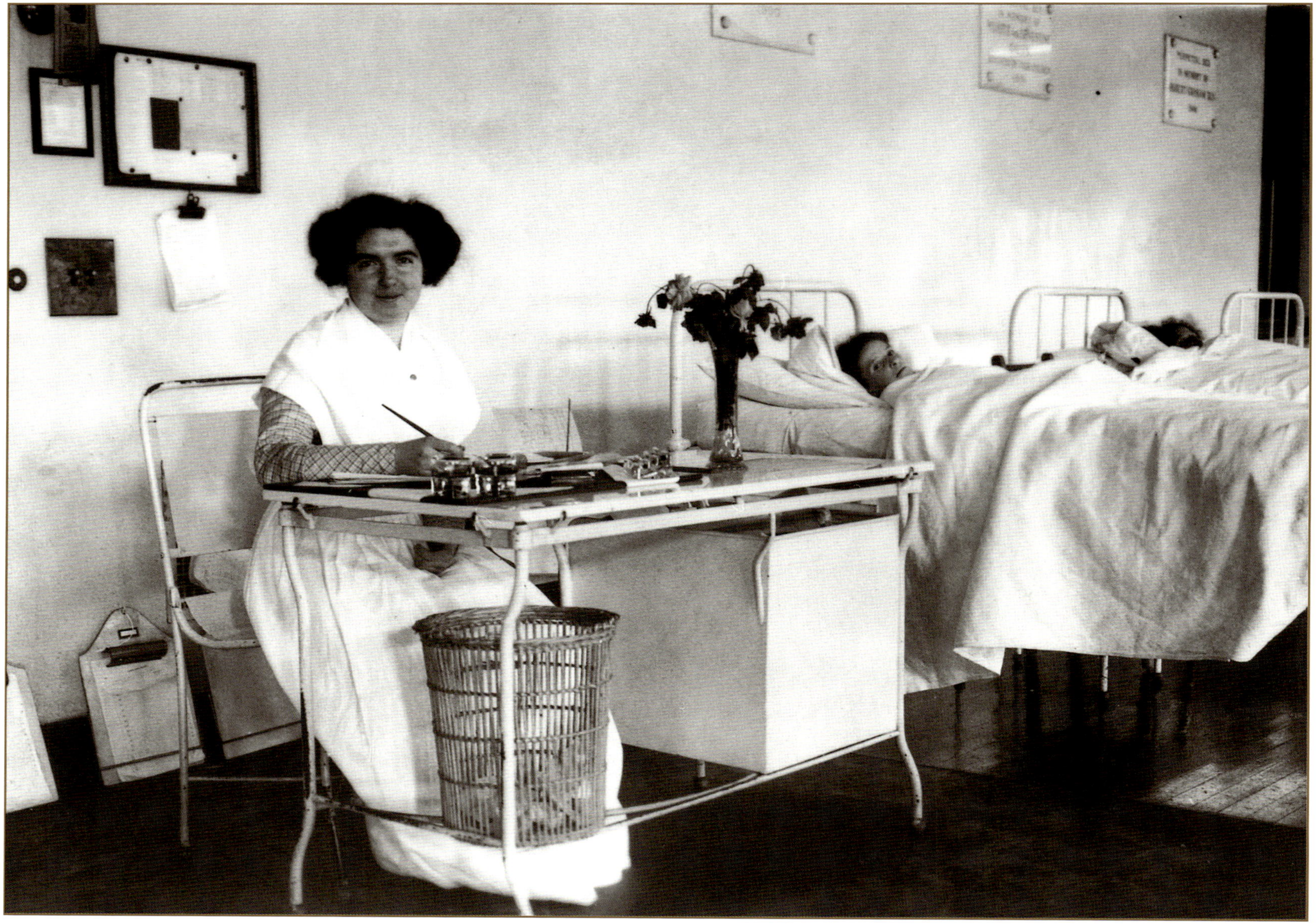

Until the 1920s, nurses' uniforms continued to have long, ample skirts. *Courtesy the Archives of the Mount Sinai Medical Center.*

TEXT

1. Annie W. Goodrich, "The Need of Orientation," *American Journal of Nursing* 13 (February 1913): 335–36.

2. *Ninth and Tenth Annual Meetings of The New York State Nurses' Association* (Syracuse, N.Y.: Lyman Bros., 1912), 55; and Sophia F. Palmer, "Editorial Comment," *American Journal of Nursing* 7 (October 1911): 3.

3. *Ninth and Tenth Annual Meetings,* 80–87.

4. Ibid., 88–103. Nutting was unable to attend the meeting, but the paper was read by her assistant, Isabel Stewart.

5. Ibid., 112. The Nurses' Associated Alumnae became the American Nurses Association (ANA) in 1911.

6. *Eleventh Annual Meeting of The New York State Nurses' Association* (Syracuse, N.Y.: Lyman Bros., 1913), 5. Later in the proceedings it was noted that the 1912 ANA convention attendees had discussed registration and emphasized the need for compulsory registration laws (p. 35).

7. Ibid., 39–41.

8. Driscoll, *Legitimizing the Profession,* 23; and *Eleventh Annual Meeting,* 11–12. Other provisions to be included in the bill were the addition of a reciprocity clause and elimination of the re-registration requirement. These provisions were recommended to delegates in a report distributed well before the meeting by the Committee on Legislation, composed of Anna Maxwell, Sophia Palmer, and Annie Goodrich. The bill eventually also included a waiver for "all reputable women doing nursing work at the present time." (Sophia F. Palmer, "Editorial Comment," *American Journal of Nursing* 13 [April 1913]: 492.)

9. *Twelfth Annual Meeting of The New York State Nurses' Association* (New York, N.Y.: Styles & Cash, 1913), 53.

10. Palmer, "Editorial Comment," April 1913, 493.

11. Sophia F. Palmer, "Editorial Comment," *American Journal of Nursing* 12 (April 1912): 545. The 1910 State Department of Education's preliminary requirement of one year of high school was what hospital administrators believed restricted the admission of "probationers" and worked a hardship on hospitals.

12. *Twelfth Annual Meeting,* 54.

13. Ibid., 57.

14. Sophia F. Palmer, "Editorial Comment," *American Journal of Nursing* 14 (April 1914): 503; and "Nursing News and Announcements," *American Journal of Nursing* 13 (February 1913): 391. The grading proposal had been debated at a December 1912 meeting of the New York Academy of Medicine devoted to nursing education. Papers were presented by physicians, nursing leaders Adelaide Nutting and Annie Goodrich, and NYSNA President Twiss.

15. *Thirteenth Annual Meeting of the New York State Nurses' Association* (New York, N.Y.: McIlroy & Emmet, 1914), 158.

16. Beatrice V. Stevenson, "The Law and the Nurse" (n.d., handwritten), Stevenson Collection, Foundation of NYSNA, Guilderland, N.Y., 7.

17. Hearing Transcript, (24 March 1915, stenotype transcript), NYSNA Archives, Foundation of NYSNA, Guilderland, N.Y., 5–8.

18. Stevenson, "Law and the Nurse," 14.

19. *The Sixteenth-Seventeenth Annual Meetings of the New York State Nurses' Association* (n.p., [1918]), 273.

20. *Eighteenth Annual Meeting of the New York State Nurses' Association* (n.p., [1919]), 42–52.

21. Driscoll, *Legitimizing the Profession,* 35.

22. *Some Reasons for the Proposed Amendment to the Nurse Practice Act* (Albany, N.Y.: NYSNA, n.d.); and Elizabeth C. Burgess, "A Brief Survey of Results in New York Arising From the Amendment to the Nurse Practice Act in 1920," *American Journal of Nursing* 22 (September 1922), 1075–78.

23. Driscoll, *Legitimizing the Profession,* 35–37.

24. Twentieth Annual Meeting of the New York State Nurses' Association (n.p., [1921]), 31–44.

25. Ibid., 27.

26. Sophia F. Palmer, "Editorial Comment," *American Journal of Nursing* 17 (August 1917): 1034. When the Surgeon General of the Army called for one thousand nurses per week in the summer of 1918, the age requirement was lowered from 25 to 21, and the ANA membership requirement was temporarily discontinued. (Mary M. Roberts, *American Nursing: History and Interpretation* [New York: MacMillan Company, 1954], 151.)

27. "Official Reports of Societies," *American Journal of Nursing* 10 (December 1909): 206. Nurses had provided care to victims of fire, flood, earthquake, and shipwreck, including that of the *Titanic.* (Henry P. Davison, *The American Red Cross in the Great War* [New York: The MacMillan Co., 1920], 78–79.) There was no formal agreement with the Navy Nurse Corps, but unofficially the Red Cross became its reserve also. (Roberts, *American Nursing,* 145.)

28. Sophia F. Palmer, "Editorial Comment," *American Journal of Nursing* 14 (September 1914): 1040. As a neutral country, the U.S. sent relief to Germany as well as England, Russia, France, Austria, Bulgaria, Serbia, and Belgium. (Davison, *Red Cross in the War,* 79.) Anticipating the war would last only a few months, it was believed that the total U.S. enrollment of over five thousand nurses was "enough to supply all demands." *(Thirteenth Annual Meeting,* 32–33.) The nurses sent abroad in 1914 returned a year later. Jane Delano and three of the returning New York nurses presented papers on their experiences at the 1915 convention. *(Fourteenth Annual Meeting of the New York State Nurses' Association* [New York, N.Y., Macgowan & Slipper, 1915],129.)

29. Davison, *Red Cross in the War,* 80–81. The first base hospital unit was established in New York in 1916. Later in the war, base hospital units were required to accommodate a thousand beds, and included a hundred nurses. (*Fifteenth Annual Meeting of the New York State Nurses' Association* [Buffalo, N.Y.: n.p., 1916], 26–28; and Roberts, *American Nursing,* 147.)

30. Sophia F. Palmer, "Editorial Comment," *American Journal of Nursing* 17 (May 1917): 673.

31. Davison, *Red Cross in the War,* 82–83.

32. *Sixteenth-Seventeenth Meetings,* 30–31.

33. Minutes of the Executive Committee, NYSNA, 1917–18, NYSNA Archives.

34. Roberts, *American Nursing,* 134; Marie Louis, "Report of the Nursing Resources in the State of New York as of November and December, 1917," *The Modern Hospital* 10 (June 1918): 436–40.

35. Palmer, "Editorial Comment," August 1917, 1033; and M. Patricia Donahue, *Nursing, The Finest Art: An Illustrated History* (St. Louis, Mo.: Mosby — Year Book, 1996), 355–61. The May 1918 ANA convention delegates became embroiled in an intense debate over the establishment of the Army School of Nursing as a demonstration school, a plan developed and promoted by Annie Goodrich. A faction led by Jane Delano advocated a plan to tap the eager labor reserve of "women of the leisure class" by training them as nurses' aides rather than as nurses. Delegates voted to support the Army School of Nursing, which eventually enrolled thousands of young women. (Kalisch and Kalisch, *Advance of American Nursing,* 222–27.)

36. Kalisch and Kalisch, *Advance of American Nursing,* 228–29. Eighty-two percent of Army deaths during the war were due to influenza, pneumonia, and other respiratory diseases. (Roberts, *American Nursing,* 152.)

37. Donahue, *Nursing, The Finest Art,* 365. See also Palmer's "Editorial Comment," *American Journal of Nursing* 19 (May 1919): 577–85 for a thorough discussion of this issue.

38. *Sixteenth-Seventeenth Meetings,* 146–48.

39. Minutes of Executive Committee, 1917–18.

40. *Sixteenth-Seventeenth Meetings,* 145, 281.

41. Donahue, *Nursing, The Finest Art,* 365.

42. "Proceedings of the Seventeenth Annual Meeting of the New York State Nurses' Association" (Rochester, N.Y., 1918, stenotype transcript), 111. Many nurses' service continued following the war's end. For four years, nurses from the Red Cross and other agencies provided civilian relief and health programs, and promoted the development of schools of nursing in Europe. (Roberts, *American Nursing,* 155.)

43. Flanagan, *One Strong Voice,* 72.

44. Edward Robb Ellis, *The Epic of New York City* (New York: Kondansha International, 1997), 510–11.

45. Teresa K. Lehr and Philip G. Maples, *To Serve the Community: A Celebration of Rochester General Hospital 1847–1997* (Virginia Beach, Va.: Donning Co./Publishers, 1997), 71–72.

46. Minutes of Executive Committee, 1917–18. The annual meeting was convened on October 21 as scheduled. Rochester nurses attended and officially adjourned the meeting to December 4. (*Sixteenth-Seventeenth Meetings,* 104–5.)

47. *Sixteenth-Seventeenth Meetings,* 16; and Ellis, *Epic of New York City,* 511.

48. *Eighteenth Annual Meeting,* 13.

49. Flanagan, *One Strong Voice,* 423; and M. Adelaide Nutting, "The Outlook in Nursing," in *Proceedings of the Twenty-Sixth Annual Convention of the National League of Nursing Education, Atlanta, Georgia, April 12–17, 1920* (Baltimore: Williams and Wilkins Co., 1921), 310.

50. Nutting, "Outlook in Nursing," 313–23.

51. Existing county or city associations merged into the district associations. (*Sixteenth-Seventeenth Meetings,* 156–59; *Eighteenth Annual Meeting,* 30; and *Nineteenth Annual Meeting,* 15–18.) See Appendix 2 for a complete list of New York's district nurses' associations.

52. *Fourteenth Annual Meeting,* 129.

53. *Eleventh Annual Meeting,* 20–21; *Twelfth Annual Meeting,* 85–91, 115–21; *Thirteenth Annual Meeting,* 206–8; and Ellis, *Epic of New York City,* 392.

54. "Proceedings of the Nineteenth Annual Meeting of the New York State Nurses' Association" (Albany, N.Y.,1920, stenotype transcript), 9.

55. *Nineteenth Annual Meeting,* 35–36; and *Twentieth Annual Meeting,* 75–78. Twiss, former hospital superintendent, devoted herself to nursing organizations following her marriage in 1904. She was elected NYSNA president for four terms, served as District 13's president, and was ANA's treasurer for twelve years.

FEATURES

ANNIE WHARBURTON GOODRICH

1. *Twelfth Annual Meeting,* 130.

2. Annie W. Goodrich, "The Past, Present, and Future of Nursing," *American Journal of Nursing* 31 (December 1931): 1387.

MARY L. KEITH

1. Lehr and Maples, *To Serve the Community,* 74–75; and *Fourteenth Annual Meeting,* 67.

EXCERPTS

1. *Eleventh Annual Meeting,* 66.

2. "Nursing News and Announcements," *American Journal of Nursing* 11 (January 1911): 305.

3. *Fifteenth Annual Meeting,* 13-14.

4. *Fourteenth Annual Meeting,* 126.

5. *Sixteenth-Seventeenth Meetings,* 273.

6. "Letters to the Editor," *American Journal of Nursing* 4 (December 1903): 243-44.

CHAPTER THREE

Nursing in 1925

BY 1925 MANY NEW FIELDS OF PRACTICE HAD OPENED UP FOR NURSES, but private duty nursing dominated, employing 54 percent of nurses. Less than one-quarter of active registered nurses were employed by hospitals or other health institutions. The rate of many contagious diseases such as typhoid had declined, and the severity of others, such as pneumonia, had lessened. Smaller homes, advances in medicine, and improved medical equipment contributed to a sharp increase in hospitalization, and private duty nurses now cared for more patients in hospitals than in homes.

NYSNA surveys in 1925 and 1926 provide a great deal of information on the working conditions of nurses. The average private duty nurse in New York had been out of school five years or less. Although over half of the nurses worked the full seven days of the week surveyed, the average nurse worked five days. She cared for one case, which she got through a registry, and did not refuse any cases. She "registered against" (that is, she wouldn't accept) contagious and maternity cases. The average nurse worked a twelve-hour shift, though many continued to work twenty-four-hour duty. Average earnings were $31.26 a week, comparable to that earned by charwomen, servants, and other unskilled laborers. Even this, however, did not represent the average weekly salary for the private duty nurse, since there were intervals between cases (often five or six weeks during July and August) when there was no income.

The private duty nurse worked in isolation, with few opportunities to develop new nursing skills or outside interests. She received no supervision, and rarely could take time away from waiting for calls or resting to engage in educational pursuits or the development of colleagial relationships. Even if she was able to upgrade her skills, it was considered unethical to increase her fees. Thus, the skilled, experienced nurse received the same compensation as the newest graduate.

During a time when the public was being more and more encouraged to live a well balanced life, the private duty nurse focused on her career. With transportation time added to twelve-hour duty, the work day left time for little else. Time off was broken up into "irregular bits"—a day, a week, or more, confined to her quarters anxiously waiting for the registry to call with her next case. She was in no way compensated for this waiting time, nor did she enjoy paid vacations or sick leave. The nurse paid for every day of waiting for a call or resting after a particularly tiring case, or isolating herself after a contagious case. The average nurse had to plan on about four months of such unpaid time during the year. If she did choose to refuse a case for a much needed break, she usually lost her place on the registry list.

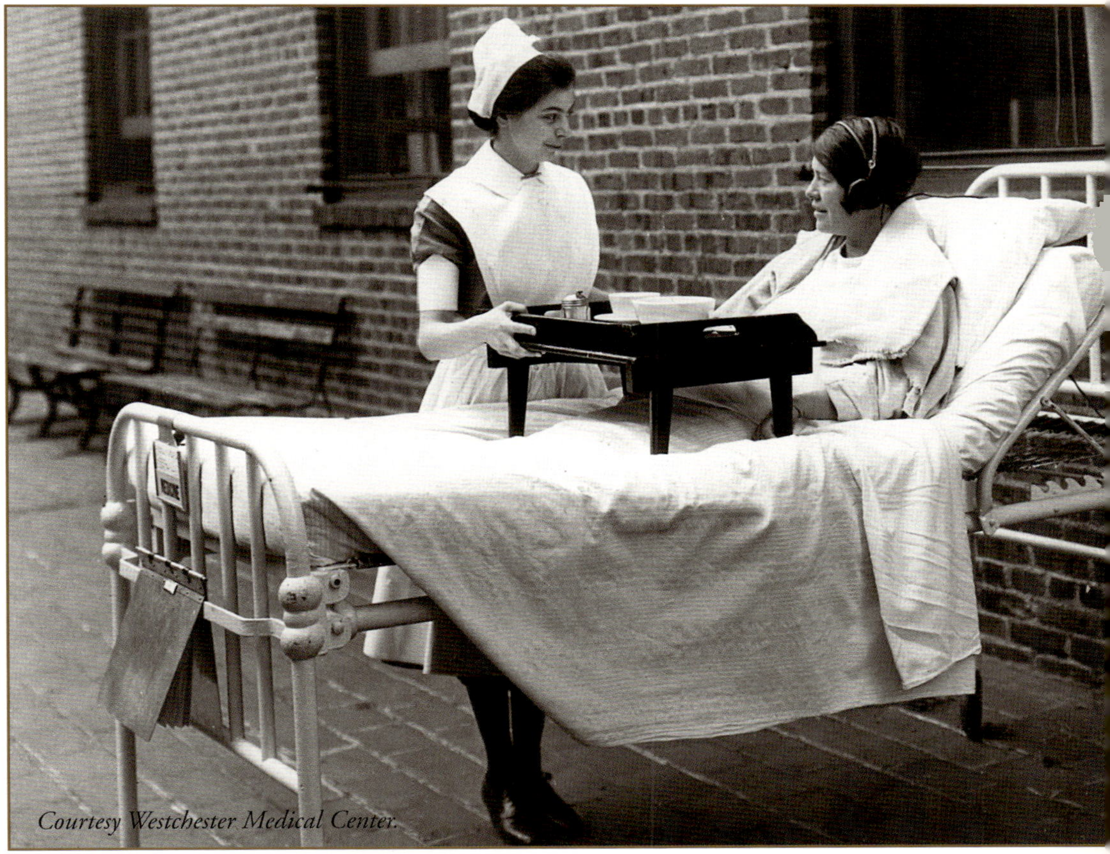

Courtesy Westchester Medical Center.

The demands of private duty nursing included having to cope with the monotony of being available to the patient for twelve hours when only a fraction of that time was needed to provide the necessary nursing care. This, combined with the irregularity of the work, and the social isolation, took a heavy toll. The private duty nurse rarely practiced past age 50.

Despite all these difficulties, and constant criticism, private duty nurses cherished the independence and freedom, and the challenge and stimulation of new cases. The average private duty nurse loved bedside nursing.[1]

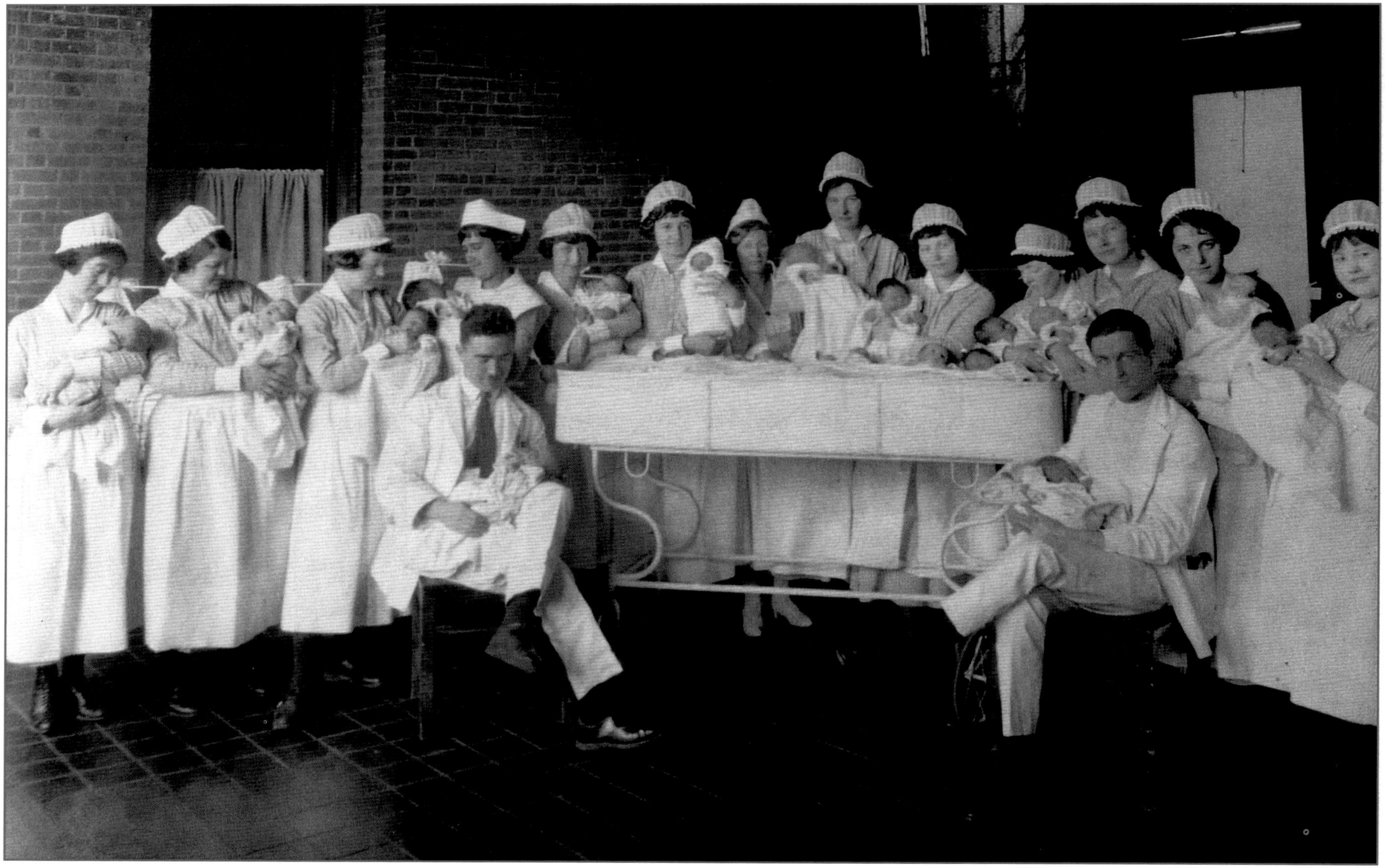

Following World War I, student enrollments increased, unemployment declined, and the economy surged.
Courtesy Bellevue Alumnae Association.

A DECADE OF FIRSTS
1920–1929

As the ravages of war and epidemic slowly faded from memory and the restlessness of the early postwar period gave way to the exuberance of the Roaring Twenties, NYSNA entered a period of organizational growth and maturation and engaged in thoughtful study of the problems of the profession. Nurses looked back with satisfaction that during the crises of war and epidemic, nursing school enrollments increased substantially, and "this person called a nurse has found a place for herself in every community . . . "[2] Across the country, unemployment was declining, and wages and the standard of living were on the rise as the United States entered "the greatest economic boom the world had yet seen."[3] NYSNA's 1922 convention opened on a decidedly optimistic note with Adelaide Nutting's welcome to delegates. "We are meeting tonight, it seems to me, under happier conditions than at any time for many years. Our long anxiety over the scarcity of applicants for admission to our schools of nursing, has given way to confidence and hope under the encouraging reports from many quarters, of the steady increase in well-qualified applicants. Some schools have admitted this autumn the largest and best equipped classes in their history, and one or two schools are in such a position as to be able to write that their classes are full and they can admit no more students until autumn, 1923."[4]

During the prosperous 1920s, the developing association began to take risky, yet important steps toward organizational maturity. It established a headquarters, hired staff, broadened its organizational structure, and initiated nationally significant research on the profession.

GROWTH AND PROSPERITY: The need for full-time staff had been discussed as early as 1913, when President Louise Twiss recommended that a capable member be hired to travel throughout the state promoting membership, emphasizing it would "require great perseverance and tact and a wide and definite knowledge of our aims to reach results . . ."[5] In 1924 President Anne Hansen noted the need for a permanent headquarters as well as staff, but neither could be supported financially unless revenue was increased. "Must New York be behind? Shall we surrender prestige to numerically and financially poorer States? It would indeed be a crying shame. With our membership we ought to be able to very comfortably support a Headquarters and a Field Secretary, and we need it in this State more than in any other."[6] Delegates responded by approving a substantial increase in dues.[7]

In November 1926 Mae Woughter, a 1915 graduate of Mt. Sinai Hospital School of Nursing, accepted the position of field secretary. She quickly secured office space and hired Elizabeth Van Fleet to provide secretarial support. The first headquarters office was established at 370 Seventh Ave, New York, where the association shared space with members of the National Health Council, including the ANA, AJN, and the NLNE.[8] These matters taken care of, Woughter turned her attention to promoting the work of the association. In her first report to delegates — complete with slides — Woughter reported visiting seventy-one alumnae groups, seventy-eight graduating nursing classes, fifty-four combined groups, and fourteen districts.[9] Although she only served as executive secretary for one year, she ". . . initiated and successfully carried on a brilliant task of organizing the districts and alumni associations for cooperative action."[10]

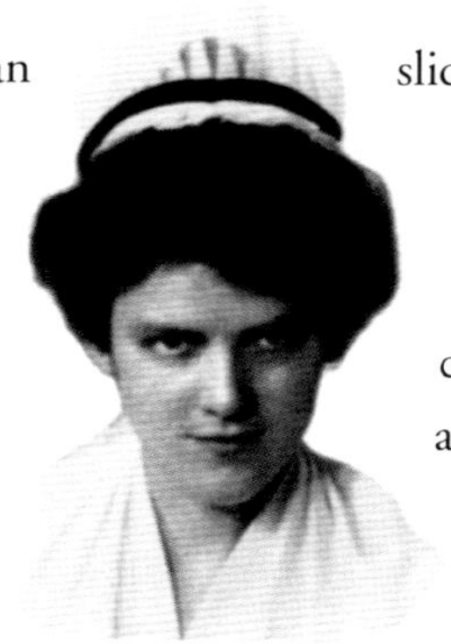

Mae Levine Woughter was experienced in organizational work before becoming NYSNA's first full-time staff member. After just a year, she married and resigned, but continued to be involved as an active NYSNA member. *Courtesy the Archives of the Mount Sinai Medical Center.*

NYSNA's Board of Directors urged the State Organization for Public Health Nursing and the New York State League of Nursing Education to share in the use and support of staff and office space. Following Woughter's resignation, the organizations formed a Committee on Common Activities to identify qualifications and prepare a detailed job description for the position of executive secretary. In addition to numerous administrative tasks, an "aggressive as well as responsive program" of fieldwork was outlined: semi-annual visits to each of the fourteen districts, and visits to as many as possible of the 144 alumnae associations and 124 student bodies. The committee appointed Caroline Garnsey as the new executive secretary.[11] Garnsey, too, remained with the association for only a short time.[12] When she resigned to marry in 1929, Emily J. Hicks of Utica was appointed.

Hicks' objectives for her first year were to increase membership and the interest of alumnae associations. She organized a meeting of the newly elected district presidents to provide information and discuss common concerns. This "President's Day" was later expanded to include district secretaries, and later still, district legislative chairs. In 1933 the event included attendance at a session of the legislature.[13] The district presidents were also members of the Advisory Council, along with NYSNA officers and ex-presidents, chairmen of the standing committees, presidents of the

"Any nurse that is actively engaged in nursing should be registered. If she is not, she is breaking the law which we worked so hard to have passed."

— *Ella F. Sinsebox*[1]

alumnae associations, presidents of other state nursing organizations, and the executive secretary of the State Board of Nurse Examiners. The Advisory Council, established about 1921, met in conjunction with each annual meeting, "to consider and promote the interests of the New York State Nurses Association." The Advisory Council was a very active group which made frequent recommendations to the House of Delegates for action, and provided a forum where state nursing leaders could discuss important issues.[14]

Even before the association established a headquarters and hired staff, a newsletter was published to keep members better informed of association activities. The first issue of the *State Bulletin of the New York State Nurses Association* was published in April 1924. The two-page newsletter included information on committee activities, excerpts from Board of Directors' meeting minutes, and a message from the State Board of Nurse Examiners on re-registration. Following publication of the second issue, the newsletter ceased.[15] A committee continued to explore efficient and effective means of publishing an association newsletter. Woughter and Garnsey both emphasized the importance of an association publication, and in July 1929 NYSNA published the first issue of the *Quarterly News.* The quarterly journal was a joint publication of the three state nursing organizations, and provided members with information on each organization, news items from the districts, and articles on nursing issues. Regular publication of the *Quarterly News* continued until 1938, when the name was changed to *The New York State Nurse,* and was sponsored solely by NYSNA.

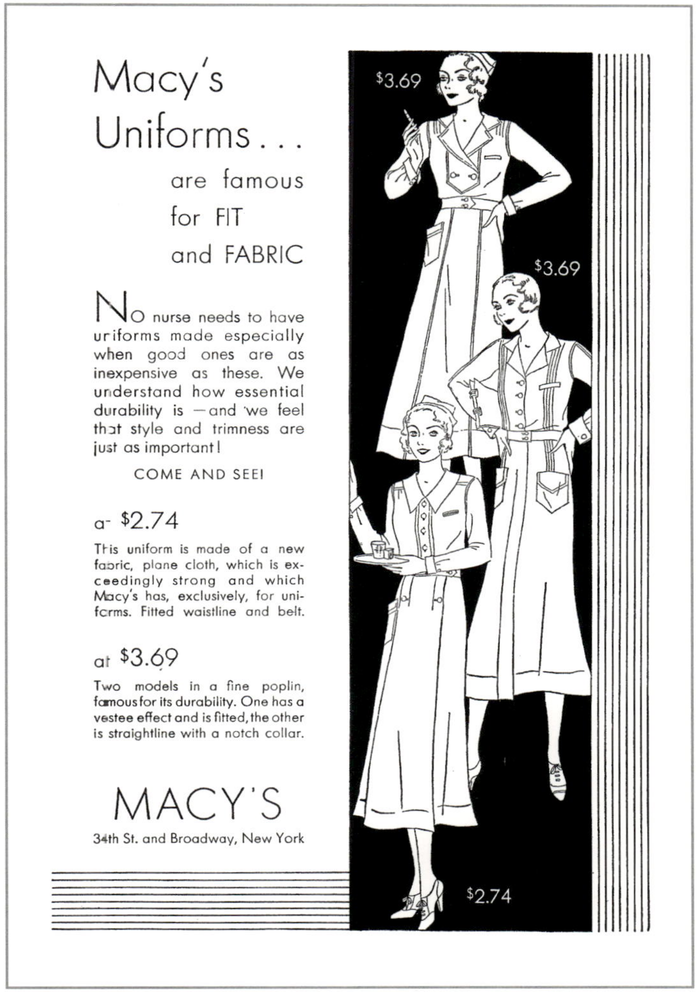

This uniform advertisement from the *Quarterly News* demonstrates the modern look of the 1920s.

THE FIRST STUDY OF THE PROFESSION: During World War I, the nation was shocked to learn that 29 percent of men drafted were physically unfit for duty. In response, there was rapid development of programs to improve the nation's health. The demand for public health nurses increased dramatically, and the lack of qualified public health nurses became a concern.[16] Nursing leaders turned to surveys and studies in an attempt to delineate and solve this and other emerging problems. As Adelaide Nutting told NYSNA delegates, "What is of supreme importance to us is that we should not fail to search for the truth concerning any part of our work; that we should not fail in courage to follow where that truth leads us."[17] Nutting persuaded the Rockefeller Foundation to finance an investigation of "the proper training of public health nurses." Known as the Goldmark study, it was expanded into a comprehensive survey of the entire field of nursing, and is generally considered to be the initial major landmark study of the profession.[18]

> "It seems to me that something might be done to make the rural nursing more attractive. It is almost impossible to get nurses no matter how great our supply is, to go out into the small town."
>
> — *Luia E. Payne*[2]

Miss Nutting discussed preliminary findings with delegates at the 1922 convention, describing the study as, "By far the most important event in nursing." The report substantiated the long-standing belief of many leaders that nursing schools needed to be funded separately from hospitals. "The Committee sees clearly the insuperable conflict of interest between the school and the hospital, due to the difference in their fundamental aims and purposes." Nutting also reported that the investigation found no evidence of a shortage of nurses "in normal times" except in rural areas, and did "not think the remuneration of private nurses is too high, considering the conditions of their work."[19]

FACING PAGE: Nurses assisted in this Harlem Hospital operating room in the 1920s. *Courtesy Alumni Association of Harlem Hospital Center School of Nursing.*

THE NURSING PROBLEM: Despite the Goldmark study's evidence to the contrary, the cry of "nursing shortage" grew louder. Trained nurses had become indispensable to patients and physicians alike. With business and industrial production booming, the public wanted more nursing services as it wanted more automobiles, more money, better homes, and more luxuries of every sort. The increased use of hospitals required more private duty nurses for in-hospital special duty nursing. At the same time, new opportunities for nurses in public health, industry, and government opened, diminishing the number of private duty nurses. Nonetheless, the largest group of nurses remained those engaged in private duty. The increasingly accepted twelve-hour day forced families wanting twenty-four-hour coverage to hire two nurses. This removed graduate private duty nursing from the financial reach of the average family, and increased demand for the untrained, less expensive nurse.[20]

The "nurse shortage" (also known as "The Nursing Problem" or "The Nursing Situation") was widely discussed in the medical and nursing communities, and in the popular press. "From the public we hear the cry that nurses are charging too much, that the twelve-hour nursing day works a hardship on the patient, that the nurse is less interested in her patient than formerly, that there are too few nurses. The medical profession is giving considerable thought to the matter . . . The nurse herself is depressed and perplexed."[21] Nurses were particularly hurt by physicians' charges that educational standards were too high and fees were exorbitant.[22] In 1923 NYSNA President Anne Hansen commented, "We have resented the injustice of the attacks, some of us with exceeding bitterness . . ."[23] NYSNA leaders met with numerous medical groups to discuss "the need for a short

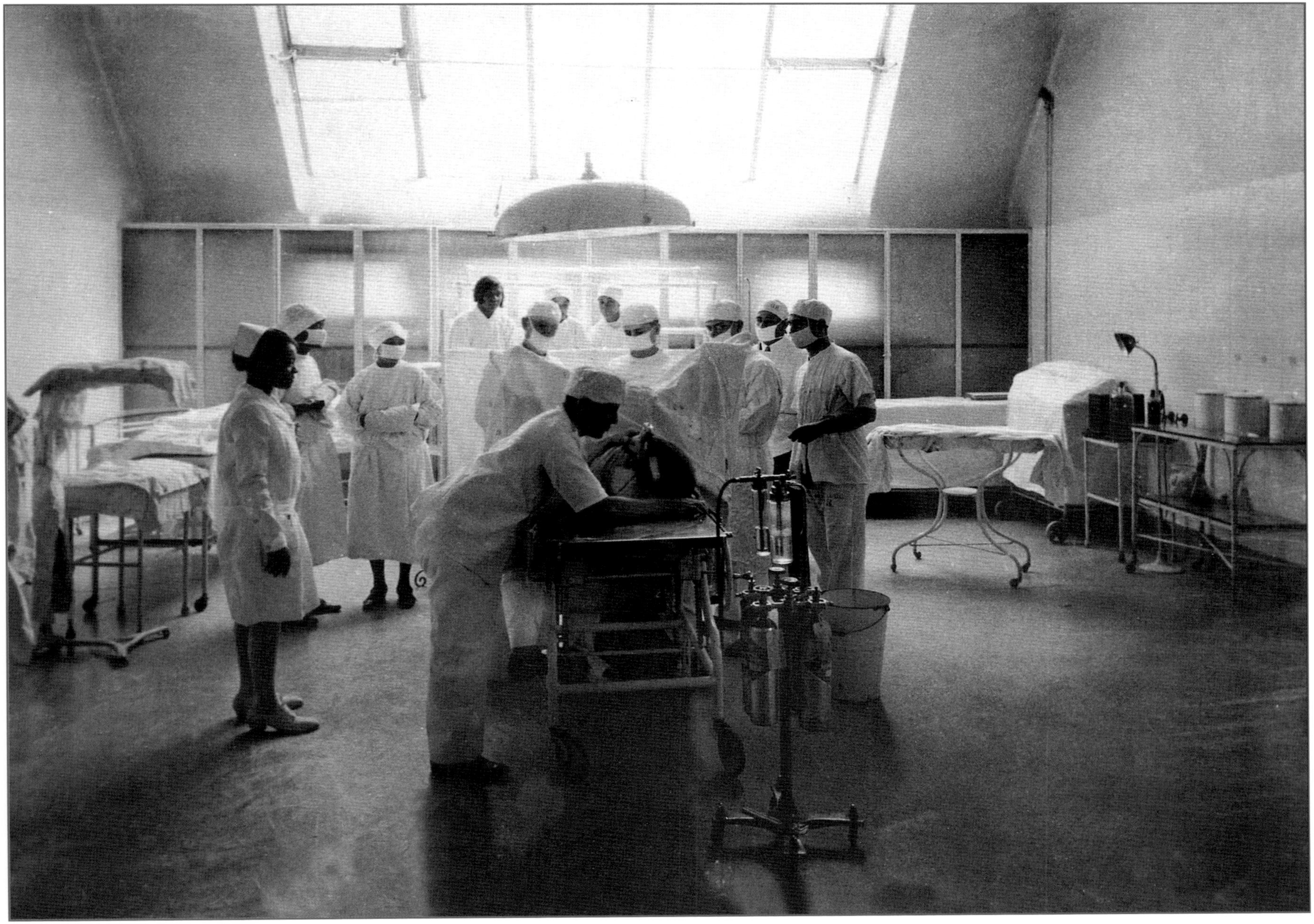

course nurse; over-education of the nurse; the shortage of graduate nurses; the exorbitant fee of the private duty nurse and nurses' refusal of certain types of cases. With some embarrassment because of lack of facts and accurate figures we argued against some of the reforms in the nursing system suggested by the medical profession, but could use only the well-known woman's reason, *because.*"[24]

> "It is the protection of the public that we are ultimately interested in; and it is the public that is suffering from the use of the nurses from the commercial registry."
>
> — *Miss Hughes*[3]

Private duty nurses had complaints of their own. The spirit of self-sacrifice of the Progressive Era had diminished, and employers in business and industry began to provide insurance, recreational facilities, and other benefits to employees.[25] These social trends highlighted the inequities of private duty nurses' working conditions. They had suffered in numbers and morale from the campaign to recruit "the very best nurses" for administrative and public health positions. The more desirable working conditions and higher salaries for these positions only emphasized their grievances: "long hours of work, over fatigue, monotony, inadequate salaries, no opportunities for advancement in work or for self improvement, bearing the blame for doctors' mistakes, unnecessary and unappreciated self-sacrifice."[26] The decade of the 1920s was a period of rapid social change, and women "came into their own" as never before. Their hair was bobbed, their skirts were shortened, and rouge and lipstick became acceptable. In contrast, the system of private duty nursing functioned much as it had for decades.

In 1924 NYSNA's Board of Directors responded to concerns of private duty nurses by suggesting the ethics committee study the economic conditions of private duty nurses. NYSNA's first Committee on Professional Ethics was established by the House of Delegates in 1922 to assist in the enforcement of the Nurse Practice Act by identifying and investigating nurses practicing as registered nurses without licensure or registration. In 1923 committee chair Elizabeth Burgess presented a broader statement of purpose, "To promote and maintain ethical standards among our members and to raise our standard of service as individuals as well as an association and a profession." The committee was charged by delegates to formulate a code of ethics. However, ANA began work on a code soon thereafter, and the committee did not wish to duplicate the national effort.[27] The committee, now charged with another important task, joined forces with a committee of the Kings County Medical Society. It was agreed that private duty was "sick," and a survey was proposed to gather data. "The prescriptions written to date such as 'lower the entrance requirements,' 'go back to 24-hour duty,' etc., are based on symptoms and not on a diagnosis. A correct diagnosis must be based on a large body of <u>facts</u>, not on opinions or guesses."[28] Janet Geister, a public health nurse with extensive research experience, including the Goldmark study, and May Ayres Burgess, PhD., an experienced statistician, were engaged to prepare a questionnaire entitled "Your Money and Your Life — For One Week." The questionnaire was sent to private duty nurses in District 13 (New York City) and District 1 (Buffalo). Nurses were asked to report on income, expenses, hours worked, and attitudes for one week in September 1925.[29]

> "We are really interested in the good of the public, because the good of the public is dependent on the type of person that is taking care of the sick in the community."
>
> — *Miss Hilliard*[4]

Geister reported on the survey to delegates at NYSNA's 1925 convention. The data confirmed what nurses already knew, "there is something seriously wrong with private duty nursing." She blamed an "out-dated system" which created wasted service and bad distribution. "The world about us has changed its clothes, its method of organization, its method of work . . . private duty nursing has kept on its old clothes."[30] The survey clearly indicated that the majority of respondents did not like the long hours, did not like idle periods *between* cases, did not like idle periods *on* cases, did not earn enough to permit saving, but most emphatically, *did like nursing.*[31] Ethics Committee chairman Elizabeth Burgess recommended further study, and delegates unanimously passed a motion to conduct an expanded statewide survey.[32]

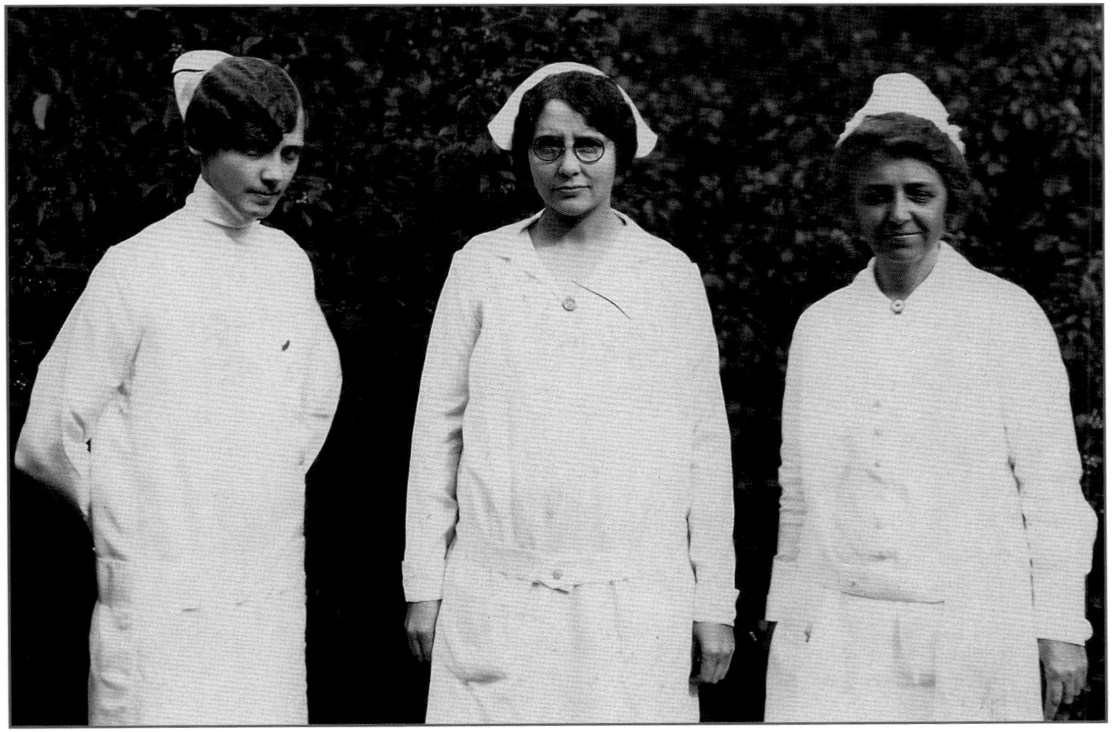

These head nurses from Ellis Hospital, Schenectady, demonstrate the new look of the 1920s — short hair and more streamlined uniforms. *Courtesy Ellis Hospital School of Nursing Collection, Foundation of NYSNA Archives.*

In 1926 questionnaires were distributed for one week in February, traditionally a time of high illness rates. Geister brought national attention to the study when she published a detailed report and analysis of the findings. Again, the results corroborated what many leaders had already concluded, that shortages were "seasonal and occasional," and what was needed was better use of nursing resources, not more nurses.[33] Twenty-five percent of the nurses surveyed worked three days or less, while at the same time, doctors reported a shortage of nurses.[34]

The survey was repeated in June, and a third was planned for later in 1926. Meanwhile, the National Committee on Grading of Nurse Training Schools was organized. The committee hired Dr. May Ayres Burgess, familiar with nursing issues through her experience with NYSNA, to direct the program. Although the primary task of the committee was to formulate a national classified list of nursing schools, the committee agreed that before actual grading of schools could be undertaken, it first had to determine whether the country continued to experience a nursing shortage. Thus, the first project focused on issues of supply and demand of nursing service, and quickly became focused on the private duty nurse.[35] The work of the committee was financed by contributions from individuals and organizations, including NYSNA. At the 1926 convention, President Louise Sherwood

Anne Lyon Hansen

1878 - 1938

Anne Hansen was one of NYSNA's most vigorous and outspoken leaders during the 1920s. A graduate of the Buffalo Children's Hospital School of Nursing, Hansen began a long career as a public health nurse with the Visiting Nurse Association of Buffalo in 1905. In 1915 she became its director, a position she held until her death in 1938. Mrs. Hansen was a charter member of the National Organization for Public Health Nursing, and served as its president from 1926 to 1930, and as a board member from 1930 until her death. When the New York State Organization for Public Health Nursing was formed in 1913, Mrs. Hansen served for four years as its first president.

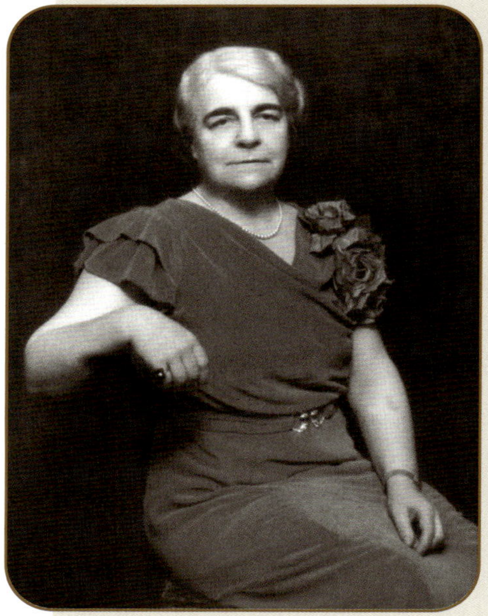

Courtesy Nurses House Collection, Foundation of NYSNA Archives.

Mrs. Hansen held the office of president of NYSNA from 1922 to '25, and continued to serve on the board until 1937. She was a strong proponent of hiring full-time staff and establishing a headquarters office, and spearheaded a complete reorganization of the association's administration. She chaired the Headquarters Committee, which directly supervised administrative and personnel activities. During her presidency she was a staunch defender of nurses and nursing and represented NYSNA at numerous meetings with physicians on "The Nursing Problem." In 1925 she urged delegates to give careful attention to the many professional issues being raised. "We have sidestepped all these questions in the past; we may no longer do so. We are faced today with the necessity of making some plan for a complete redistribution of nursing service." She advocated for "an adjustment of nursing service through group, hourly and visiting nursing, so as to bring trained nursing care within the reach of all. It is time for nurses to wake up and face changing conditions, throw off complacency and become alert."[1]

Hansen served on many national committees, including the critical Committee on the Distribution of Nursing Service. She was an outspoken participant in NYSNA conventions, and her counsel seemed always to be respected. In 1937 NYSNA named the "Anne L. Hansen Loan Fund" in recognition of her untiring efforts. At her death, she was nationally respected as a brilliant leader and beloved friend.[2]

reported that NYSNA "was the first state organization to join cooperatively with the Committee on the Grading of Schools."[36] In fact, NYSNA turned over the remaining work on its series of private duty surveys to the Grading Committee, which Sherwood referred to as a "foster child . . . it was the New York State Nurses Association which gave it it's start in life."[37] A comprehensive report of the study of supply and demand, *Nurses, Patients and Pocketbooks,* was published in 1928. The report of this study, considered to be another landmark study of nursing, was widely read and generated a great deal of interest and constructive thinking.[38]

"It seems to me that in many of our institutions many of our professional women are being used not as professional women, but, as it were, jobs."

— *Miss Selfridge*[5]

Dr. Burgess, now a familiar figure to NYSNA delegates, reported on the study at the 1927 and 1928 conventions. Contrary to the widespread perception that a shortage of nurses existed, the study demonstrated there was a serious overproduction of nurses, causing chronic unemployment among private duty nurses, and there was uneven distribution, with most nurses residing in urban areas.[39] "We have the paradox of too many nurses, and at the same time people who believe they can prove there is a shortage of nurses because it is impossible for them to find a nurse to fill their particular position."[40] This conclusion was startling to many, even to members of the committee, but it could not have come as much of a surprise to members who had been paying attention to the results of NYSNA's earlier studies. Burgess also reported that those entering the nursing profession were less intelligent and "well equipped" than previously. "It is well known that anyone who drops out of high school can't get a position as a clerical worker in an office, or cannot work in a department store, but is limited to two sources. She can go into factory work, or she can go into a school of nursing . . . the nursing profession is enticing a class of girls into it today that would not have been able to enter it thirty years ago."[41]

The Grading Committee found dissatisfaction with salaries and working conditions among private duty nurses throughout the country. "There are particularly four things that private duty people are missing which the public health and institutional people pretty largely have, and those four things are reasonable hours, adequate income, constructive leadership and opportunity for professional growth . . . Because of the free-lance nature of the work, private duty nurses were 'lonely, separate people.' "[42]

Presented with voluminous information, delegates were challenged by Dr. Burgess, "What are you going to do about it? . . . You have in this state, one-eighth of all the graduate nurses in the country, and the thing to do is to start right here and see that the majority of these nurses do not stand still, but advance."[43] She urged nurses to keep up to date on nursing issues, and to encourage all graduate nurses to register. President Clifford asked members to carefully study Burgess' report, and challenged districts and committees to consider experiments in hourly and group nursing, the development of central community nurse registries, and other innovative activities.[44] These concepts were not new. Leaders had been promoting them for years, but there was now the incontrovertible evidence that the distribution of nursing services was seriously flawed, and that nurses were poised to leave the field of private duty.[45]

GROUP AND HOURLY NURSING: Group nursing in hospitals was described in a 1922 convention paper as a system whereby a group of patients received care by one nurse at a reduced cost.[46] Dr Burgess recommended that these nurses be regular, full-time hospital employees working an eight-hour day, and a forty-hour week with annual vacation pay; that the staff include enough nurses to provide adequate care; that supervision be provided; and that the patient pay for nursing services directly to the hospital. This plan was in contrast to the traditional method of hospital nursing care, whereby students provided nursing services unless the patient hired a private duty nurse to provide exclusive care, and where nurses often had difficulty collecting fees when hospitals required that patients pay special duty nurses directly for their services.

Hourly nursing was care provided in the home by the hour rather than by the shift. This allowed the nurse to provide care to more patients, reduced patient costs, and eliminated the problem of "idle time" on a case. Services included bathing, massage, and various treatments such as enemas, ear irrigations, and dressing changes. Organized hourly nursing services had been sporadically utilized throughout the state, first by visiting nurse associations, and later through central registries. Implementation was not widespread, and in 1938 the "need for a more concentrated effort in the development of hourly nursing service" was still described as "urgent."[47]

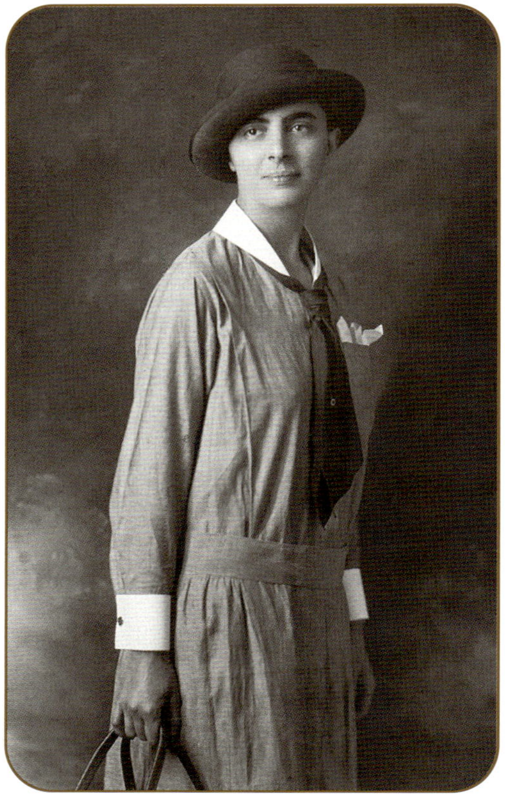

The demand for public health nurses soared in the 1920s. *Courtesy Brooklyn VNA.*

REGISTRIES — THE GREAT SOLUTION: Early private duty nurses received patients largely through the recommendation of physicians, friends, and former patients. By the late 1920s, however, most private duty nurses were linked with patients through registries. Many hospitals and alumnae associations established registries to provide work for their graduates through the hospital's doctors and patients in need of a private duty nurse. Some medical societies also sponsored registries, and "commercial registries" and employment agencies sprang up. Registries maintained a list of nurses available for home or hospital private duty. When a call for a nurse came into the registry, nurses were called on the basis of their position on the list rather than on skills and abilities. Many nurses found it necessary to register with more than one commercial agency in addition to the hospital registry in order to make an adequate living.[48]

The desire of nurse leaders to eliminate the commercial registries was a frequent topic of consideration. In 1922 President Alice Gilman strongly urged delegates to undertake a survey of the commercial registries. "To my mind the commercial registry is one of the worst enemies of the nursing profession and one of the greatest detriments in securing the confidence of the public, because it is the women going out from these registries that are largely responsible for the criticism which has come upon us as members of a profession."[49] A committee, under the leadership of Anna Maxwell, surveyed both commercial and professional registries in New York.[50] However, no results of the registry surveys were reported. Anne Hansen later revealed that "When the report was brought to us by the nurse we employed . . . it was so dreadful we never published it; we couldn't. Where it is at the present time I don't know, I know it is in somebody's vault under lock and key, because it had so much dynamite in it, it exposed things in this city of New York that were so dreadful — and I doubt very much if there is any change today — that we couldn't use the material for which we paid. It was perfectly dreadful."[51]

"One of our nurses is trying out hourly nursing and she has an enclosed car and she is now making calls on a similar basis as a physician."

— *Miss Faust*[6]

The committee promoted the development of official registries, operated by professional nurses, in each district. President Hansen commented that "I think you will find as time goes on that that is going to be the great solution of many problems."[52] Leaders believed official registries would be able to solve problems by consistent application of ethical principles, and united cooperation with the medical and hospital associations to set and maintain high standards. By the end of 1929 official registries had been established in Albany, Brooklyn, Buffalo, New York, Rochester, Syracuse, and Watertown.[53]

The results of NYSNA's study of private duty nursing, and the studies of the Grading Committee placed additional emphasis on the registries. Geister recommended the organization, broadening, and strengthening of central registries, which would bring together all the registries in a community, as the first step in solving the distribution problem.[54]

"The current of unfavorable public opinion directed against nurses in recent years, has been proof of the difficulty in maintaining professional standards in a group, so many of whom are surrounded by the ethics of the business world."

— *Emma L. Collins*[7]

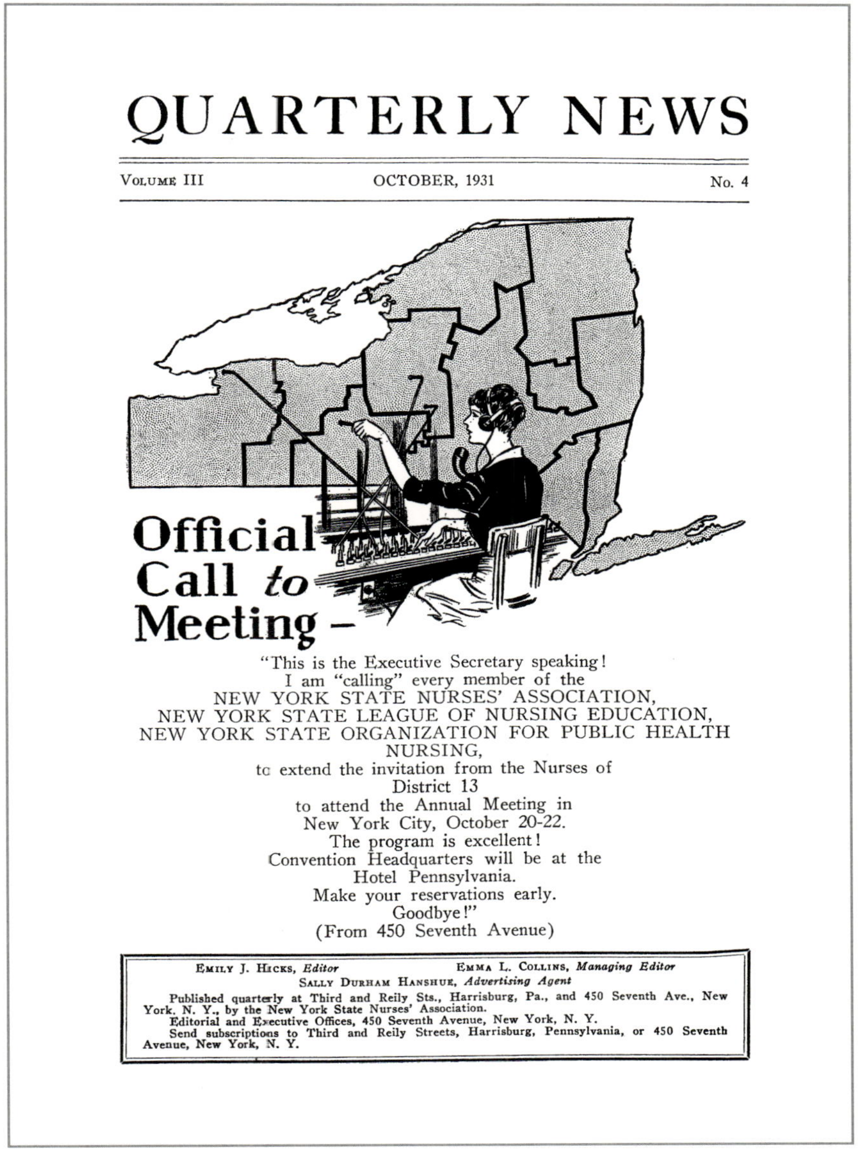

QUARTERLY NEWS

VOLUME III OCTOBER, 1931 No. 4

"This is the Executive Secretary speaking!
I am "calling" every member of the
NEW YORK STATE NURSES' ASSOCIATION,
NEW YORK STATE LEAGUE OF NURSING EDUCATION,
NEW YORK STATE ORGANIZATION FOR PUBLIC HEALTH NURSING,
to extend the invitation from the Nurses of District 13
to attend the Annual Meeting in New York City, October 20-22.
The program is excellent!
Convention Headquarters will be at the Hotel Pennsylvania.
Make your reservations early.
Goodbye!"
(From 450 Seventh Avenue)

EMILY J. HICKS, *Editor* EMMA L. COLLINS, *Managing Editor*
SALLY DURHAM HANSHUE, *Advertising Agent*

Published quarterly at Third and Reily Sts., Harrisburg, Pa., and 450 Seventh Ave., New York, N. Y., by the New York State Nurses' Association.

Editorial and Executive Offices, 450 Seventh Avenue, New York, N. Y.

Send subscriptions to Third and Reily Streets, Harrisburg, Pennsylvania, or 450 Seventh Avenue, New York, N. Y.

This call to meeting from NYSNA's *Quarterly News,* uses the familiar image of a registry calling private duty nurses.

The registry of the future was seen as a coordinating body for community nursing needs and services, providing traditional private duty nursing services in homes and hospitals, as well as hourly nursing services. In 1927 the Medical Association and NYSNA successfully sponsored the Webb-Lattin bill mandating that registries provide to each patient a card indicating qualifications and fees of the caregiver. In effect, the bill disclosed to the patient whether the caregiver was a graduate registered nurse, a "practical" nurse, or a trained attendant. It was believed such a measure was an important step toward the development of "officially controlled certified registries which may prove a most practical help in the solution of the nursing problem."[55]

"A convention is . . . to give the nurses and people who attend the convention the thing that they need to give them — the facts, the information, the discussion, the inspiration which they need for carrying on their work during the year."

— *Miss Conroy*[8]

Reforms Do Not Come Through Miracles: Activities of NYSNA during the 1920s clearly focused on private duty nursing. Considerable frustration was expressed, however, over the lack of participation of private duty nurses themselves in the association. Survey returns were disappointing. "I believe in all of our meetings with the hospital people and with medical men, at least 75 percent of all discussions are devoted to the private duty nurse. The private duty nurse is the one whom the doctor is having trouble with at the present time. We are trying to fight their battle and we get no help from them. They look on the questionnaires as a sort of advertisement, they do not seem to realize its vital importance. If the private duty nurses do not help they cannot expect to get anywhere and they cannot expect to win the fight."[56]

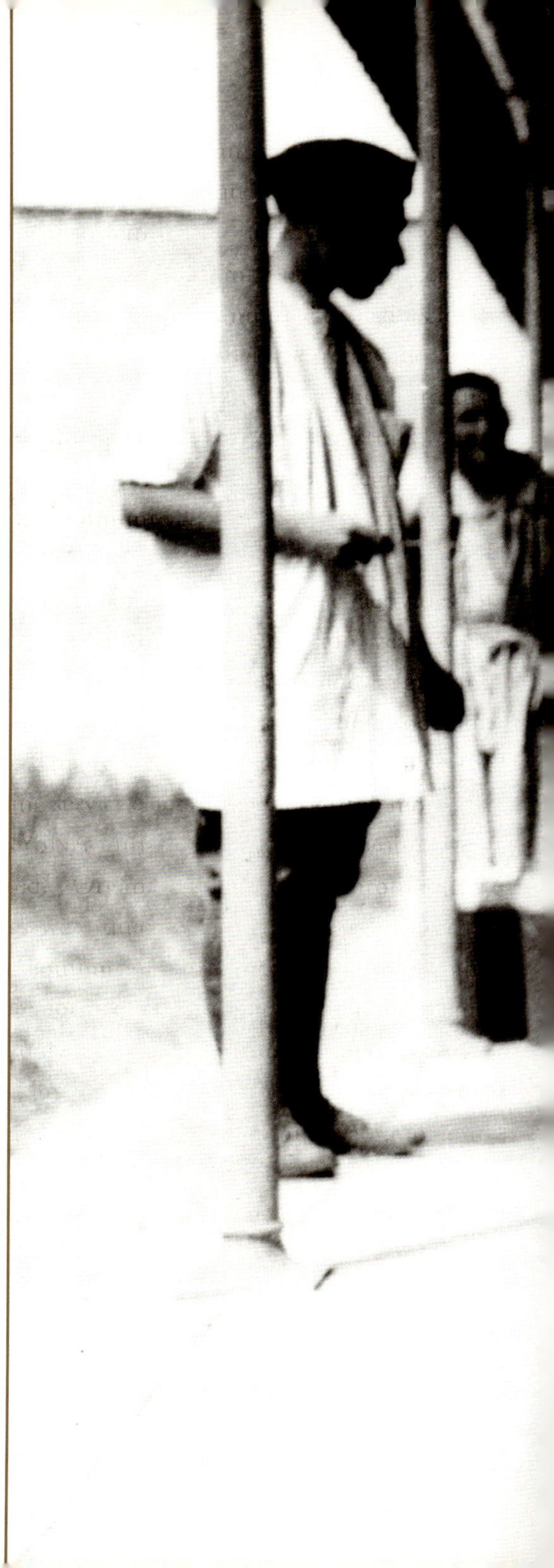

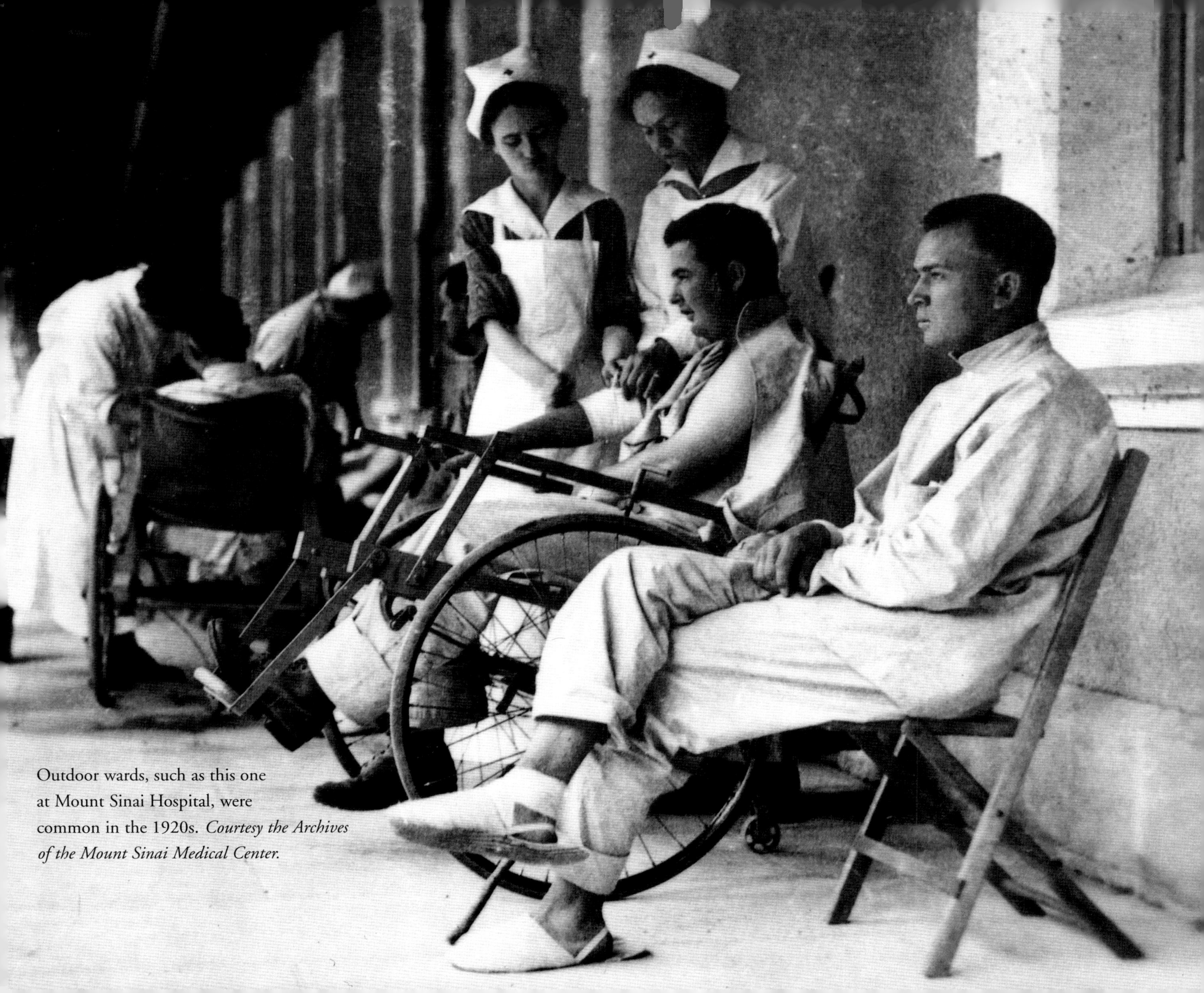

Outdoor wards, such as this one at Mount Sinai Hospital, were common in the 1920s. *Courtesy the Archives of the Mount Sinai Medical Center.*

When the first private duty survey was discussed at the 1925 convention, a plea was made that private duty nurses be given an opportunity to organize. In fact, private duty nursing had been made a standing committee the previous year, but involvement of the nurses was minimal.[57] Part of the problem, of course, was the working conditions themselves — the isolation and long hours of the private duty nurse hampered participation in professional activities. A great deal of time and effort had been expended in "searching for the truth" about nursing. However, the effort had to be continued, and sacrifices accepted if improvement was to be expected. "Reforms do not come through miracles. Somebody has to work for them . . . If private duty nurses will get together, work together, and join in experimenting with the different solutions which are now being urged, they can remake their jobs . . . The big problem for private duty nurses is how much of this cherished independence of action are they willing to give up, in order to get the other things they want."[58] In the end, however, it was neither nurses nor miracles that precipitated change as much as it was the severe economic depression that followed the dramatic stock market crash in October 1929.

A DECADE OF FIRSTS: During the 1920s the association experienced dramatic change. The opening of its first headquarters office, the hiring of its first executive secretary, and the publication of its first newsletter established NYSNA as a mature organization. The extensive work with districts, the development of an Advisory Council and other events for district presidents, and the appointment of the first Committee on Professional Ethics marked the beginning of long-standing, continuing association practices. By 1929 NYSNA was stable, growing, and prepared to face new challenges.

CHAPTER NOTES
TEXT

1. May Ayres Burgess, "The Private Duty Nurse in New York State — What the February Study Showed" (1926, mimeographed), NYSNA Archives; Janet M. Geister, "Hearsay and Facts in Private Duty," *American Journal of Nursing* 26 (July 1926): 515–28; and Kalisch and Kalisch, *Advance of American Nursing*, 370.

2. "Proceedings of the Twentieth Annual Convention of the New York State Nurses' Association" (Utica, N.Y.,1921, stenographic transcript), 15–16.

3. Robert S. McElvane, *The Great Depression* (New York: Time Books, 1993), 16; and Howard Zinn, *The Twentieth Century: A People's History* (New York: HarperPerennial, 1998), 106.

4. M. Adelaide Nutting, "Address of Welcome," 1922, NYSNA Archives, 2.

5. *Twelfth Annual Meeting*, 20–21. Part-time secretarial help had occasionally assisted association leaders.

6. "Address of the President" (Albany, N.Y.,1925, typewritten), NYSNA Archives, 13. In early 1926, NYSNA paid ANA for the services of its field secretary to assist NYSNA for one month. (Board of Directors Minutes, NYSNA, 25 October 1926, NYSNA Archives.)

7. "Proceedings of the Twenty-Fourth Annual Meeting of the New York State Nurses' Association" (Albany, N.Y., 1925, stenotype transcript), 196. "The move was opposed by Roosevelt Hospital, Fifth Avenue, Post Graduate and Mount Sinai . . . This opposition was brought, not against the measure itself, but rather in an effort to have the program for state headquarters explained and mapped out more thoroughly before it was undertaken. Several delegates felt that the bulk of the assessment would fall upon the graduate private duty nurses, yet this large group of supporters felt that national development thus far had exclusively developed nursing schools and had not followed the interests of those already in the work, and they wished to see their problems considered in a state plan." ("New York Decides on a State Secretary with Headquarters," *Trained Nurse and Hospital Review* 75 [December 1925]: 622.) The scope of work was comprehensive: "The functions of a Field Secretary are to represent the State Association; to know it's ideals and policies; to study the needs of the nursing service and profession as a whole; to familiarize herself with the public opinion toward nursing; to present the nursing question as a whole to the District Associations and their Alumnae Associations and their sections as well as to student bodies and Boards of Directors; to take over some of the duties of the Officers; to readjust organizations to meet new needs, new ambitions and new opportunities." (Advisory Council Minutes, NYSNA, 1926, NYSNA Archives, 11–12.)

8. "Headquarters Office Moves," *Quarterly News* 3 (April 1931), 42. In April 1931, these offices were moved to 450 Seventh Avenue. Van Fleet served under the first three executive secretaries until she resigned to marry in 1933. She provided sorely needed continuity during the years of frequent executive secretary turnover. (Board of Directors Minutes, NYSNA, 29 April 1933, NYSNA Archives.)

9. [Mae Woughter, First Annual Report of Headquarters Office,] 1927, NYSNA Archives, 4.

10. "Mrs. Henry Strack," *New York State Nurse* 14 (April 1942): 77. Mae Woughter Strack died October 26, 1941.

11. Common Activities Committee Minutes, 12 November 1927 and 14 December 1927, NYSNA Archives. The other two state organizations expressed a desire to make use of the office and the services of the executive secretary, but were unable to contribute financially. At its first meeting, committee members agreed on desirable qualifications for the executive secretary, ". . . education, personality, health, ability for public speaking, a broad contact with the nursing profession, good professional standing," and state registration. A sub-committee submitted a detailed outline of the executive secretary's duties, which included office management — rental and upkeep of office and equipment, hiring, directing and dismissing of staff, administration of funds, maintenance of membership lists and files (district, alphabetical, correspondence and individual leaders, board meeting, minutes, and reports), correspondence, meeting arrangements, and minutes.

12. At the 1928 convention Garnsey reported on her activities (visited 13 of the 14 districts, met four thousand nurses, received 1,176 pieces of mail, and sent 14,029 pieces of mail) and urged membership recruitment activities to increase membership by one-third in 1929. She also touched on other activities, such as visits by foreign nurses "just off the boat. They are entering an already overcrowded field with a foreign training that New York State does not feel it can be held responsible for. Conditions are not as they were represented in their home country." (Report of the Executive Secretary, NYSNA, 1928, NYSNA Archives, 3–4.) Garnsey was injured in an auto accident in late fall and worked "under great difficulty" until September 1929. She died suddenly in childbirth August 14, 1930. ("In Memoriam," *Quarterly News* 2 [October 1930]: 6.)

13. Board of Directors Minutes, NYSNA, 24 October 1929, NYSNA Archives; "President's Day," *Quarterly News* 5 (April 1933): 38.

14. "Articles of Incorporation and By-Laws of the New York State Nurses' Association," 1926, NYSNA Archives. The earliest known minutes of the Advisory Council are from 1921. No copies of NYSNA bylaws are available from 1910 to 1925.

15. The only clue to the demise of the newsletter was provided by Anne Hansen at the 1928 Advisory Council meeting. She indicated hundreds of copies of the bulletin were returned, presumably because of incorrect addresses. "Some members have said they never knew we had such a thing as a bulletin." ("Annual Meeting of the New York State Organizations of Nurses" [Brooklyn, N.Y., 1928, stenotype transcript], 87.)

16. Roberts, *American Nursing,* 164.

17. Nutting, "Address of Welcome," 17–18.

18. Susan B. Bastable, "Landmark Studies-Stimuli for Change in Nursing," in *Prologue to Professionalism: A History of Nursing,* ed. M. Louise Fitzpatrick (Bowie, Md.: Brady Communications, 1983), 216–17. Social worker and author Josephine Goldmark was the chief investigator and secretary of the Committee for the Study of Nursing Education. The committee, composed of nineteen professional and lay representatives, had overall responsibility for the project. New York nurses M. Adelaide Nutting, Lillian Wald, Annie Goodrich, and Mary Beard were committee members.

19. Nutting, "Address of Welcome," 7–10. The report of the Goldmark study, *Nursing and Nursing Education in the United States,* was published in 1923.

20. Emma L. Collins, "What the Registry Means to the Private Duty Nurse," *American Journal of Nursing* 28 (July 1928): 677.

21. Geister, "Hearsay and Facts," 515.

22. "The Viewpoint of the Nurse," *Trained Nurse and Hospital Review* 67 (November 1921): 427. The medical community persisted in its attempts to reduce the length of nurse training as well as the theoretical content of the coursework. A study of the hospital nursing situation in New York City hospitals completed by the New York Academy of Medicine in 1921 concluded that the teaching of nursing "is often carried out haphazardly, and is always secondary to the exigencies of the hospital service," yet recommended the length of nurse training be shortened. (E.H. Lewinski-Corwin, "The Hospital Nursing Situation," *American Journal of Nursing* 22 [May 1922]: 604–5.)

23. *Proceedings of the Twenty-second Annual Meeting of the New York State Nurses' Association* (n.p., [1923]), 15.

24. Genevieve M. Clifford, "Knowing Ourselves," *Quarterly News* 3 (October 1931): 109. Nurses not wishing to care for certain types of cases, usually maternity, "nervous disorders," and communicable diseases, "registered against" them.

25. McElvane, *Great Depression,* 12–15.

26. Katherine DeWitt, "Editorial Comment," *American Journal of Nursing* 21 (January 1921): 209.

27. Board of Directors Minutes, NYSNA, 27 October 1924, NYSNA Archives; *Proceedings of the Twenty-first Annual Meeting of the New York State Nurses' Association* (n.p., [1922]), 186; and *Twenty-second Annual Meeting,* 100–16.

28. "Your Money and Your Life for One Week of Private Duty Nursing," *American Journal of Nursing* 25 (December 1925): 952.

29. Burgess had worked as a statistician during World War I. From 1920 to 1923 she was the director of the Joint Statistics Bureau of the Commission on Dispensary Development in New York City, where Janet Geister was also employed. ("May Ayres Burgess," in *American Nursing: A Biographical Dictionary (Volume 1),* ed. Vern L. Bullough, Olga M. Church, and Alice P. Stein [New York: Garland Publishing, 1988], 52.)

30. "Twenty-Fourth Annual Meeting," 78.

31. "Your Money," 996. One respondent commented, "Can anybody conceive of anything more tiring than sitting in an uncomfortable chair and looking interested hour after hour?" ("Twenty-Fourth Annual Meeting," 112.)

32. "Twenty-Fourth Annual Meeting," 119-25.

33. Katherine DeWitt, "Team Work," *American Journal of Nursing* 25 (May 1925): 392-93. Dewitt also recommended "More group nursing in hospitals, more hourly nursing in homes, administered by visiting nurse associations or by highly organized central registries . . ." She urged nurses to work cooperatively with the medical community to solve these problems.

34. Geister, "Hearsay and Facts," 522.

35. Roberts, *American Nursing,* 185.

36. *Synopsis of Proceedings of the Twenty-fifth Annual Meeting of the New York State Nurses' Association* (n.p., [1926]), 19.

37. "President's Address," 1927, NYSNA Archives, 3. Burgess herself told delegates, "It is because you people got interested in the problems of private duty nurses two years ago that I happened to get entangled with the grading committee." ("Proceedings of the Twenty-Sixth Annual Meeting of the New York State Nurses Association" [Rochester, N.Y., 1927, stenotype transcript], 71.)

38. Bastable, "Landmark Studies," 223–26. The committee adopted a five-year plan of study, divided into three separate projects. The first project was a study of supply and demand for nursing service. The work of the committee ultimately ran for eight years.

39. "Too Many Nurses — Where?" *American Journal of Nursing* 29 (March 1929): 293. For instance, in New York County, one out of every 234 people was an active, registered nurse, in Albany county, one out of 394, and in Schoharie County, one out of 5,391.

40. "Annual Meeting of Organizations of Nurses," 6.

41. Ibid., 10.

42. "Proceedings of the Twenty-Eighth Annual Meeting of the New York State Nurses Association" (Buffalo, N.Y., 1929, stenotype transcript), 75–76.

43. "Twenty-Sixth Annual Meeting," 75–76.

44. Genevieve Clifford, "Annual Address," 1928, NYSNA Archives, 1–7.

45. The 1925 survey of private duty nurses in Districts 1 and 13 reported, "A startling number of nurses indicated their desire to leave the field of private duty at the first opportunity." Thirty-three percent of respondents in District 13 and 46 percent of respondents in District 1 stated they were not planning to remain in private duty. ("Your Money," 994.)

46. *Twenty-first Annual Meeting,* 291–301. The presenter commented, "I remember being rather startled at the Atlanta Convention when Miss Nutting, with her usual foresight, made the statement that the time was fast approaching when one nurse would no longer care for one patient in the hospital or in the private duty field."

47. Ella F. Sinsebox, "Hourly Nursing," 1922, NYSNA Archives; and Margaret L. Rogers, "By the Hour," *Trained Nurse and Hospital Review* 100 (May 1938): 580–81.

48 Collins, "What the Registry Means," 678.

49. *Twenty-first Annual Meeting,* 13.

50. Board of Directors Minutes, NYSNA, 24 October 1922 and 19 January 1923, NYSNA Archives.

51. "Advisory Council Proceedings," (Binghamton, N.Y., 1928, stenotype transcript), 67–68. In April 1925 the board passed a motion regarding this study, directing "that after submitting to legal advice, a resume of commercial registries be made and a report be sent to Miss Burgess." Elizabeth Burgess was secretary to the State Board of Nurse Examiners. (Board of Directors Minutes, NYSNA, 17 April 1925, NYSNA Archives.)

52. "Twenty-Fourth Annual Meeting," 176.

53. "District and Alumnae News," *Quarterly News* 3 (January 1931): 18.

54. Geister, "Hearsay and Facts," 525–26.

55. Nathan B. Van Etten, "The Lattin Bill," *American Journal of Nursing* 27 (April 1927): 277–78.

56. Advisory Council Minutes, 1926, 4. Anne L. Hansen is quoted.

57. "Twenty-Fourth Annual Meeting," 119–25.

58. May Ayres Burgess, "Preliminary Studies of Private Duty," *American Journal of Nursing* 27 (August 1927): 640.

FEATURE

ANNE LYON HANSEN

1. Anne L. Hansen, "President's Address," 1925, NYSNA Archives, 9.

2. "Anne Lyon Hansen," in *American Nursing: A Biographical Dictionary (Volume 1),* ed. Vern L. Bullough, Olga M. Church, and Alice P. Stein (New York: Garland Publishing, 1988), 163-64; and "In Memoriam," *Public Health Nursing* 30 (May 1938): 308.

EXCERPTS

1. Advisory Council Minutes, 1926, 8.

2. "Annual Meeting of Organizations of Nurses," 109.

3. *Twenty-first Annual Meeting,* 161.

4. Ibid.

5. "Twenty-Fourth Annual Meeting," 116.

6. Ibid., 181.

7. Emma L. Collins, "The Co-operative Movement Among Nurses Which is Called the Official Registry," 24 October 1928, NYSNA Archives.

8. *Twenty-Second Annual Meeting,* 132.

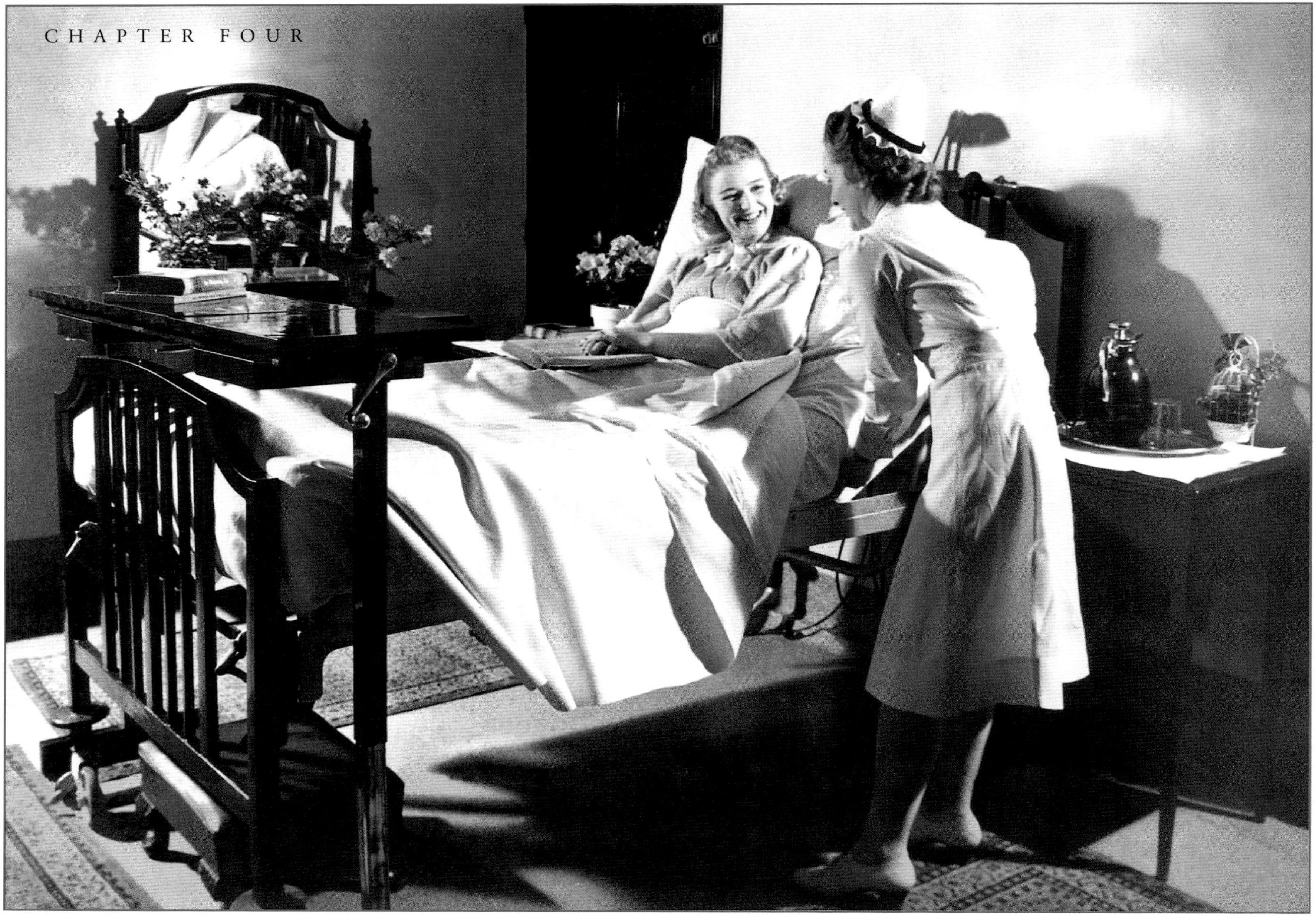

CHAPTER FOUR

HARD TIMES
1929–1938

Despite the rise in consumption of goods in the 1920s, mass demand was ultimately unable to keep up with the rapid increase in industrial production. Overproduction and speculation resulted, and the October 1929 stock market crash brought the seemingly endless prosperity to an abrupt end. The overproduction of nurses identified by the Grading Committee became an even greater problem during the worldwide economic depression that followed. Unemployment on "an unimagined and unprecedented scale" lasted longer than anyone could have predicted.[1] The alarming rate of unemployment among nurses added a sense of urgency to NYSNA's efforts to solve the distribution problems identified by studies in the 1920s.

FACING PAGE: As hospitals became more established, many developed patient rooms with home-like amenities, such as this room at Mount Sinai Hospital. *Courtesy the Archives of the Mount Sinai Medical Center.*

UNEMPLOYMENT: With the advent of the depression, the chronic unemployment among private duty nurses escalated. A speaker at NYSNA's 1930 convention stated, "Workers in every community have been affected this year by hard times; that term so full of menace, which may mean a reduced purchasing power of the public or a feeling of apprehension that turns normal spending into hoarding."[2] This widespread unemployment, the overproduction of nurses, and medical advances which reduced infectious disease and hastened recovery following childbirth led to a serious reduction in the demand for nursing services.

A 1930 study of reports of registries throughout the state revealed "there was no shortage of nurses anywhere," and nurses were urged to remain in their own communities. "Do not go elsewhere in the expectation of finding something better. Almost certainly you will meet in the next town conditions similar to your own."[3]

As the depression deepened, the number and duration of private duty cases steadily declined. In a District 3 survey, private duty nurses reported an average of only 122.5 days of employment in 1931, with average earnings for the year of $644.33. (Institutional and public health nurses, on the other hand, reported 365 days of employment, with earnings of $1,600-$1,700.) The situation was no better downstate, where the Nursing Bureau of Brooklyn reported employment during the first third of 1932 declined 36 percent.[4]

In 1932 a committee on nursing of the Hospital Association of New York State recommended that nursing schools reduce enrollment and carefully consider the justification of continuance of the school. Many schools closed, including one of New York City's pioneer schools, the City Hospital School of Nursing. By and large, however, changes were minimal, and large classes of students continued to be admitted. Executive Secretary Emily Hicks chastised hospitals for ". . . admitting each year, a large class of students, and graduating each year, more nurses than the community could have used, in the days of prosperity . . . One is forced to believe that the implications of the Goldmark Study, Grading Committee Reports . . . and others have been wholly lost on a Board of Directors and Hospital Executives."[5] Indeed, there was growing frustration that the problems identified by the Grading Committee persisted. "To what use is this material being put? Is it merely to be filed with other statistics? As Dr. Burgess has shown, over-production is the greatest evil of our nursing schools and is on the increase . . . The private duty group suffers from this thoughtless over-production more than any other."[6]

BELOW: Emily J. Hicks was NYSNA's executive secretary from 1929 to 1944. She came to the association with a varied background in supervision, private duty, education, and U.S. Army Nurse Corps service, and was a former officer of NYSNA's District 7. Hick's long tenure with the association provided badly needed continuity of leadership. *Courtesy Nurses House Collection, Foundation of NYSNA Archives; photograph by Bachrach.*

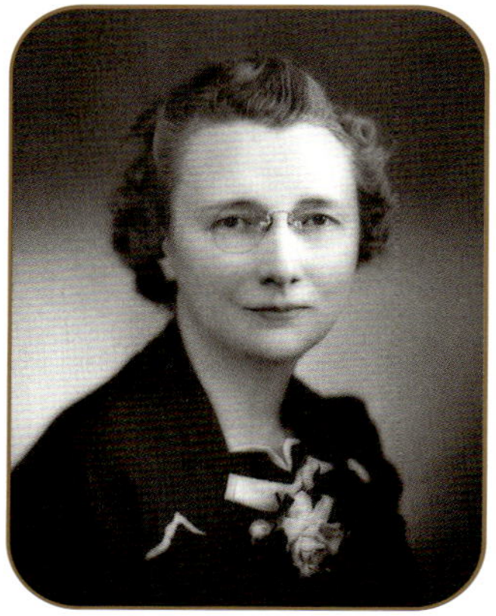

"Our nursing problems are so inextricably involved with community and national health that to be a member of NYSNA should be synonymous with good citizenship."

— *Emily J. Hicks*[1]

Government relief programs initiated in 1931 gradually began to reverse the unemployment, hopelessness, and despair of the depression. By 1935 there were reports of a steady increase in calls for private duty nurses, and the Social Security Act, which provided funds for the development of state and local health services, increased the demand for public health nurses.[7]

RELIEF: With more and more nurses out of work, efforts were stepped up to provide assistance to nurses in need. The ANA had started a Relief Fund in 1911 to assist nurses "overtaken by some great calamity."[8] Following World War I, an appeal was made for contributions so "we should be able to care for those of our members who have sacrificed their health in the service of our country. In this way no nurse need be cared for through the charity of strangers, but through the provision of the members of her own professional family, from a fund to which she herself had contributed during her days of prosperity and health."[9] Each state had a Relief Fund Committee that solicited contributions, investigated applicants, and maintained direct contact with recipients of aid. NYSNA's committee solicited funds, and provided detailed reports at each convention, giving information on New York nurses helped by the fund, and the status of pledges and contributions. The number of nurses aided increased each year until contributions could not keep up with demand, and investment income had to be used. At the 1930 ANA biennial convention, it was decided that the fund would be discontinued after 1932, at which time the state associations would assume responsibility for any necessary relief work.[10]

NYSNA's Board of Directors asked each district to discuss the type of program needed in New York. Committee chair Alta Dines stated, "At this time of unemployment and consequent distress, it is peculiarily fitting that the nurses of New York consider together the problem of a State Fund that may be called upon by any member of the State Association if for some reason she finds herself in real need of financial help and with no one to whom she can turn."[11] At the 1931 convention, delegates approved the formation of a Service Committee to plan for assisting the twenty New York nurses receiving benefits from ANA's fund, advise district committees, and administer a fund. The state committee provided $100 to each District Service Committee to be used as a revolving fund for any emergency. Services not of an emergency nature were referred to the state committee. "The important thing to remember is that no member of our Association should go without service which her District Committee can render." During its first year, the state and district service committees helped 102 nurses in need.[12]

The service committees became important links to broader relief programs. In the early days of the depression, private charitable organizations provided most of the care for the needy, with local governments stepping in when private agencies could no longer keep up. By mid-1931, most local governments were nearly bankrupt because of the burden of relief programs, and Governor Franklin D. Roosevelt urged state government to extend aid, "not as a matter of charity but as a matter of social duty." In 1931 legislation embodying Roosevelt's proposals created the Temporary Emergency Relief Administration (TERA) to distribute aid to communities for relief programs. TERA was a pioneering venture, and set the pattern for state and federal government relief programs nationwide during the depression. Medical care was included as a component of the relief program for families of the unemployed, and in 1932 NYSNA member Marion Sheahan developed a program to hire unemployed nurses to provide public health nursing services to public relief recipients — what Sheahan termed "an experiment in double relief."[13]

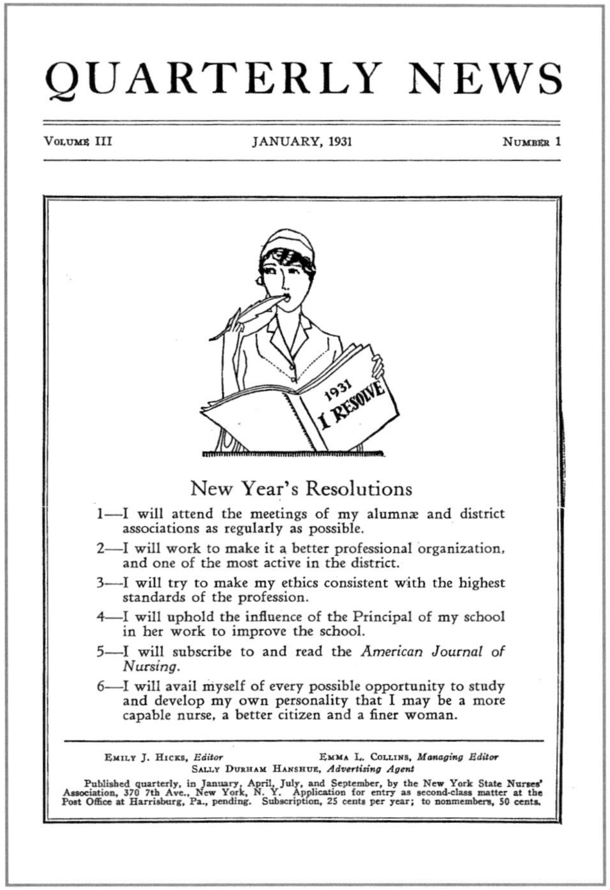
QUARTERLY NEWS

VOLUME III — JANUARY, 1931 — NUMBER 1

New Year's Resolutions

1—I will attend the meetings of my alumnæ and district associations as regularly as possible.

2—I will work to make it a better professional organization, and one of the most active in the district.

3—I will try to make my ethics consistent with the highest standards of the profession.

4—I will uphold the influence of the Principal of my school in her work to improve the school.

5—I will subscribe to and read the *American Journal of Nursing.*

6—I will avail myself of every possible opportunity to study and develop my own personality that I may be a more capable nurse, a better citizen and a finer woman.

EMILY J. HICKS, *Editor* — EMMA L. COLLINS, *Managing Editor*
SALLY DURHAM HANSHUE, *Advertising Agent*

Published quarterly, in January, April, July, and September, by the New York State Nurses' Association, 370 7th Ave., New York, N. Y. Application for entry as second-class matter at the Post Office at Harrisburg, Pa., pending. Subscription, 25 cents per year; to nonmembers, 50 cents.

With the advice and assistance of NYSNA's Service Committee, nurses throughout the state were surveyed. Over 90 percent of the respondents, many of whom supported dependents, indicated an immediate or approaching need for relief. The Service Committee sent letters to respondents who indicated interest in work relief, and through the district committees identified other nurses in need of employment. In 1933 TERA hired two hundred unemployed nurses at reduced rates to provide health services to families in need. The project was so successful that nurses' salaries were increased, and in 1934 more than seven hundred nurses were employed. Experts cited care provided through TERA as the primary factor in all time low rates of maternal mortality, still births, and infant deaths reported in 1935.[14]

The Service Committee continued assisting nurses in need even after the worst of the depression passed. NYSNA established a Loan Fund which was available to members for post-graduate education, and developed educational programs on insurance, savings, pensions, and other "prevention" topics. Funds used by the Service Committee program were contributed by NYSNA members, district associations, and alumnae groups. The $13,500 received as New York's share of ANA's Relief Fund was contributed to Nurses House, a Long Island facility that provided convalescent services to nurses.[15]

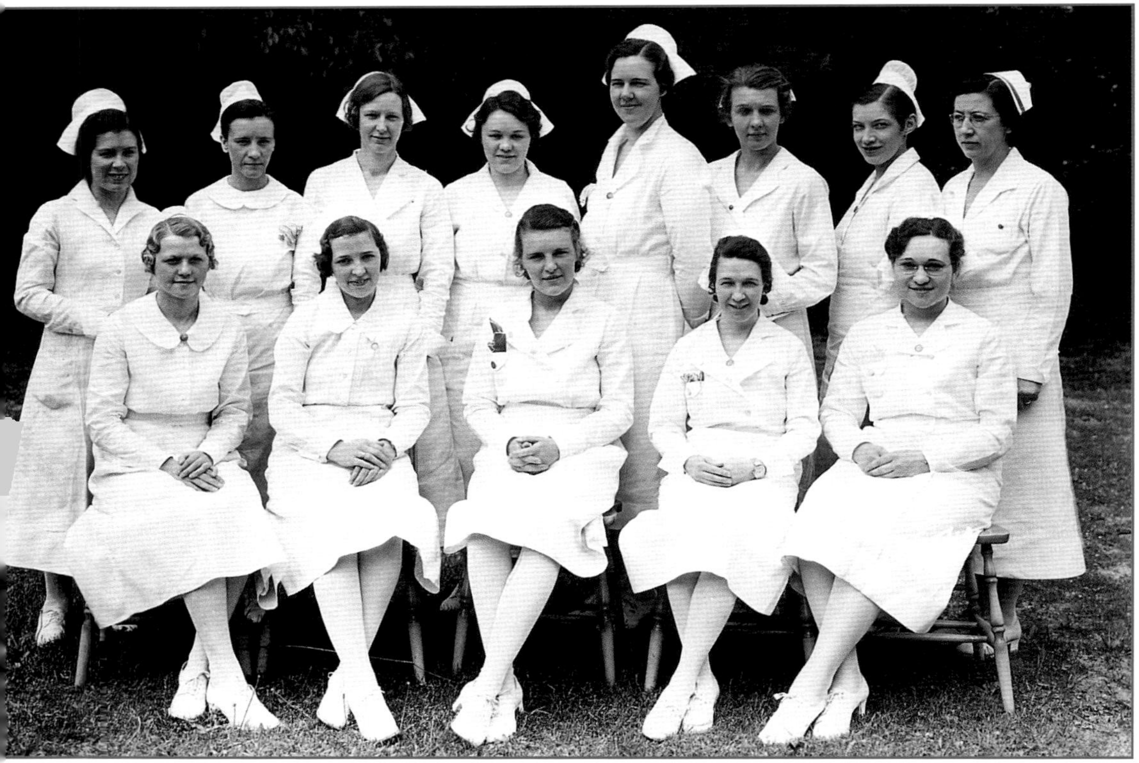

Hospitals required additional graduate nurses during the 1930s. The nurses shown here were head nurses and supervisors at Ellis Hospital, Schenectady, 1934. *Courtesy Ellis Hospital School of Nursing Collection, Foundation of NYSNA Archives.*

EIGHT-HOUR DUTY: The eight-hour work day was a frequent topic for discussion at NYSNA conventions. In 1911 the American Nurses Association urged schools of nursing to limit students' clinical hours to eight per day, but it wasn't until 1917 that schools in New York State began implementing the plan. As labor leaders began promoting the eight-hour work day in industry, nursing leaders started to think about the eight-hour day for all nurses employed by hospitals and in homes.[16] In 1929 a national movement began promoting eight-hour duty as beneficial to both nurse and patient because of the improved care provided by a rested and more efficient nurse. The real impetus for the plan's popularity, however, was the need for hospitals to provide more economical care during the deepening depression and the contribution the eight-hour day made to the spread-the-work movement.

In 1932 District 14 formed a committee to study ways of stimulating employment in response to private duty nurses' question, "What are you going to do to help us earn a living?" The committee met with over three hundred private duty nurses, and developed a plan whereby special duty nursing would be provided at the rate of $5 for eight-hour duty instead of the usual $7 for twelve-hour duty. When the plan was offered to the Hospital Council of Brooklyn, there was concern over the loss of income from the meals nurses bought during extended workdays. Nonetheless, there was gradual acceptance of the plan. By February 1934 over half of District 14's alumnae groups had secured the eight-hour day and the Hospital Council approved a resolution for the adoption of eight-hour duty for hospital special duty nurses.[17]

District 13 formed a Committee on Eight Hours for Nurses specifically to work for adoption of eight-hour duty in hospitals. The committee hired staff, produced numerous publications, and conducted an intensive campaign. A symposium held in March 1934 to discuss the issue drew an audience of nearly two thousand nurses, physicians, and hospital administrators.[18] New York City's French Hospital was one of the first to institute the eight-hour day for private duty nurses. Nurses accepted a reduced fee for eight-hour shifts. Thus, three nurses rather than two provided care to the patient over a twenty-four hour period at no increase in cost to the patient. The hospital reported employing 100 percent more private duty nurses. Nurses continued to work a six-day week, but immediately reaped the benefits of a shortened workday. One nurse stated, "Heretofore, I have simply worked, traveled, and slept. Now I have time for rest, for normal hours of recreation, and for study at the University. I should never want to return to twelve-hour duty!"[19]

In 1935 the movement made steady progress. An editorial in the *New York Herald Tribune* urged readers to "do their part toward hastening the complete acceptance of the change."[20] Twenty-six hospitals in District 13, twenty-one in District 14, and a few others scattered throughout the state offered "8-hour special nursing service." However, 60 percent

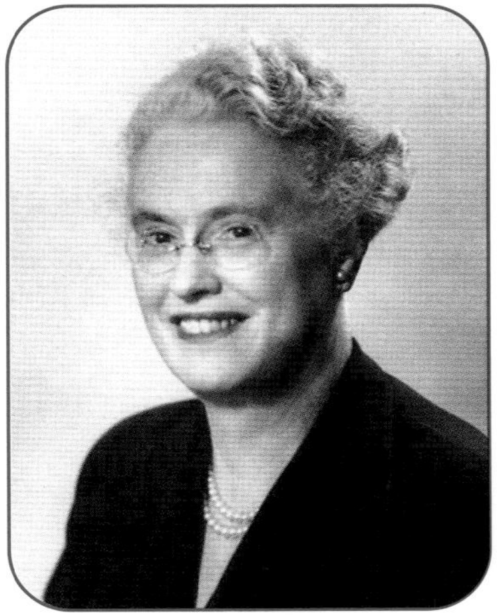

RIGHT: Ethel G. Prince was elected NYSNA President in 1934 and continued in that office until 1939. As president she was deeply involved in the association's efforts to enact new nursing legislation. Prince was a former private duty nurse, and had been active in the establishment of District 14 and the achievement of the eight-hour day for nurses. In 1936 she became District 14's first executive secretary, a position she held until 1957. Mrs. Prince was an active, visible leader in the district, and inspired a generation of nurses. *Courtesy the District 14 Collection, Foundation of NYSNA Archives; photograph by Paul Parker.*

of nurses statewide still worked twelve-hour days, and some hospitals continued to have twenty-hour duty. ". . . it is breathtaking to realize that any hospital sanctions and permits a plan of duty involving 160 hours a week."[21]

Implementation of eight-hour duty was credited with increasing the number of calls to registries and a more even distribution of employment. However, while eight-hour duty eased the unemployment of private duty nurses, it exacerbated a growing shortage of nurses for hospital general duty nursing. In 1937, when a local law went into effect which established the eight-hour day for all New York City public hospital employees, 1,289 nurses were added to the staff of the Department of Hospitals. Nonetheless, even more nurses were needed, and once again, the cry "nursing shortage" was heard.[22]

> "We old girls here haven't even scratched the surface of the work that is to be done and I have no doubt if we are mentioned at all by future historians somebody will say that, considering the times we did as well as could have been expected . . ."
>
> — *Lillian Wald*[2]

HOSPITAL SHORTAGES: The rapidly alternating reports of unemployment, overproduction, and nursing shortage led a Joint Committee on Community Nursing Service to prepare a questionnaire to determine "What Is The Real Status of Nurse Employment in New York State? . . . very conflicting reports are in circulation about employment conditions in the nursing profession. Some REGISTRIES have stated they cannot fill vacancies; some have reported that many of their registrants are leaving the profession because they cannot find work. HOSPITALS . . . report that nurses are unavailable . . . NURSES continue to state that they cannot find enough nursing work . . . they must either seek other work or starve." Questionnaires were included in an issue of the *Quarterly News,* and were sent to five hundred hospitals and sanatoria. Survey returns indicated there were more graduate nurses than ever before.[23]

Since the height of the depression in 1932, when one out of every four employable New Yorkers was jobless, hospitals had been suffering from a loss of income due to the decreased number of paying patients. More than ever before, hospitals needed to find the most economical way of providing nursing care. Many hospitals closed schools of nursing or cut enrollments, and hired more graduate nurses. These factors, together with implementation of eight-hour duty, contributed to a marked shift from private duty nursing to general duty hospital nursing. Between 1927 and 1937, the number of nurses employed in institutions more than doubled. Nonetheless, hospitals were in desperate need of general duty staff nurses.[24]

The staff nurse was quickly becoming accepted and sought after as a permanent member of the hospital staff, but nurses were not eager to take advantage of these new opportunities. Hospital nursing had long been viewed as not quite respectable, and nurses were not eager to re-enter the paternalistic atmosphere of their student days. It was clear that conditions had to be improved if hospitals were to provide adequate nursing service. Poor working and living conditions, inadequate salaries, and lack of other benefits needed to be addressed. Nurses wanted challenging programs of staff education, recognition of ability through promotion and salary increases, and paid vacations and sick leave. Unable to fill staff positions, many hospitals began to employ nurses who were not registered. Nursing leaders feared that hospitals would increase the size of their schools to provide the necessary patient care, thus exacerbating the overproduction of nurses. NYSNA members were encouraged to cooperate with the Hospital Association to enhance working conditions to attract qualified graduates and stabilize hospital nursing services.[25]

CONSTANT LEGISLATIVE WARFARE: In 1930 the Nursing Committee of the New York County Medical Society discussed opening up the Nurse Practice Act to impose a classification of nurses for the "better protection of the sick public, and to meet the growing demand of the public unable to pay the highly specialized registered nurse."[26] The committee proposed additional classes of nurses (graduates of non-registered schools, students who had not completed training programs, and other groups of "practical nurses") who they proposed would be registered without examination. NYSNA opposed opening up the Nurse Practice Act, favoring instead legislation to control commercial registries. Association leaders became alarmed when an alliance developed between the New York County Medical Society and a coalition of New York City commercial registries, the American Nurses' Association, Inc. (ANA, Inc.)[27] In response, NYSNA assembled a formidable Legislative Committee, and hired its first full-time lobbyist, Louise Arnold.[28]

When delegates at NYSNA's 1931 convention celebrated the thirtieth anniversary of the association's founding, President Elisabeth Greener commented, "Those of us who are more or less familiar with the work and progress of the Association feel that its life and history has been one constant legislative warfare ever since the passage of this first nurse practice act. The nurses of New York State have learned many bitter and costly lessons through their 30 years of legislative effort. Possibly the one that has been most deeply impressed upon our consciousness is the menace of the ever recurring Waiver when for any reason it becomes necessary to open the bill . . . there is in the heart of each New York State registered nurse a very real dread and fear of the possible result or outcome of further legislative efforts."[29] Greener went on to acknowledge the need to improve the Nurse Practice Act, and recommended the formation of a committee to prepare a new bill should any other group introduce nursing legislation.

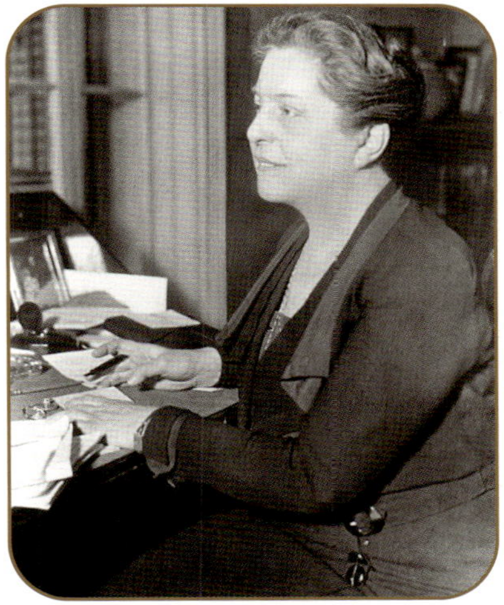

RIGHT: Lillian Wald founded the famous Henry Street Settlement on New York City's lower east side in 1893, and is considered to be the founder of public health nursing. By the 1930s Wald was a prominent nurse and social activist. After a passionate speech calling for disarmament at NYSNA's 1931 convention, delegates voted to send a telegram to President Herbert Hoover, expressing support of disarmament. *Courtesy Nurses House Collection, Foundation of NYSNA Archives.*

Association staff closely monitored legislative activities in Albany. Of special concern were any attempts to open the Nurse Practice Act, but the association followed a wide variety of bills, including health, education, social welfare, and employment agency legislation. Staff and leaders also offered testimony when necessary. In 1931 Assistant Executive Secretary Marguerite Jacobsen was appointed, freeing Hicks to spend more time in Albany. NYSNA maintained combined living quarters and offices for Hicks in Albany during the legislative session for two years, until the headquarters office was moved from New York City to Albany in 1934. It was during this period that staff began to prepare weekly digests of legislative news which were sent to members of the board and Legislative Committee, chairs of district legislative committees, and alumnae associations.[30]

A Committee to Study the Nurse Practice Act was appointed in 1933 to quickly propose a new bill if it became necessary to sponsor "defensive" legislation. The ANA, Inc. was thriving, and the association believed "the consequences in the Legislature may be serious . . . under the guise of a commercial registry, with immense power behind it politically in the City of New York, this thing is flourishing. They openly boast that we cannot do anything to them and they are going to lead nursing."[31] NYSNA leaders believed the political power of the ANA, Inc. was responsible for failure of an association-backed bill to control the commercial nurses' registries, and feared the consequences if the group submitted a nurse practice bill.[32]

> "It is evident that a revision in our Nurse Practice Act is necessary to keep our profession attuned to changing society."
>
> — *Mary Creed*[3]

Under the leadership of chairman Marion Sheahan, the Committee to Study the Nurse Practice Act examined the law in relation to other professional practice acts, and identified deficiencies in the existing law. The 1920 act contained no definition of nursing, no definition of violations, no mechanisms to enforce the law or discipline nurses, and most importantly, no prohibition of anyone practicing as a nurse. The law protected titles, but did not control the practice of nursing. The "vicious saving clause" in the 1920 legislation permitted anyone to provide nursing services as long as the terms "registered, trained, or certified nurse," or "trained attendant" were not used. For several days, the committee fiercely debated the issue of licensure for "all who nurse for hire," and finally concluded that there was a need for a worker trained in simple nursing procedures and household tasks to care for chronic and convalescent patients, and that the practice of these workers must be controlled through licensure.[33]

> "The subsidiary worker is needed, and whether or not we are willing to recognize her, we are going to have her."
>
> — *Marian R. Fleming*[4]

In 1934 the Department of Education issued a report by Dr. Harlan Hoyt Horner, assistant commissioner for Higher Education. The report, "Nursing Education and Practice in New York State with Suggested Remedial Measures," was based on a three year study conducted by NYSNA member Lenore Bradley. The association cooperated in distribution of the publication and facilitated widespread discussion. The Horner report strengthened NYSNA's resolve to craft a new Nurse Practice Act, and provided data and rationale to support many of the committee's proposals. The report recommended the elimination of the trained attendant and the establishment of two classes of licensed nurses, the registered nurse and the practical nurse.[34]

The committee prepared a new bill which included a definition of nursing practice; licensure of all who provide nursing care in two groups, the practical nurses and the graduate registered nurses; specificity regarding violations; and procedures for discipline and prosecution. The central issue — and most controversial — continued to be whether a new bill should be patterned after the existing law, which was a protection of title, or designed to truly control the practice of nursing. Licensing everyone who practiced nursing was the basis for a "real" practice act, but opposition to the licensure of practical nurses was fierce. The highly respected Annie Goodrich and Beatrice Stevenson, both

MARION W. SHEAHAN
1892 - 1994

Marion Sheahan graduated from St. Peter's Hospital School of Nursing in Albany in 1913. Early in her career, she worked as a public health nurse at the famous Henry Street Settlement and in several state and local public health programs. In the 1920s she began working for the State Department of Health's Bureau of Public Health Nursing. As the Bureau's director during the depression years, Sheahan was instrumental in shaping the Temporary Emergency Relief Act to identify nursing care as a "necessity of life." Organizations throughout the country replicated her innovative model programs to provide work for unemployed nurses and deliver essential health services to families on relief.

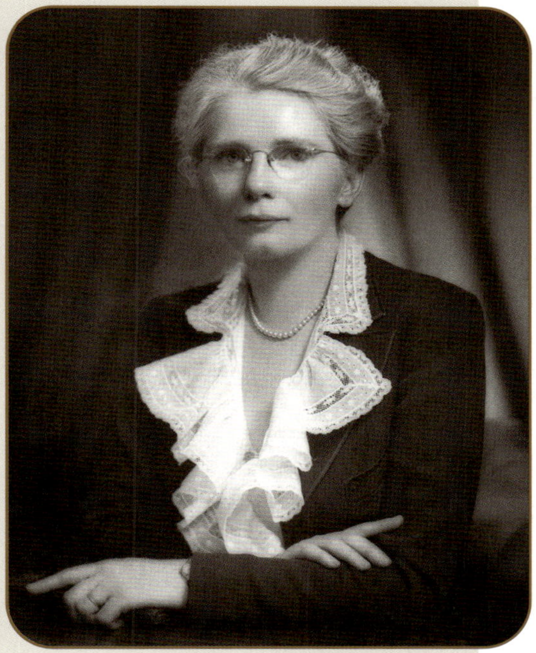

Courtesy the Sheahan Collection, Foundation of NYSNA Archives; photograph by Bachrach.

Marion Sheahan began a lifetime of organizational involvement in the 1920s when she became active in NYSNA. In 1933 she was appointed to chair NYSNA's Nurse Practice Act Committee, and worked tirelessly for the enactment of legislation mandating licensure for "all who nurse for hire." Sheahan guided the committee in the drafting of legislation and met with representatives of state agencies and other health professions to build consensus. Most importantly, year after year, she was able to lead discussion on the controversial provisions of the proposed legislation at meetings of NYSNA's House of Delegates, the Advisory Council, and special forums. Her clear explanations and forthright opinions enabled the association to gain the support of its members for this landmark legislation.

Experience gained during these years of involvement in NYSNA prepared her for national roles in the decades to come. In the 1940s, as president of the National Organization for Public Health Nursing, she was a member of the National Nursing Council, and served on several of the council's most important committees. In the 1950s she was appointed director of the Division of Nursing Services of the newly formed National League for Nursing, and in the 1960s she was the first nurse elected president of the American Public Health Association. She received numerous honors and awards including honorary doctoral degrees from Adelphi College and Case Western Reserve University, the Lasker Award, the Florence Nightingale Medal, the Sedgwick Memorial Medal, NLN's Distinguished Service Award, ANA's Pearl McIver Award, and Honorary Recognition from NYSNA. Throughout her long career, Marion Sheahan kept the needs of the individual nurse and the patient in the forefront of her efforts to improve the public's health.[1]

so instrumental in the passage of earlier legislation, were both strongly opposed. Goodrich believed "that there is no nursing except the best nursing," and Stevenson argued that the number of "properly qualified nurses" should be increased to meet existing needs. Many members expressed fear that competition with licensed practical nurses would eliminate registered nurses completely.[35] District 1 formally opposed licensure of practical nurses, as did NYSNA's Private Duty Section. Several districts and the Men's Section were supportive, while many districts remained divided. Sheahan noted that the opposition was primarily based on fear. "They fear that the practical nurse will be elevated and will be in further competition."[36]

"I myself believe that the test of nursing and the nursing profession lies in the quality of the nursing done by the private duty nurse."

— Mary Gladwin[5]

For four years Sheahan reported to convention delegates and led discussion, and delegates authorized the board to introduce legislation if conditions warranted. An intensive program of study and discussion was implemented in the districts. Opinion remained divided, but delegates at the 1936 convention finally voted to introduce a bill.[37]

The ANA, Inc. never developed into the powerful threat the association feared, but opposition to NYSNA's proposed legislation gained strength elsewhere. The National Nurses Association (NNA) was established specifically in response to the proposed legislation. Its primary focus was to secure more rights, including registration by waiver, for nurses denied registration in New York, primarily out-of-state graduates. In order to obtain New York licensure, out-of-state nurses had to be graduates of an approved school. The State Board of Nurse Examiners, lacking staff to make on-site inspections, had hundreds of applications from out-of-state schools pending. Thus, large numbers of nurses registered in their own states were unable to be licensed in New York. The NNA, funded by substantial initiation fees and dues, was able to hire an office staff of six, and formed local groups in Syracuse, Utica, Albany, Rochester, Niagara Falls, Buffalo, and Middletown. The NNA sponsored the Feld-Byrne Bill, which provided for licensure without examination for any nurse registered in another state or foreign country, and licensure by practical exam for graduates of any non-accredited school. A similar bill, the McCaffrey Bill, was sponsored by the Association of Hospital and Medical Professionals, a local of the American Federation of Labor.[38]

NYSNA's bill was introduced in the Senate by Joseph A. Esquirol in January 1937. Although the association had secured the support of the Medical Society of the State of New York (MSSNY), the Hospital Association of New York State, the New York State Departments of Education, Health, Mental Hygiene, and Social Welfare, and various other groups, opposition was formidable. In addition to the rival nursing organizations, NYSNA leaders were shocked to learn that the Board of Regents opposed the bill. The association had worked very closely with Assistant Commissioner Horner, and had assumed his report, published by the Department of Education, was endorsed by the regents. However, at a February 1937 meeting, Sheahan learned that the regents believed the bill was too radical a step, and that they had never given approval to the Horner report. The Board of Regents did acknowledge the need for a stronger law, and agreed to oppose the Feld-Byrne and McCaffrey bills. One can imagine the deflating effect of this on the association's enthusiasm. NYSNA leaders surely realized there was little chance of their bill's passage without the regents' support.[39]

A hearing on the Esquirol and Feld-Byrne bills was held in March. The NNA had planned a variety of activities in Albany, including a march of uniformed nurses to the hearing. The hearing, moderated by Senator Feld, sponsor of the NNA bill, apparently went badly. Marion Sheahan commented, "the less said about the conduct of the public hearing, the better . . . There was certainly a great deal of misrepresentation, and a great deal of misinterpretation." The Feld-Byrne bill was strengthened at the hearing by the endorsement of the labor group. Nonetheless, all nursing bills were killed in committee.[40]

NYSNA's Board of Directors voted to further educate the public and be prepared to introduce another bill. They were particularly concerned about the rival nursing organizations, which they believed were jeopardizing the very existence of ANA and NYSNA. The board appealed to ANA for financial assistance to fight these opposing groups and secure legislation. ANA agreed to provide an interest-free loan of $10,000 for three to four years for NYSNA to "carry on its work regarding the NNA, and extending other service."[41]

"If the patient is sick enough to have a doctor, that patient is sick enough to have a trained nurse."

— Miss Schultz[6]

A newly drafted bill presented at the 1937 convention reflected an effort to offer a compromise in hopes of reducing opposition from the Board of Regents and the NNA. Following advice from the regents, the definition of nursing practice was rewritten, and after meetings with Virginia Mirabella, president of the NNA, and Luciel McGorkey of the Associated Hospital and Medical Professionals, measures to facilitate registration of out-of-state graduates were strengthened. The increased difficulty in securing registered nurses for hospital duty and public health positions provided added incentive for this modification.[42] President Prince reported to delegates, "Hospitals want to employ only registered nurses. But, if this is impossible with our present number, then these institutions must nurse their patients with unregistered out-of-state graduates unless our law is changed to admit qualified nurses, meeting standards, to the licensing examinations."[43] The House of Delegates voted to reintroduce a bill as soon as possible.

Cognizant of the failure of the previous year's strategy of engaging an attorney to prepare and promote the bill, the board voted that funds be expended to employ professional speakers to interpret the bill rather than to engage an attorney.[44] Staff were hired to prepare pamphlets, articles, radio talks, information for speakers, and newspaper releases. Irene Hellen, a private duty nurse, was employed as a full-time lobbyist, and members from each district were trained to teach their committee members to lobby for the bill in their local communities.[45]

NYSNA held additional meetings with representatives of the NNA and the Hospital and Medical Professionals, now affiliated with the CIO. NYSNA and the NNA joined forces, and Senator Feld and Assemblywoman Jane Todd introduced a new bill. Organized labor remained unalterably opposed to licensure of any subsidiary group, and continued to oppose the bill. Nonetheless, the Todd-Feld Bill passed and Governor Lehman signed the bill on April 6, 1938. With the passage of this bill, New York State became the first to legislate licensure of "all who nurse for hire." Passage of this landmark legislation set a national precedent. The three national nursing organizations went on record as favoring similar legislation for all states.[46]

REGISTRIES AND BUREAUS: In 1930 the ANA Inc. convinced the New York City Bureau of Licenses to prohibit the term "official" in the names of registries, thus necessitating changing the name of district sponsored registries to "professional registries." When the ANA Inc. changed its name to Registries of New York, Inc. in 1934, registries were advised by legal counsel to again change their name, this time to "nursing bureaus."[47]

NYSNA's Registry Committee worked to develop minimum standards for all the nursing bureaus. "If we are to help the private duty nurse solve her problem, we must focus attention on Registries as the central factor in distribution." Leaders hoped that nursing bureaus would offer communities more diversified, complete, and economical nursing service, and change private duty nursing from an "unsatisfactory free lance occupation" to a "stabilized, organized profession, comparable in its hours, income, and chance for specialization and advancement with the other branches of nursing."[48]

> "The results of the licensing examination as well as over-production of nurses in the country lead us to believe the time has surely come when we should choose our candidates most carefully."
>
> — *Clara Quereau*[7]

In 1935 the Registry Committee recommended that NYSNA sponsor a demonstration community nursing council which would serve as a clearinghouse for all types of nursing services and which might supplement other health demonstrations to improve, extend, and make available nursing service to the community. National and state committees on Distribution of Nursing Service, chaired by New York's Anne Hansen, urged the development of these local councils of nursing.[49] Despite enthusiasm by the board for comprehensive community nursing bureaus such as these, the project was postponed and never came to fruition.[50]

Another initiative sought to enhance the placement services of nursing bureaus. During the depression years the headquarters office received an increasing number of calls from nurses seeking employment and from hospitals seeking nurses to fill staff vacancies. Many of the official registries provided placement services, but in 1934 a specially appointed committee recommended the development of a statewide professional placement bureau to supplement registry services. The committee recommended a bureau be established in connection with the headquarters office to provide services to educational directors, instructors, and supervisors as well as general duty nurses. When ANA announced plans for a national placement service, no further steps were taken. In 1937 the committee turned its focus back to the districts, recommending adding a field secretary to assist districts in organizing nursing bureaus, planning institutes for registrars, and centralizing all professional registries in each community.[51]

AN ERA OF CONTRASTS: The activities of NYSNA during the depression years were marked by both confusion and a growing sophistication and maturity. The association took many steps in an attempt to solve the problems of distribution of nursing services, yet changes occurred more as a result of external factors than NYSNA initiatives. Recommendations were made but rarely implemented. Organizational units proliferated. Committees and sub-committees were quickly formed and were often as quickly disbanded. Many joint committees with medical, hospital, and other nursing organizations were formed to work on mutual problems. Special committees of NYSNA, the state league for nursing, and the State Organization for Public Health Nursing (SOPHN) often had overlapping purposes and frequently duplicated efforts. A joint committee attempted to sort out responsibilities and tasks and recommended "amalgamating" the three state groups by making the state league and the SOPHN strong NYSNA committees on education and public health respectively. In 1937 the SOPHN became the Public Health Section of NYSNA, but the state league for nursing continued to function independently.[52]

Despite confusion and chaos in some areas, the association showed growing strength and maturity. Sections were formed when two hundred or more members requested a section on a common interest, usually an occupational group. By 1938 three sections, representing private duty, public health, and male nurses, were active. A committee was formed to study district boundaries in response to complaints that the "district centers" were often inaccessible to some members, and the fifteenth district was formed in Olean and Chenango Counties. As staff increased, more services were provided to the districts. A committee formed to study the needs of districts and alumnae associations recommended planned educational programs, and staff responded by developing year-long programs for districts on a single topic. Membership grew steadily, dropping only in 1932 at the height of the depression. Districts and alumnae associations were encouraged to make every effort to assist "economically handicapped nurses" to maintain their membership, and the following year membership was again on the rise.[53] Membership in 1938 was 17,883 — 45 percent of the total number of registered nurses in the state.

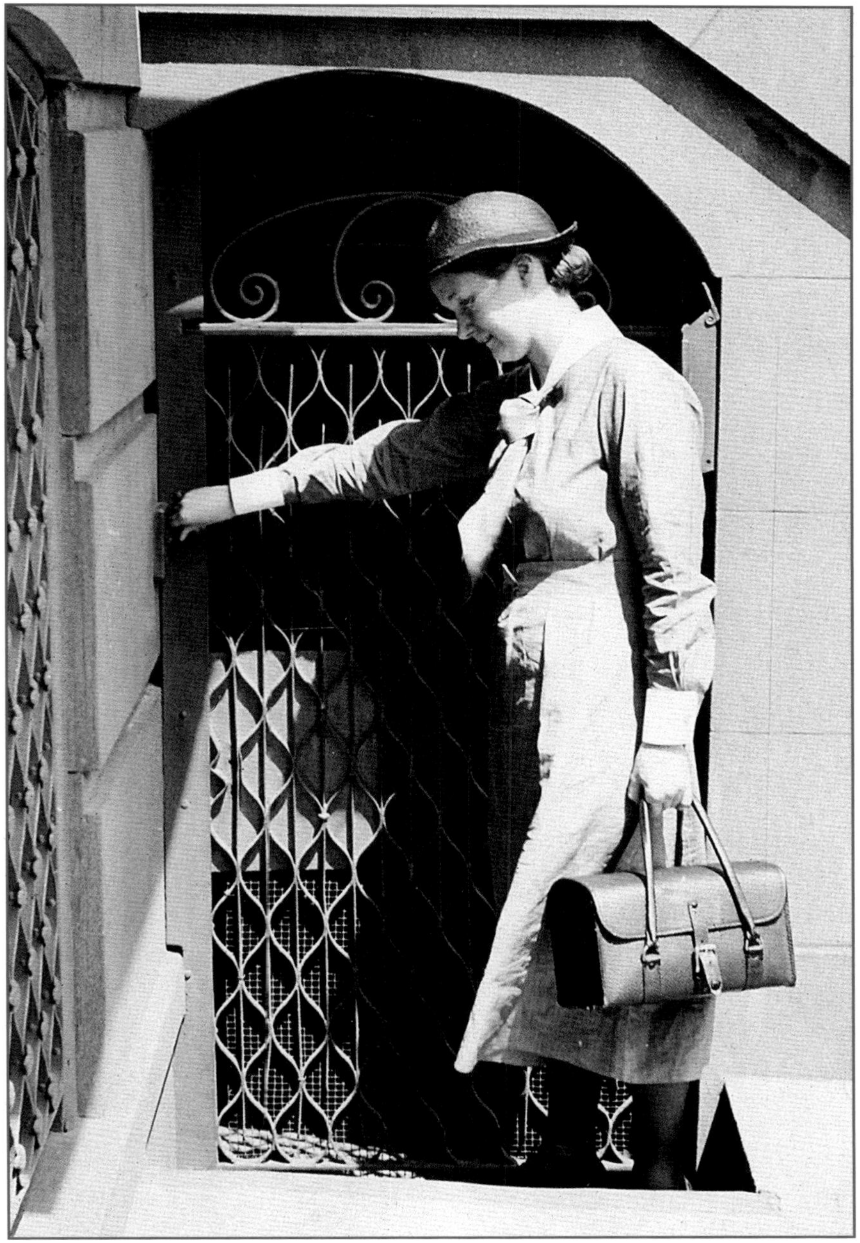

RIGHT: The demand for public health nurses accelerated during the 1930s as relief programs developed and federal grants became available for local and state health departments. *Courtesy Brooklyn VNA.*

Perhaps the most significant example of the association's growing sophistication was the passage of the Nurse Practice Act, guided by the experience of thirty years of "legislative warfare." While prepared to act quickly if necessary, NYSNA did not act precipitously. The Committee to Study the Nurse Practice Act focused on weaknesses in the 1920 law and carefully prepared new legislation. Years were devoted to careful study, discussion, and consensus building. The association developed support in the medical and hospital communities and utilized professionally prepared materials. Districts and alumnae associations raised funds through appeals and "assessments," and NYSNA poured resources into lobbying and educating both nurses and the general public.[54] Compromises were reached without sacrificing goals, and New York legislation again provided a model for the rest of the nation. The exhilaration of legislative success was soon tempered, however, by growing international unrest that postponed implementation of the law.[55]

> "When nursing becomes recognized as an economic necessity as well as a social necessity, we will have more opportunity for our schools than we have yet had . . . How can we, with the knowledge we have — prepare nurses as we know they should be prepared to meet the demands made upon us when we are controlled by the economic situation of hospitals in such an extraordinary measure as we still are?"
>
> — *Mary M. Roberts*[8]

CHAPTER NOTES
TEXT

1. Eric Hobsbawm, *The Age of Extremes: A History of the World, 1914–1991* (New York: Vintage Books, 1996), 92–100.

2. "New York Association of Nurses" (Syracuse, N.Y., 1930, stenotype transcript), 148.

3. Baer, *Editor's Notes*, 49; "Nurses, Stay Home," *Quarterly News* 3 (January 1931): 6.

4. "Report of a Survey of Economic Conditions Among the Members of District Number 3," *Quarterly News* 4 (April 1932): 37–9; and "District No. 14," *Quarterly News* 4 (July 1932): 82. District 3 was made up of nurses in the Elmira, N.Y. area.

5. "Editorials," *American Journal of Nursing* 32 (August 1932): 871; "Vital Issues of the Nursing Question and Ways to Meet Them," *Modern Hospital* 39 (November 1932): 58–59; "Hospital Association of New York State," *Quarterly News* 4 (July 1932): 64; and Emily J. Hicks, "Editorial," *Quarterly News* 6 (January 1934): 6.

6. Teresa Rutledge, "The Private Duty Section," *Quarterly News* 5 (April 1933): 34.

7. Kalisch and Kalisch, *Advance of American Nursing*, 310–11.

8. *Ninth and Tenth Annual Meetings*, 106.

9. Sophia F. Palmer, "Editorial Comment," *American Journal of Nursing* 19 (March 1919): 419.

10. Genevieve Clark, "Thoughts from the Biennial," *Quarterly News* 2 (July 1930): 17. One of the problems was that once accepted, recipients received assistance until death or return to duty. In fifteen years, 543 nurses were helped (nearly 50 percent with TB), with 50 percent receiving help before age 40. ("Nurses' Relief Fund of the American Nurses' Association," *American Journal of Nursing* 30 [September 1930]: 1119–24.)

11. Alta Elizabeth Dines, "What Do You Think?" *Quarterly News* 2 (October 1930): 15; Alta Dines, "The Relief Fund," *Quarterly News* 3 (October 1931): 96; and Alta E. Dines, "A Special District Meeting to Discuss Relief Fund," *Quarterly News* 3 (April 1931): 35–36.

12. "The Service Fund and You," *Quarterly News* 5 (July 1933): 63–64; "Convention Report," *Quarterly News* 4 (January 1932): 19; and "Proceedings the New York State Nurses' Association Thirty-Second Meeting" (Rochester, N.Y., 1933, stenotype transcript), 47.

13. Ellis, et al. *History of New York State*, 416–18; and Marion W. Sheahan, "An Experiment in Double Relief," *Public Health Nurse* 25 (July 1933): 378–81.

14. Sheahan, "Experiment in Double Relief," 378–81; and "Unemployed Nurses Aid 62,857 Families Under T.E.R.A. Work Projects," *Quarterly Nurse* 6 (April 1934): 55–56.

15. *Annual Reports of Officers and Committees* (Lake Placid, N.Y.: NYSNA, 1937), 22; and Board of Directors Minutes, NYSNA, 1937–38, NYSNA Archives. In 1937, two loans were granted to nurses for post-graduate study, and the fund was renamed the "Anne L. Hansen Loan Fund."

16. *Ninth and Tenth Annual Meetings*, 104–6; *Sixteenth-Seventeenth Meetings*, 26. In 1919, twenty-four-hour duty was only beginning to give way to twelve-hour duty. (Sophia F. Palmer, "Editorial Comment," *American Journal of Nursing* 19 [January 1919]: 260–61.)

17. Ethel G. Prince, "How Brooklyn Established the Eight Hour Plan," 14 March 1934, Nurses Association of the Counties of Long Island (NACLI) Archives, Foundation of NYSNA, Guilderland, N.Y.; and Emma L. Collins, "Progress Notes on Eight-hour Duty," *American Journal of Nursing* 34 (May 1934): 453. Despite these advances, very little progress was made on eight-hour private nursing in the home.

18. Anna L. Tittman, "The Eight Hour Plan Progresses," in *Nurses' Hobby Show Souvenir Program* (New York, N.Y.: Committee on Eight Hours for Nurses, 1935), 17; and Anna L. Tittman, "New York's on the Way to the Eight-Hour Day," *Quarterly News* 6 (July 1934): 78–79. The committee "platform" included eight reasons for the eight-hour day: "improves service to the patient," "costs the same," "spreads the work," "gives the nurse time for rest," "gives the nurse time for human interests,"

"gives the nurse time for study," "improves morale," and "proves its own success."

19. "The Eight-Hour Day," *Quarterly News* 5 (July 1933): 80. See also, Helen M. Moir, "Another Successful Eight-Hour Plan," *American Journal of Nursing* 33 (August 1933): 775–76. The cost to patients was $17 per 24 hour period — $5 per shift per nurse, plus $2 for meals for the nurses.

20. "Eight Hour Duty for Nurses," *Quarterly News* 7 (July 1935): 97.

21. Emily J. Hicks, Report of Headquarters Office, 27 May 1935, NYSNA Archives, 3; and "Eight-hour Duty Throughout the State," *Quarterly News* 7 (April 1935): 62.

22. *Annual Reports*, 1937, 34; and Mary Ellen Manley, "The Eight-hour Day," *American Journal of Nursing* 38 (January 1938): 26.

23. Insert, *Quarterly News* 8 (April 1936); and Minutes of the Joint Committee on Nursing Problems, 9 November 1936, NYSNA Archives.

24. Ellis, *Epic of New York City*, 533; and Stella Hawkins, "Summary of Study of Clinical Services," *Quarterly News* 9 (October 1937): 120–21.

25. "Private Duty Problems," *Quarterly News* 8 (July 1936): 83–84; "Allies!" *Quarterly News* 7 (October 1935): 121–22; and *Annual Reports,* 1937, 3–4.

26. Emily J. Hicks, Report of Headquarters Office, 28 January 1933, NYSNA Archives.

27. This group incorporated in New York, taking advantage of the American Nurses Association's incomplete incorporation in Washington, thus initiating several years of legal proceedings. It was not until 1934 that the ANA, Inc. was forced to change its name to the Registries of New York, Inc. Meanwhile, the ANA, Inc. took delight over and credit for the closing of the District 13 registry. (Hicks, Report of Headquarters, 28 January 1933; and Report of Meeting of "American Nurses" Association of New York State, Inc., 13 December 1932, NYSNA Archives.)

28. "Legislation," *Quarterly News* 3 (April 1931): 38. Louise Arnold was formerly superintendent of the Samaritan Hospital, Troy and Ellis Hospital, Schenectady. The Legislative Committee was composed of Helen Young, Marion Sheahan, Anne Hansen, Genevieve Clifford, Grace Allison, Elizabeth Burgess, Cassie Rogers, Mary Rogers, Louise Arnold, and Emily Hicks.

29. "Proceedings, Annual Meeting of the New York State Organizations of Nurses" (New York, N.Y., 1931, stenotype transcript), 1–2.

30. Board of Directors Minutes, 28 January 1933; "Proceedings Advisory Council Dinner and Meeting" (Rochester, N.Y., 1933, stenotype transcript), 20–21; and *Annual Reports of Officers and Committees* (Albany, N.Y.: NYSNA, 1934), 13. Many members believed the headquarters "belonged to New York City." There were definite advantages to working in such close proximity to the ANA, NLNE, and AJN staff, but it was much more economical to move the headquarters to Albany.

31. "Advisory Council," 1933, 8–9.

32. "Proceedings Advisory Council of the New York State Nurses' Association" (Buffalo, N.Y., 1934, stenotype transcript), 52.

33. Ibid., 52–62; and "Nursing Laws to Safeguard the Public," 1938, NYSNA Archives. As a part of the discussion at the 1934 meeting, Anne Hansen commented on the 1920 bill. ". . . when I thought back to the last time when we put our Bill through, the trouble that we got into was because we were terribly badly advised. We could have withdrawn that Bill when they demanded a waiver. When the Governor of the State demanded a waiver be extended we could have withdrawn the Bill entirely. But we had nothing to go back on, and we didn't know. We are not in that position today and we have learned by the experience of the past that it would have been better even in that day to have waited a few years, and withdrawn the Bill then, rather than put through that tremendous waiver. But we had not had that experience then. However, some of us are still alive to tell the tale of the trouble, and as long as we are alive, we are going to prevent a waiver even if we have to withdraw the Bill from the Governor's desk." ("Thirty-Second Annual Meeting," 71–77.)

34. Harlan H. Horner, "Looking the Facts in the Face," *American Journal of Nursing* 33 (January 1933): 13–30; and "Advisory Council," 1934, 50–51. Only 1,070 persons had been trained as trained attendants under the 1920 legislation, and only 250 had renewed their registration. The few schools training attendants discontinued their programs within a few years of the law's passage. Other recommendations made by Horner included placing a moratorium on nursing school enrollment, and reorganizing the system of training nurses, including a preliminary requirement of one year of college. Board members were not in favor of a moratorium, approved one year of college as a preliminary educational requirement, and approved "fitness tests" for applicants in order to raise standards. They also recommended no registration of new schools until new standards were established, noting that some schools were now "wisely closing."

35. "Advisory Council," 1934, 52–56; B. Stevenson to A.S. Feld, 29 January 1938, NACLI Archives; and [1938 Nurse Practice Act], n.d., NYSNA Archives, 9. Goodrich met with the board to discuss her objections. (Board of Directors Minutes, NYSNA, 9 March 1935, NYSNA Archives.)

36. "Proceedings Advisory Council of the New York State Nurses Association" (New York, N.Y., 1936, stenotype transcript), 67–70. The term used in the proposed bill was very controversial and changed several times from "practical nurse" to "nursing aide" to "licensed domestic nurse" and finally back to "practical nurse."

37. "Proceedings New York State Nurses Convention" (New York, N.Y., 1936, stenotype transcript), 431. A minimum of $1 per capita from each district (up to $30,000) was requested as a "legislative assessment" to fund the legislative initiative. (Board of Directors Minutes, NYSNA, 8 November 1936, NYSNA Archives.)

38. Driscoll, *Legitimizing the Profession,* 48; National Nurses Association, Inc. flyer, n.d., NYSNA Archives. NNA's motto was "ONE Woman can be Forceful; One HUNDRED Women can be Helpful; One THOUSAND Women can be Powerful but TEN THOUSAND WOMEN, UNITED, are Invincible; THEREFORE HELP US TO HELP YOU." The initiation fee was $15 and dues were $12 per year. In contrast, NYSNA dues in 1935 were $2 per year.

39. Memo from Emily Hicks to Board of Directors, Nurse Practice Act Committee, Legislative Committee, 1 March 1937, NYSNA Archives. There had been other indications that the regents supported the concept. In June 1933 Miss Hicks attended a meeting of the Advisory Council of the Board of Regents and reported to President Elizabeth Greener. "One of the most interesting developments of the discussion yesterday was the fact that the Board of Regents would consider the possibility of licensing under the Department of Education practical nurses and all who nurse for hire. Both Mrs. Hansen and I expressed our gratification on this change of attitude on the part of the Department." (Excerpt from letter of 22 June 1933, sent by Miss Emily Hicks to Miss Elizabeth Greener, then President of the New York State Nurses Association, n.d., NACLI Archives.)

40. "Proceedings, Thirty-Sixth Annual Meeting of the New York State Nurses Association" (Lake Placid, N.Y., 1937, stenotype transcript), 87–90. See also "Hearing Held on Nurse Practice Bills," *Quarterly News* 9 (April 1937): 42.

41. Board of Directors Minutes, NYSNA, 24 May 1937, NYSNA Archives. No other references to this loan were found.

42. "Proceedings Advisory Council Meeting of the New York State Nurses Association" (Lake Placid, N.Y., 1937, stenotype transcript), 110; and Nancy W. Walburn, "The Nurse's Place in the Sun," *Trained Nurse and Hospital Review* 100 (February 1938): 146. Marion Rottman, director of nursing for the New York City Department of Hospitals was a strong supporter of NYSNA's legislation. She expressed the need for qualified out-of-state graduates to fill the many nursing staff positions opened by the adoption of eight-hour duty. ("Convention," 1936, 425).

43. *Annual Reports,* 1937, 3.

44. Board of Directors Minutes, NYSNA, 27 September 1937, NYSNA Archives.

45. [1938 Nurse Practice Act], 10.

46. "Todd Nurse Bill Becomes Law . . . Signed by Governor April 6" *Quarterly News* 10 (April 1938): 16–17; [1938 Nurse Practice Act], 11; and "All Those Who Nurse for Hire," *American Journal of Nursing* 39 (March 1939): 275.

47. Emily J. Hicks, Report to the Board, 6 October 1934, NYSNA Archives; and "Change of Registry Name," *Quarterly News* 3 (January 1931): 18.

48. Clifford, "Knowing Ourselves," 110.

49. "Distribution of Nursing Service," *Quarterly News* 3 (January 1931): 8; and Board of Directors Minutes, NYSNA, 23 January 1936, NYSNA Archives.

50. *Annual Reports of Officers and Committees* (New York, N.Y.: NYSNA, 1936), 29.

51. *Annual Reports,* 1937, 28.

52. The SOPHN had originally been NYSNA's Committee on Public Health. When it became the Public Health Section in 1937, it reverted to NYSNA organizational unit status.

53. "Convention Report," *Quarterly News* 4 (January 1932): 19.

54. Board of Directors Minutes, NYSNA, 19 March 1937, NYSNA Archives. From 1913 to 1922, pledges and contributions for the legislative fund were secured at every annual meeting. During the 1930s special appeals were made.

55. "Licensure for Those Who Nurse," *American Journal of Nursing* 49 (May 1949): 272.

FEATURE

Marion W. Sheahan

1. "Marion Sheahan Bailey," in *Professionalization of Nursing in New York State: Oral History Interviews With Six Leaders Who Helped to Advance the Mission of NYSNA,* ed. Elizabeth Carter and Jane Fielding (Guilderland, N.Y.: NYSNA, 1988), 6–28. Although Sheahan married Frank Bailey in 1937 she continued to use her maiden name for professional purposes.

EXCERPTS

1. "Meeting of the State Organization of Nurses," 10.
2. Ibid., 296.
3. "Advisory Council," 1936, 68.
4. "Convention," 425.
5. "New York Association of Nurses," 166.
6. "Thirty-Sixth Annual Meeting," 221.
7. "Meeting of the State Organization of Nurses," 19.
8. Ibid., 153.

CHAPTER FIVE

Nursing in 1939

THE EFFECTS OF THE DEPRESSION LED TO A RAPID RISE IN THE number of graduate nurses hired by hospitals for general duty nursing. For the first time, there were nearly as many general duty staff nurses as private duty nurses. General duty nurses contributed maturity and experience to hospitals formerly staffed solely by students. Nursing services stabilized and patient care improved. Hospital work offered both advantages and disadvantages to graduate nurses. It replaced the irregular work schedule of the private duty nurse with the security of regular employment, but nurses sacrificed their independence and autonomy. In return, they discovered a newfound source of professional support and stimulation in small work groups and communal living arrangements.

Most general duty staff nurses were expected to live in hospital quarters, with room, board, and laundry services ("maintenance") included in their compensation. When the trend to employ general duty nurses intensified during the depression, nurses were so desperate for work, they were willing to accept the rock bottom salaries and poor working conditions offered by many hospitals. Even after the depression receded, however, salaries remained poor. In 1938 an ANA survey reported the average general duty staff nurse received an $825 annual cash salary, plus full maintenance, for a forty-eight-hour work week. Eight-hour duty was now common, but usually the eight hours were not consecutive. A typical eight-hour day shift was 7 a.m. to 7 p.m. with four hours off sometime during the shift. Time off amounted to one day per week, often scheduled with less than twenty four hours' notice. Two weeks of annual paid vacation were expected, but there was typically no paid sick leave. No provisions were made for staff education, staff meetings, or time off for professional meetings. Thus, the nurse living and working in the hospital environment rarely had a chance to participate in community, recreational, or professional activities.

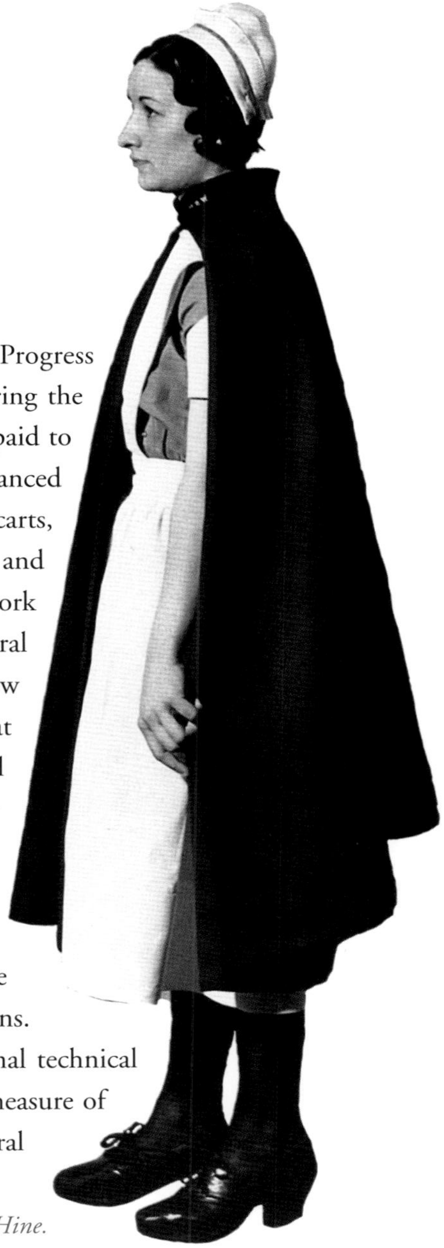

By 1939 hospitals had undergone significant changes. The Works Progress Administration, which provided funds for projects to increase employment during the depression, funded construction of many new hospital facilities. Attention was paid to making patient rooms more attractive, and better lighting and new materials enhanced the working environment. Improved castors, for instance, allowed beds, laundry carts, and other equipment to be easily moved. Adjustable beds, electronic call systems, and streamlined equipment altered patterns of care. Innovations to ease nurses' work were especially important when making the transition from private duty to general duty. Nurses accustomed to providing care to one patient in private duty were now expected to care for as many as six patients during the day, and twenty or more at night. Nurses continued to provide complete patient care, including physical therapy, nutrition, and x-ray services. In fact, nurses were often the only representatives of the hospital the patients encountered.

For many nurses, the transition to hospital nursing was a return to student life. Living and working was again under the rigid discipline of their training school days. On the ward, staff nurses were subjected to the same strict discipline as students, and in their living quarters, to curfews and other social restrictions. Nevertheless, hospital general duty offered the opportunity to develop additional technical expertise and meet the challenge of expanded responsibilities, and provided a measure of job security. Despite the poor salaries and a paternalistic atmosphere, most general duty nurses found their work satisfying.[1]

RIGHT: *Courtesy Westchester Medical Center; photograph by Lewis W. Hine.*

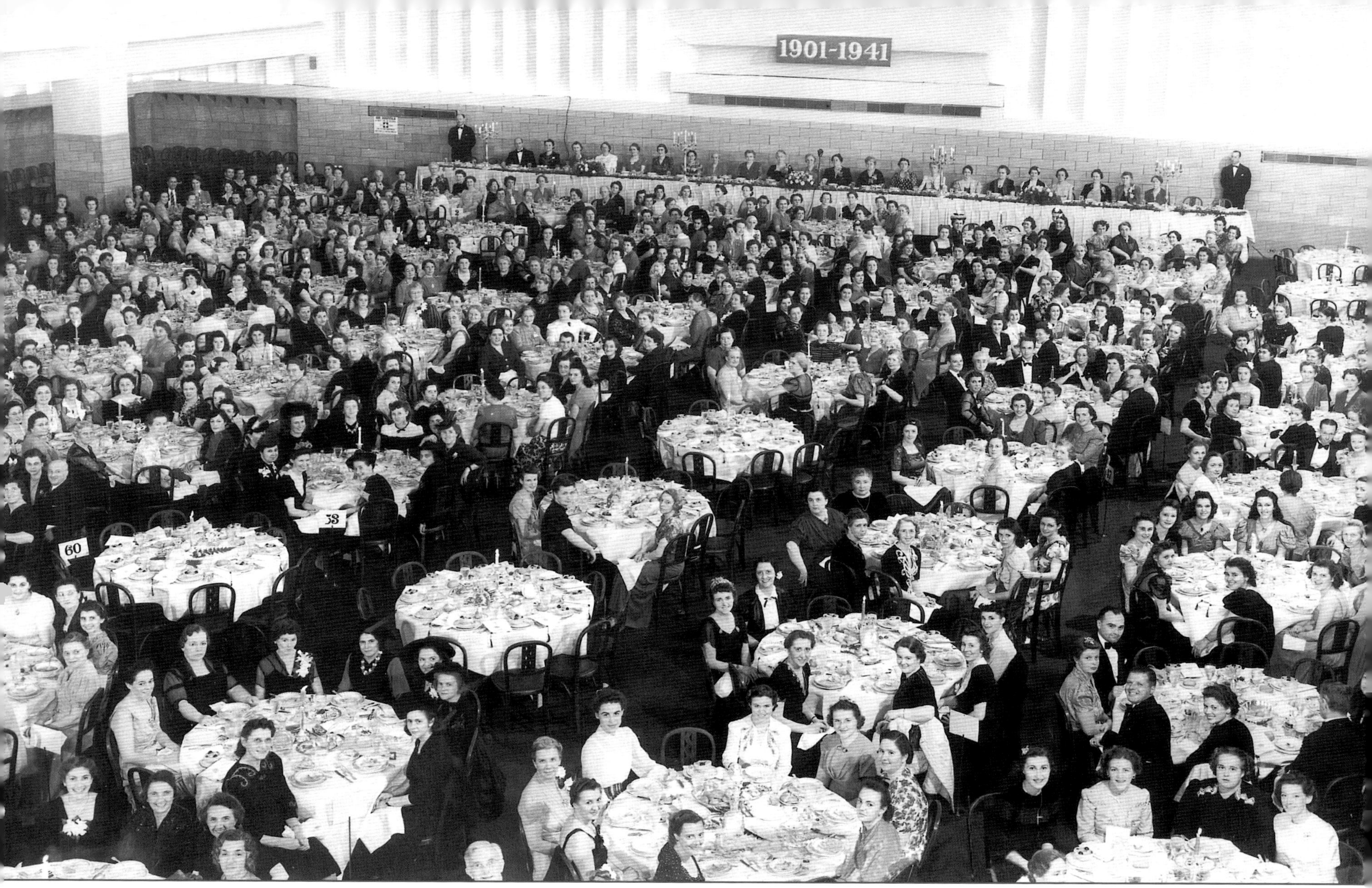

NYSNA's 1941 convention, held in Brooklyn just months before Pearl Harbor, celebrated NYSNA's fortieth anniversary and was a gala affair. *Courtesy the District 14 Collection, Foundation of NYSNA Archives; photograph by Knickerbocker photography.*

DAYS OF GREAT CHANGE 1939–1949

While the United States was recovering from the devastation of the Great Depression, fascist regimes were rising to power in both Europe and Asia. In 1939 the American Red Cross initiated an intense enrollment campaign by issuing an appeal to increase its First Reserve by ten thousand nurses. Although the Red Cross served as a reserve for the Army and Navy Nurse Corps, early recruitment efforts downplayed military service, focusing instead on "... a program devoted to the alleviation of suffering in our own country and, infrequently, to relieve victims of war."[2] When President Ethel Prince referred to "these days of great change" in her 1939 address to delegates she could not have predicted that the escalating demand for nurses would form the pivotal point around which the activities of NYSNA would revolve for nearly a decade.

Nursing in Health Defense: As the conflict in Europe worsened, concern about national defense intensified. A speaker at a 1940 NYSNA institute on "Nursing in Health Defense" noted, "The thinking of everyone on practically every subject is now conditioned by the overshadowing national emergency."[3] Despite deep divisions of public opinion over the advisability of the United States entering the European war, a draft was imposed, and industry was converted to produce aircraft, weapons, tanks, and ships. Population shifts from rural to urban areas resulting from increased industrial production created public health problems, and industrial accidents and injuries soared.

Adequate national defense depended on a healthy military and a healthy workforce, and nursing realized the importance of its role in safeguarding health.

In the spring of 1940 Hitler's armies invaded Norway, Denmark, the Netherlands, and Belgium. The impending fall of France cast a pall on ANA's biennial meeting, and the assembly sent a telegram to President Franklin Roosevelt pledging support in any nursing activities of service to the country.[4] Soon after the meeting, NYSNA's board met with the New York State Red Cross Committee to discuss ways of increasing New York's enrollment in the First Reserve. Board member Alta Dines proposed that a questionnaire be sent to all nurses in the state to determine the availability of nurses in an emergency, and to stimulate enrollment. A Committee to Plan for a Nursing Survey was appointed to prepare and distribute a questionnaire. The committee was concerned not only with identifying nurses for Red Cross service, but with identifying nurses to replace those called to service.[5]

"A new emphasis has been placed upon health, not only of armed forces but of civilians as well. With this emphasis, nursing is called upon to translate its interest and responsibility into appropriate participation in defense."

— *Ruth G. Hall*[1]

Meanwhile, Isabel Stewart, director of the Division of Nursing Education at Teachers College, Columbia University, mobilized a small group to plan and organize the profession's response to the demands of national defense. In

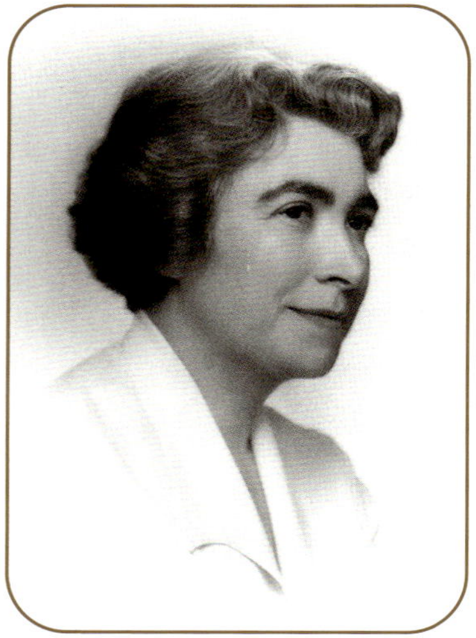

Alta Elizabeth Dines was an active NYSNA member, former Army nurse, and nationally known for her commitment to nursing preparedness. As a board member, Dines proposed and developed a survey of nurses in New York that became the model for the national inventory. Dines was also devoted to providing assistance to nurses in need. In 1941 NYSNA President Ruth Hall said, "To know Miss Dines is to touch a great spirit." *Courtesy Nurses House Collection, Foundation of NYSNA Archives; photograph by Bachrach.*

Isabel Maitland Stewart, Director of the Division of Nursing Education at Teachers College, Columbia University, played a key role in the development of nursing's response to the demands of World War II. Stewart frequently addressed delegates at NYSNA conventions to keep them appraised of developments. *Courtesy Nurses House Collection, Foundation of NYSNA Archives; photograph by Blackstone.*

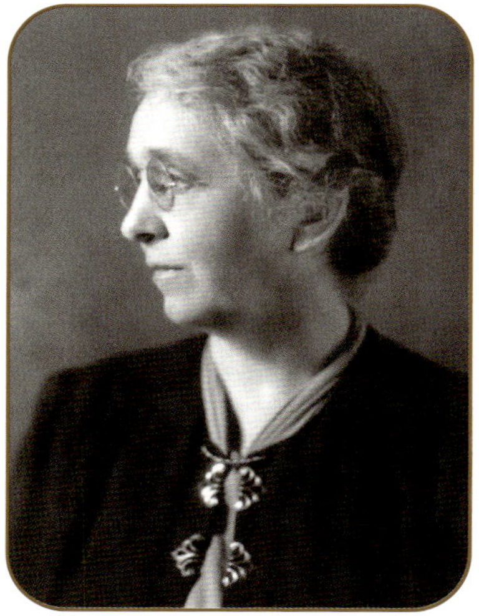

this first step toward the organization of a united, national nursing response to the threat of war, Stewart emphasized that the nursing profession had to provide the initiative to plan and organize a response that would protect the standards of the profession, thereby safeguarding the health of the nation's citizens, both civilian and military. She was extremely concerned that the demand for additional nurses in the event of a national emergency would result in compromised educational standards and poorly prepared nurses who could jeopardize the health of the nation's citizens. She predicted that if war came, "the cry of nurse shortage will become louder . . . short cuts will be tried and we shall be told that patriotism demands the sacrifice of many of our hard-won standards."[6] Representatives from seven nursing organizations met in July 1940, established the Nursing Council for National Defense (Nursing Council), and agreed to survey the nation's nursing strength. Alta Dines, representing NYSNA's Committee to Plan for a Nursing Survey, was the only participant at the meeting who did not represent a *national* nursing organization, and was presumably invited to share New York's experience in planning for a survey.[7]

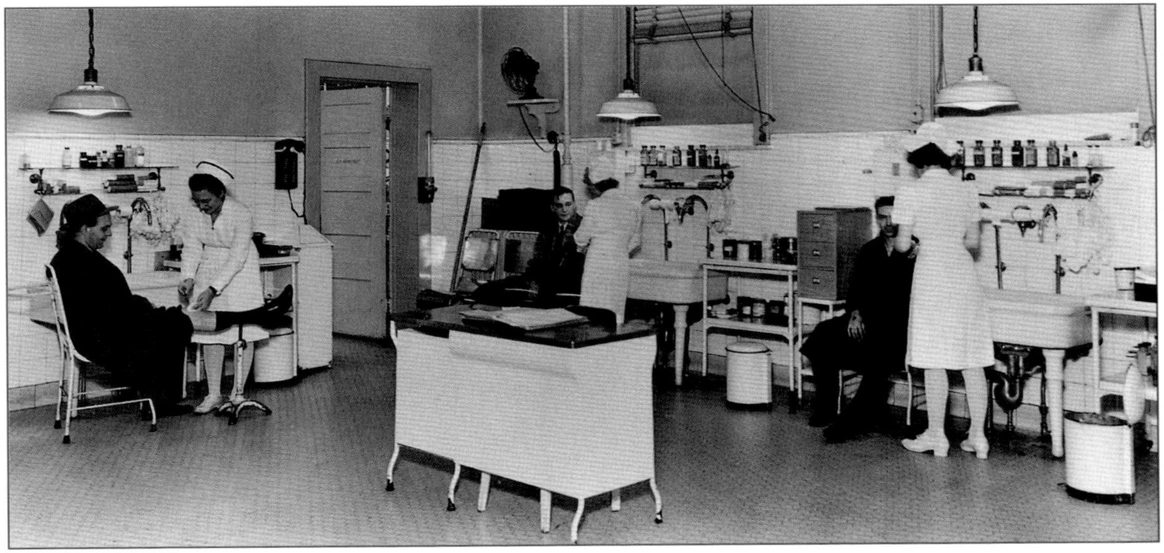

Industrial nurses at the General Electric Works in Schenectady cared for ill and injured workers. The field of industrial nursing gained importance during the war, when industries expanded rapidly and there was a marked increase in industrial accidents. During the 1940s, NYSNA formed an Industrial Nurses Section, and the American Association of Industrial Nurses was formed. NYSNA President Mary Delehanty served as president of the industrial nurse organization from 1947 to 1951. *Courtesy Schenectady Museum Archives.*

The national survey was based on NYSNA's questionnaire and the procedures developed by NYSNA's committee.[8] Although the project was sponsored by the Nursing Council, each state was responsible for publicity and processing the questionnaires. On December 10, 1940, NYSNA launched the nationwide survey by mailing one hundred thousand questionnaires to New York nurses. Mailings to district and alumnae presidents, registrars, and county medical societies spread the word on the importance of the inventory, and mass meetings, with simultaneous radio broadcasts and newspaper coverage, were held in each district. Sixty-eight percent of New York's registered nurses responded. More than twenty thousand nurses indicated willingness to serve in the military, and over thirteen thousand in their own communities in the event of war.[9]

The survey completed, NYSNA's committee changed its name to the State Committee on Nursing Participation in the Defense Program, and focused on utilization of the data. Three nurses were hired to work with districts to identify inactive nurses, plan refresher courses, and develop local preparedness programs. They prepared a comprehensive manual, *Nursing Participation in the Defense Program,* to assist in planning for the use of nurses to meet emergencies and long-range health needs.[10] The Board of Directors celebrated this achievement at its regularly scheduled meeting on December 7, 1941. By day's end, Pearl Harbor had been attacked, and the United States was at the brink of war.

MARCHING FORWARD INTO A GREAT UNKNOWN: After the Japanese attack on Pearl Harbor, enrollment in the Red Cross First Reserves soared to nearly one hundred per day, prompting the editor of the *American Journal of Nursing* to proclaim, "The disturbing and disheartening lag in Red Cross enrolment [*sic*] is over!"[11] The country united behind the war effort, and leaders within the profession called for unity. "We are marching forward into a great unknown without a clue as to what the cost of our ultimate victory will be . . . Never has unity in our profession been more important than now. Never before have we faced so great a test."[12] The Nursing Council became the vehicle through which the country's nurses united to meet the challenges of war.[13]

Elmira Wickenden, NYSNA member and executive secretary of the Nursing Council, met with NYSNA's board, urging the reorganization of the Committee on Defense into a State Nursing Council which would allow for the participation of consumers, defense officials, and representatives of other professions. While New York had provided invaluable assistance in the nursing inventory and preparedness plans, Wickenden felt New York lagged behind other states in Red Cross enrollment and student recruitment. In September 1942 the committee "laid aside its peacetime program and became the nucleus of a New York State Nursing Council for War Service which will have broad representation in coping with war nursing problems."[14] NYSNA's assistant executive secretary, Emily Creevey, was appointed to head the State Nursing Council, and NYSNA provided supplies, equipment, and thousands of dollars to support its work for the duration of the war. Dozens of local nursing councils were formed to coordinate all local nursing activities related to the war. They provided the same united front at the local level that nursing presented at the national level, thus forming a complex and very effective network.[15]

The primary task of the State Nursing Council was to secure an adequate supply of nurses. There continued to be tremendous concern that there be enough nurses to care for military personnel abroad and to protect civilian health. Nurses recruited for military service left hospitals short staffed at a time when increased industrial accidents, expansion of hospital insurance plans, polio epidemics, and general improvement in the economy and the ability to pay created increased demand for hospital care.[16] The encouraging increase in enrollment immediately following Pearl Harbor did not continue, and New York State quotas for nurses in the First Reserve were "far from being met."[17] The State Nursing Council formed local Procurement and Assignment Committees to classify nurses as to availability for service. Nurses holding positions in nursing education, nursing administration (including supervisors and most head nurses), and public health were considered essential to civilian health and the production of additional nurses, and were strongly encouraged to remain in those positions. Unmarried nurses in private duty, office duty, and general staff duty were requested to report immediately for enlistment or to present reasons for not doing so in an appeal.[18] Despite the official nature of these procedures, there was, in fact, no authority to enforce the system. Creevey later stated, "The interesting part of it all is, to me, that there was no force behind this at all. No one could compel anybody to do what we were classifying them as appropriate to do. It worked, nevertheless, to a very large extent."[19] Classification of forty thousand nurses was the largest single task accomplished by the State Nursing Council. The classification process not only increased military enrollments, but also emphasized the importance of nurses to the war effort. "We as nurses may feel a modest pride in being thus far the only woman's profession considered so essential to the winning of the war that we have been singled out for special classification procedures."[20]

Despite the ongoing cry for more nurses in military service, male nurses were barred from the military nursing services, and quotas drastically restricted the number of African-American nurses accepted. NYSNA made formal requests that the Army Nurse Corps raise the quotas of "colored nurses." The Nursing Council fully integrated all African-American nursing activities into the total program, providing every committee with minority representation, and passed a resolution that colored nurses be appointed to the Army and Navy Nurse Corps on the same basis as all other nurses. It was largely through the efforts, however, of New York nurse Mabel Staupers, that progress toward full inclusion was made. The number of African-American nurses in the Army Nurse Corps eventually increased to six hundred, but it was 1945 before the Navy accepted an African-American nurse.[21] On the recommendation of the Men's Section, NYSNA's board repeatedly urged that male nurses be commissioned, but the Army Nurse Corps consistently refused such requests.[22] It was not until 1954 that men were admitted with full rank as officers.[23]

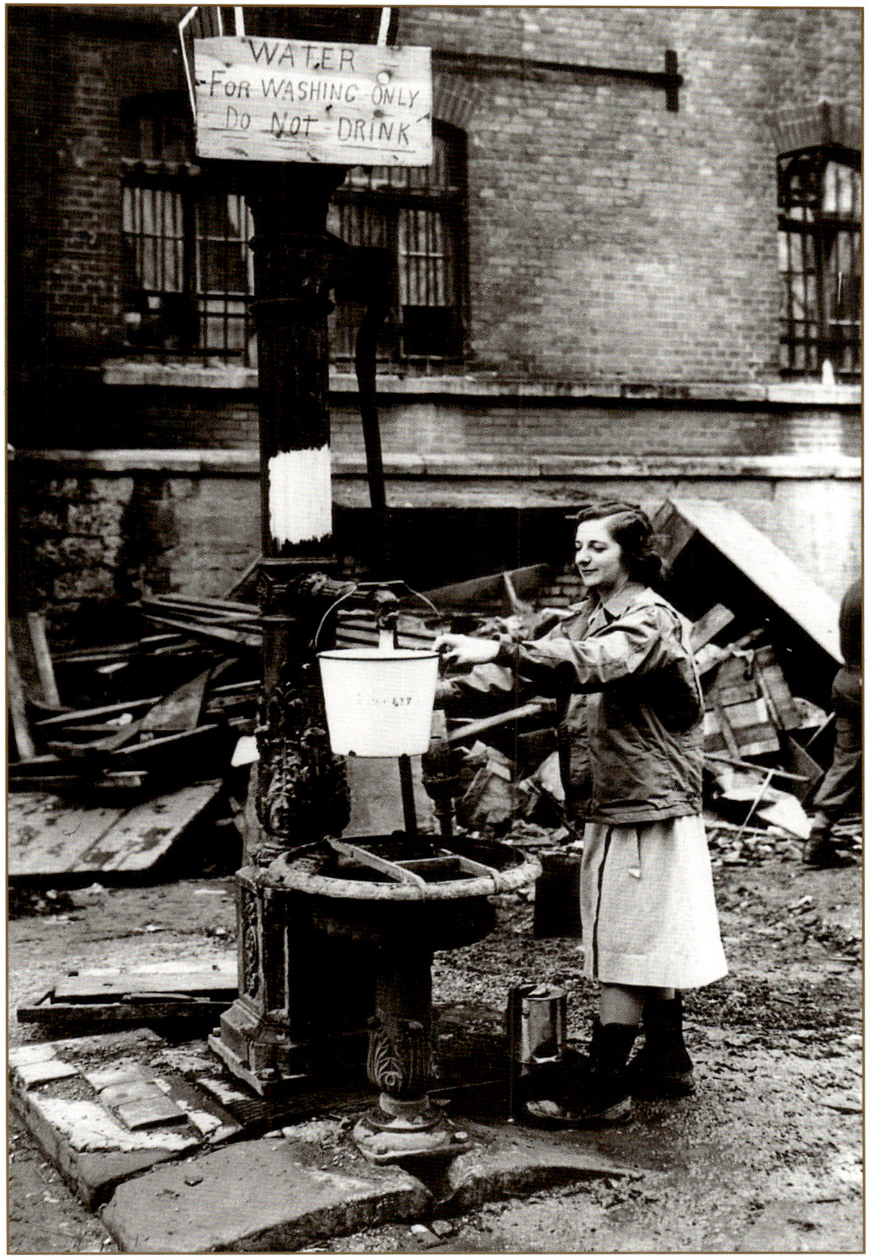

RIGHT: Military nurses like Edna Tuffley, shown here, experienced primitive conditions and many hardships during their World War II service. *Courtesy Army Nurse Corps Historical Collection.*

Mabel Keaton Staupers
1890 - 1989

Mabel Keaton Staupers was a nursing leader with extraordinary perseverance, courage, and vision. She spent most of her professional career in New York, working to break down racial barriers in the profession of nursing. In 1934 Staupers became the first paid executive secretary of the National Association of Colored Graduate Nurses (NACGN). When the threat of war intensified in 1940, Staupers was determined that African-American nurses would not be excluded from serving in the military as was the case during World War I. In meetings with War Department officials, national nursing leaders, and even First Lady Eleanor Roosevelt, Staupers struggled to gain full acceptance for African-American nurses in the military. She reluctantly agreed to quotas, but only as a stepping stone to full integration.

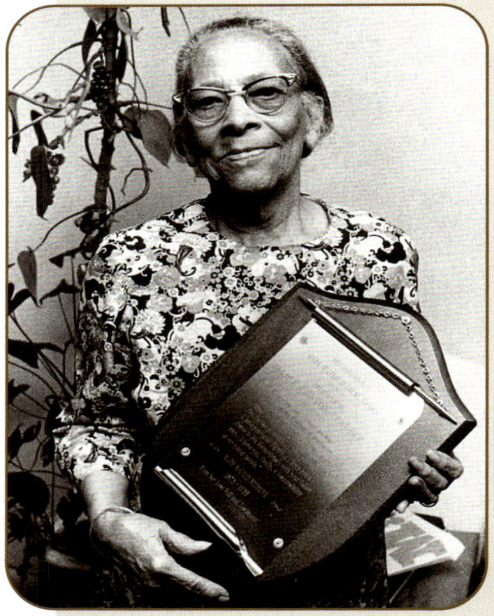

Courtesy the Staupers Collection, Foundation of NYSNA Archives.

For most of the war, small numbers of African-American nurses served in the Army Nurse Corps, providing care primarily to African-American soldiers and to German prisoners of war. The call for a nurse draft to solve the shortage of military nurses provided Staupers with an opportunity to achieve her goal. When Surgeon General Norman Kirk announced the possibility of a nurse draft to a New York City crowd, "Staupers immediately rose to her feet and pointedly asked the surgeon general, 'If nurses are needed so desperately, why isn't the Army using colored nurses?' She challenged, 'Of 9,000 registered Negro nurses the Army has taken 247, the Navy takes none.'"[1] She worked quickly to capitalize on a subsequent wave of public anger and sympathy, urging nurses and other sympathetic groups across the country to protest the exclusion and segregation of African-American nurses by contacting President Roosevelt and members of Congress. The War Department quickly responded by ending the quotas and exclusion.

Following this triumph, Mabel Staupers continued to promote minority recruitment into nursing, and provided leadership to fully integrate the ANA. In 1948, when NACGN voted to dissolve and merge with the American Nurses Association, Staupers agreed to serve as its last president to guide the transition. Without the high caliber of leadership and clear vision demonstrated by Staupers, it is unlikely that "the overall struggle for recognition, status, and acceptance of black nurses into the institutional structures of American nursing . . . would have advanced."[2]

The nursing councils expended a great deal of effort in promoting student enrollment in schools of nursing. Students eased the critical shortage of nurses in hospitals, and once graduated, were eligible for military or civilian service. The Nursing Council developed a massive publicity campaign to urge young women to become nurses, and relied upon state and local constituencies to provide leadership and distribute information. Local committees counselled prospective students, established speakers' bureaus and developed recruitment projects.[24] The Nursing Council lobbied for legislation, and in 1941, for the first time in history, federal funds were appropriated for nursing education. As always, nursing leaders were vigilant lest educational standards be sacrificed.

New York received a portion of the federal funds to organize central schools of nursing. These innovative programs provided collegiate nursing education in rural areas, utilizing a number of hospitals and other health agencies for clinical experience. NYSNA's board voted to support and promote the development of central schools, and Lenore Bradley, supervisor of nursing education for the New York State Board of Nurse Examiners, worked tirelessly to develop these schools, first on NYSNA's Committee on Nursing Participation in Defense, and later as chair of the Committee on Central Schools of Nursing of the State Nursing Council. The State Education Department was being pressured to establish new hospital schools and re-open schools that had closed, many of which had a 70 to 100 percent failure rate on licensing examinations. The Board for Nursing was receiving "daily inquiries" regarding the possibility of shortening the coursework.[25] The nursing community believed that to shorten the course of instruction would seriously compromise the quality of the education, and Bradley believed that a new and creative mechanism such as central schools was needed to increase the nurse supply and provide sorely needed nursing care, particularly in rural areas. In early 1943 Adelphi College and Keuka College opened the state's first central collegiate schools, and "set a pattern for a new type of nursing preparation." The programs aroused "keen interest in other states as well as in New York," and the movement soon spread in both rural and urban areas.[26]

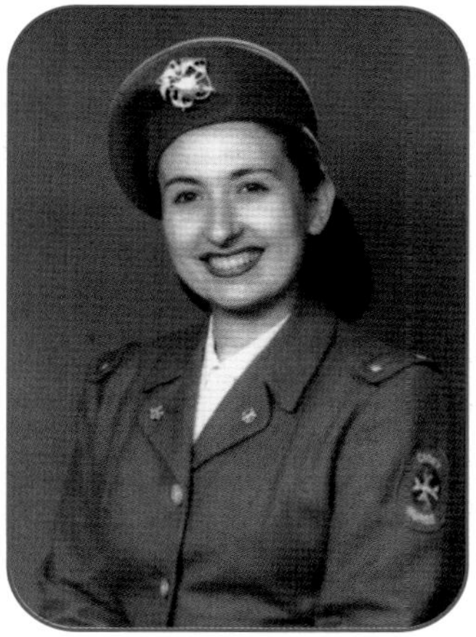

Like thousands of other young women during the war years, Nettie Birnbach, NYSNA president in the 1990s, received her basic nursing education through the U.S. Public Health Service Cadet Nurse Corps. The program offered full tuition and expenses, including the uniform, an important symbol of the student's status as a full partner in the war effort. Through extensive advertising the Cadet Nurse Corps became the focus around which all student recruitment efforts rallied. *Courtesy the Birnbach Collection, Foundation of NYSNA Archives.*

Another proposal was developed for federal appropriations to schools of nursing as a temporary emergency measure to provide additional nurses. This bill created the United States Public Health Service Cadet Nurse Corps in 1943, providing federal funds to qualified schools of nursing that shortened the length of their program, *and* maintained minimum standards. Ninety-one of New York State's 121 schools of nursing participated.[27]

The progress of the war was followed closely by the American public. New technologies allowed unprecedented reporting and information flow, flooding the airwaves and news media with massive amounts of information. When American troops suffered the heaviest casualties of the war in late 1944, well-known *Washington Post* columnist Walter Lippmann alarmed the American public, stating, "Our men are not receiving the nursing care they must have," and maintaining there were plenty of nurses in non-essential positions eligible for the military. Word that Army hospitals were being sent overseas without nurses further aroused public concern, and President Roosevelt requested a draft of nurses in his 1945 State of the Union address. Three days later, a bill was introduced providing for national registration and induction of registered nurses between the ages of 18 and 45.[28]

A draft for nurses had been discussed by NYSNA's board and the nursing councils long before Roosevelt called for a nurse draft. In 1943 NYSNA's board voted to endorse compulsory national registration of nurses and, if necessary, of all women. Nursing's concern with the draft bill was that drafting nurses exclusively into military service could lead to a crisis in civilian health care.[29] The boards of both ANA and NYSNA endorsed a plan to draft nurses only as a first step in a draft of all women, and recommended legislation to provide for civilian health needs. Information on the status of the bill "flowed continuously and swiftly from ANA headquarters through state associations to local districts" to keep nurses informed and to channel opinion.[30] Enrollment of nurses immediately increased, and Allied military successes contributed to a waning sense of emergency. The bill was not brought to a vote, and by the end of the European war in May, the Army Nurse Corps had more nurses than it needed. "The response of the nurses to the call for volunteers has been most generous and is an eloquent tribute to the nursing profession."[31]

Marion Sheahan, Alta Dines, and many other New York nurses contributed to the war effort by serving simultaneously on the Nursing Council and its committees, on government committees, and on NYSNA's board and committees. Thus, work of the national groups was personally interpreted to state and local groups. The Nursing Council relied heavily on this multiple representation to facilitate its work.[32] Hidden beneath those in the limelight were countless New York nurses whose contributions and sacrifices are unrecorded. Thousands enlisted and served in the military, gave up lucrative employment in "unessential" positions to serve where the need was greater, and patriotically enrolled in the Cadet Nurse Corps. Through local committees and nursing councils, nurses worked diligently to provide for civilian health services by seeking out inactive nurses, encouraging nurses to return to work, promoting the use of

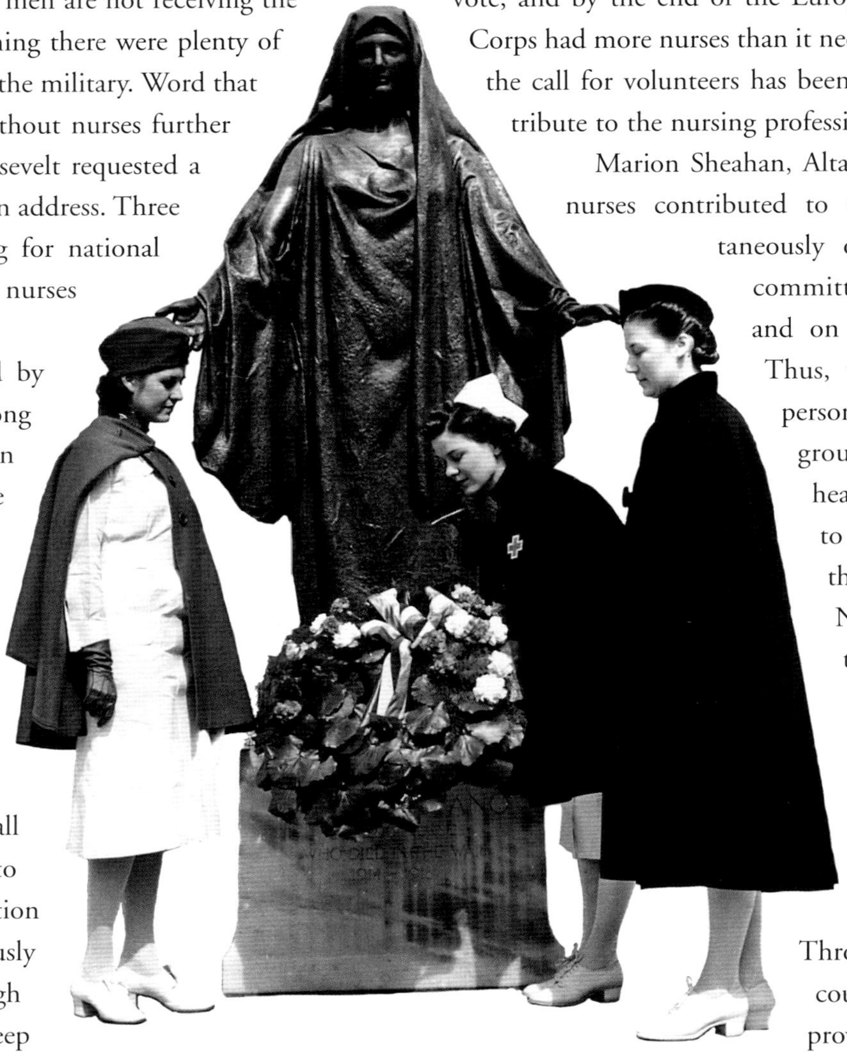

In 1941 Army, Navy, and Red Cross nurses laid a wreath at the Jane Delano Memorial in Washington, D.C. *Courtesy American Red Cross.*

volunteers, reducing "luxury nursing," and integrating Red Cross trained nurse's aides into hospitals. They developed opportunities for part-time employment and solutions to the newly created problem of child care, promoted refresher and orientation programs, and tirelessly recruited students.[33] NYSNA President Clare Casey paid tribute to New York's nurses at war's end. "Across the pages of our record . . . may be seen history weaving its design in the pattern of war. Classification of nurses, statements of availability, quota for the Armed Forces, proposed nurse draft, recruitment of student cadets, postwar planning, war bond drives — all these have had a prominent place in our schedule. We have celebrated V-E Day and now, as we go to press, there is every indication that V-J Day is fast approaching. Through such world shaking events, nursing has been and will continue to be an essential activity."[34]

"While many time-worn concepts and traditions have gone through the refining fire of a crisis which has brought necessary change and adjustment, it is equally true that the great and profound experiences of the last three years have, in many ways, made for progress and new life."

— *Elmira B. Wickenden*[2]

POSTWAR: While focusing intently on the demands of war, nursing organizations never stopped looking ahead. In 1943 both the Nursing Council and NYSNA formed postwar planning committees to plan for nurses returning from military service and other nurses who would need assistance in adapting to the changes of a postwar world. The focus of the national committee broadened to encompass the development of a single plan for the future of nursing, and became the National Nursing Planning Committee. Led by Marion Sheahan, the committee published a "Comprehensive Program for Nation-Wide Action in the Field of Nursing," formulated on the premise that coordinated action in nursing would be as important in the postwar period as it was during the emergency. The program proposed action on long-standing needs of the profession now highlighted by the war emergency, and stressed the inclusion of all nurses — professional and practical, black and white, male and female — in its plans to convert local councils to address peacetime needs.[35]

"They are extremely bewildered about what they are going to do. And you and I, who have stayed at home during the war period, we have worked hard, I admit. On the other hand, we have stayed at home . . . and we don't have to remake our lives."

— *Dorothy Wheeler*[3]

The initial exhilaration at war's end was soon replaced by uncertainty. Even experts feared a return to depression levels of unemployment, and many anticipated an oversupply of nurses. Nurse veterans, however, did not return to hospital work as expected, and the shortage of general duty staff nurses continued to be a grave concern. In 1945 a counseling service staffed by NYSNA was established at District 13 headquarters to assist the thousands of returning military nurses. In a *New York Times* article, the service was described as part of ANA's program "to assist all nurses, and especially nurse veterans, for whom war service has meant serious professional dislocation . . ."[36] NYSNA delegates to the 1945 convention accepted a statewide plan for a consultant to assist districts in the development of professional counseling and placement for all nurses —

members and non-members, professional and practical. The program assembled permanent files containing applicants' qualifications and references, developed guidance programs, counseled veterans, matched applicants with lists of employment opportunities, organized district committees, and issued monthly bulletins to employers. In its first decade, thousands of nurses were served by the program.[37]

As busy as the war years had been, in the first postwar year, association staff and activities doubled. The increasing pressure to relieve the severe shortage of nurses through improved salaries and conditions of employment and to counter attempts made by trade unions to organize nurses precipitated increased emphasis on public relations and increased the overall work load.[38]

"We believe our professional organization members should be anxious to work on these important matters and thereby obviate the need for outside trade union activity."

— *Leah Bryan*[4]

IMPROVING EMPLOYMENT CONDITIONS: During the war, the need for nurses grew to astonishing heights and the long-standing shortage of general duty staff nurses worsened when nurses flocked to higher paying non-nursing industrial positions and to military service. The issue of supply and distribution of nurses, however, was not new. The nursing shortage was a long-standing problem only exacerbated and brought into focus by the war. The real underlying issues were the poor salaries and conditions of employment under which nurses worked. Equipment and health care were being modernized while personnel practices remained firmly entrenched in tradition and past practice.

BELOW: In the late 1940s the *New York State Nurse* devoted increasing attention to the Economic Security Program.

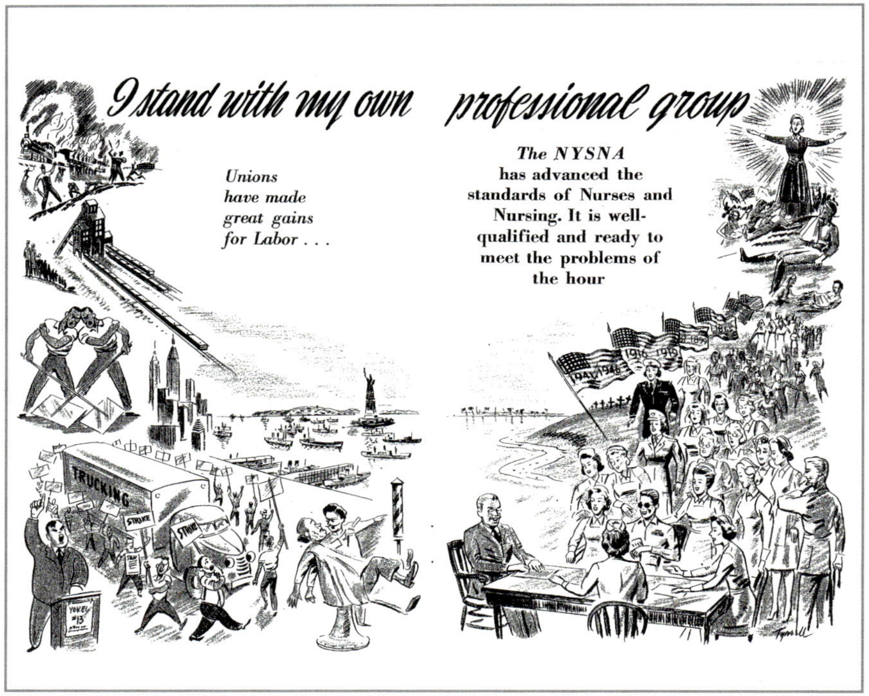

The escalating demand for nurses and the threat of a takeover of nursing by unions drove the association's personnel practices program during these years. Many nurses saw "trade unions," specifically those in the CIO and AFL, as serious threats to nursing and to NYSNA. Labor strikes during the war years, viewed as unpatriotic, strengthened middle-class anti-labor sentiment, and labor's fierce opposition to NYSNA's Nurse Practice Bill in the 1930s must have exacerbated this attitude among many NYSNA members. There was also a strong belief that the nursing profession could take care of its own affairs. When delegates to the 1939 convention voted to disapprove membership in labor organizations for registered nurses, one delegate stated, "We have our own aim, our own principles and standards to meet, and we don't need any labor organization to push them forward for us. We are able to do that for ourselves."[39]

In 1939 the boards of directors of NYSNA and the Hospital Association of New York State (HANYS) met to discuss mutual problems, and a Joint Coordinating Committee was appointed.[40] The committee identified poor salaries, non-consecutive hours of duty, non-nursing tasks, undesirable residences, poor working conditions, and the lack of merit systems and democratic staffing structures as serious impediments to securing general duty nurses. A series of institutes was developed for directors of nursing on personnel administration, where questionnaires were distributed to participants to collect data on employment conditions. NYSNA's newly formed Personnel Practices Committee summarized the data and prepared a progress report which indicated that maximum salaries for nurses were less than $1,600 per year for a forty-four- to sixty-hour work week. The report recommended starting salaries of $1,800, a maximum work week of forty-eight hours with one whole day off per week, eight *consecutive* working hours for eight-hour day duty, six holidays, vacation and sick leave benefits, grievance and termination procedures, and cash salaries rather than the traditional cash plus maintenance.[41] The Personnel Practices Committee met with representatives of HANYS and agreed on modifications to the report, which was then adopted at NYSNA's 1943 convention. Districts were encouraged to appoint local committees to enter into discussions with hospital boards and administrators to solve problems and implement the recommendations.[42]

Within months, most districts reported a general increase in salaries and improved employment conditions. The board approved an ambitious program proposed by the Personnel Practices Committee, and agreed with a State Nursing Council recommendation that the committee work to increase salaries in hospitals having difficulty in replacing nurses leaving to join the military. The board also recommended that the committee advocate for contracts between employees and employers. Not surprisingly, discussion of contracts at a meeting of the Coordinating Committee revealed that hospitals were not in favor of contracts, though nurses were "keenly interested."[43]

"I am absolutely, positively, not only not a member of the CIO, but I am most definitely afraid that the CIO or something other than we, ourselves, is going to take over our Association."

— *Mrs. Revzin*[5]

Personnel practices improved slowly. In May 1945 New York City's Department of Hospitals increased all nurses' salaries in an attempt to ease the nursing shortage, finally bringing the minimum salary to the $1,800 recommended in 1943.[44] However, only 75 percent of hospitals surveyed in 1945 had adopted the eight-hour day, and vacation time in most hospitals continued to be far less than the committee's recommendation. At the 1945 convention, increasing union activity among nurses was on the minds of delegates. Board member Agnes Gelinas was applauded when she stated, "We want to combat union activities by having a strong professional organization that will work and work and work on personnel practices and make them so satisfactory that we will scare the life right out of the CIO, and they won't want to have anything to do with us."[45] The convention adopted motions calling for nurses, not administrators, to handle personnel matters in hospitals, and that the forty-hour work week for nurses be recommended "when feasible." Following the meeting, staff visited hospitals and discussed methods to combat CIO activity. Special mailings were sent to alert districts to "broad campaigns to unionize nurses" being launched by the AFL and CIO, and to announce Assistant Executive Secretary Charlotte Seyffer's re-assignment to work full time on personnel practices. The Personnel Practices Committee believed that if district committees had successfully organized hospital "staff associations" to negotiate with hospitals on personnel issues, the union activities would not have occurred.[46]

In June 1946 President Clare Casey, speaking at the HANYS convention, recommended a revolutionary $50 for a forty-hour week and improved conditions of employment as a way to ease the nursing shortage. She noted that staff nurses used to put "ideals of service" over "rights as a human being," but because of social and economic upheavals, were no longer willing to do so. When asked why nurse veterans were not returning to civilian hospitals, Casey cited poor salaries, split shifts, and the desire of hospitals to "continue on the same old slave labor basis as before the war."[47] HANYS President McCormack was reported sympathetic to Casey's recommendations, but believed they were financially unrealistic.[48]

At ANA's 1946 convention, delegates unanimously adopted an economic security program for nurses, which included state associations representing nurses for the purposes of collective bargaining. NYSNA's board and district presidents met during ANA's biennial meeting and voted approval of this "dynamic program of the future . . . to organize nurses for the purpose of improving personnel practices." President Casey expressed to ANA the belief that NYSNA's activities to improve employment conditions constituted an effective program. She emphasized various achievements, especially the development of recommended minimum personnel practices for general duty, private duty, public health, and industrial nurses.[49]

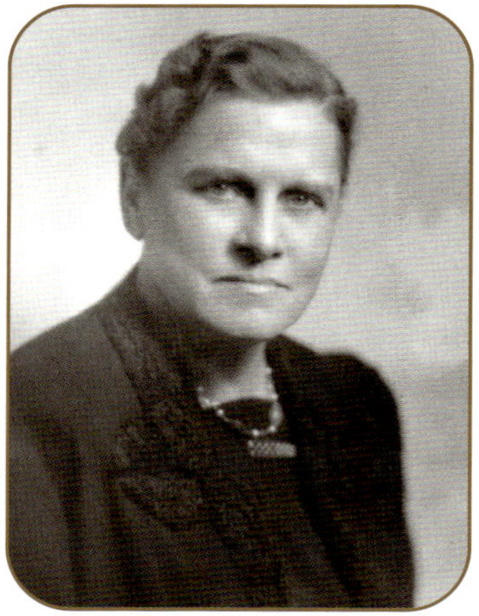

Julia Stimson received her nursing education in New York, served as superintendent of nurses at Harlem Hospital, and later was superintendent of the U.S. Army Nurse Corps. As president of ANA in 1940, she was instrumental in forming the Nursing Council for National Defense to plan nursing's response to the escalating world conflict. *Courtesy Nurses House Collection, Foundation of NYSNA Archives; photograph by Blackstone Studios.*

Despite the endorsement of ANA's program, there was strong opposition to NYSNA designating itself a labor union and acting as a collective bargaining agent. NYSNA's participation in ANA's Economic Security Program was discussed extensively in 1946 at the Advisory Council meeting and at a special House of Delegates meeting convened specifically to discuss the Economic Security Program. NYSNA attorney Edward Handelman, admittedly anti-labor, noted that if NYSNA wanted to be a labor union the charter would have to be changed — a matter he believed would be difficult. He recommended that NYSNA work as a professional association to improve conditions rather than as a collective bargaining agent.[50]

Assistant Executive Secretary Seyffer outlined for delegates the scope of needs yet to be met: the need to decrease hours of employment (some hospitals continued to demand a work week of up to sixty hours), democratic administration and supervision, salaries commensurate with other professions, increased training for nurses to properly supervise practical nurses and other auxiliary personnel, and the need for a mechanism to calculate the number of nurses needed. "We think . . . that our Association will have to study very carefully the number

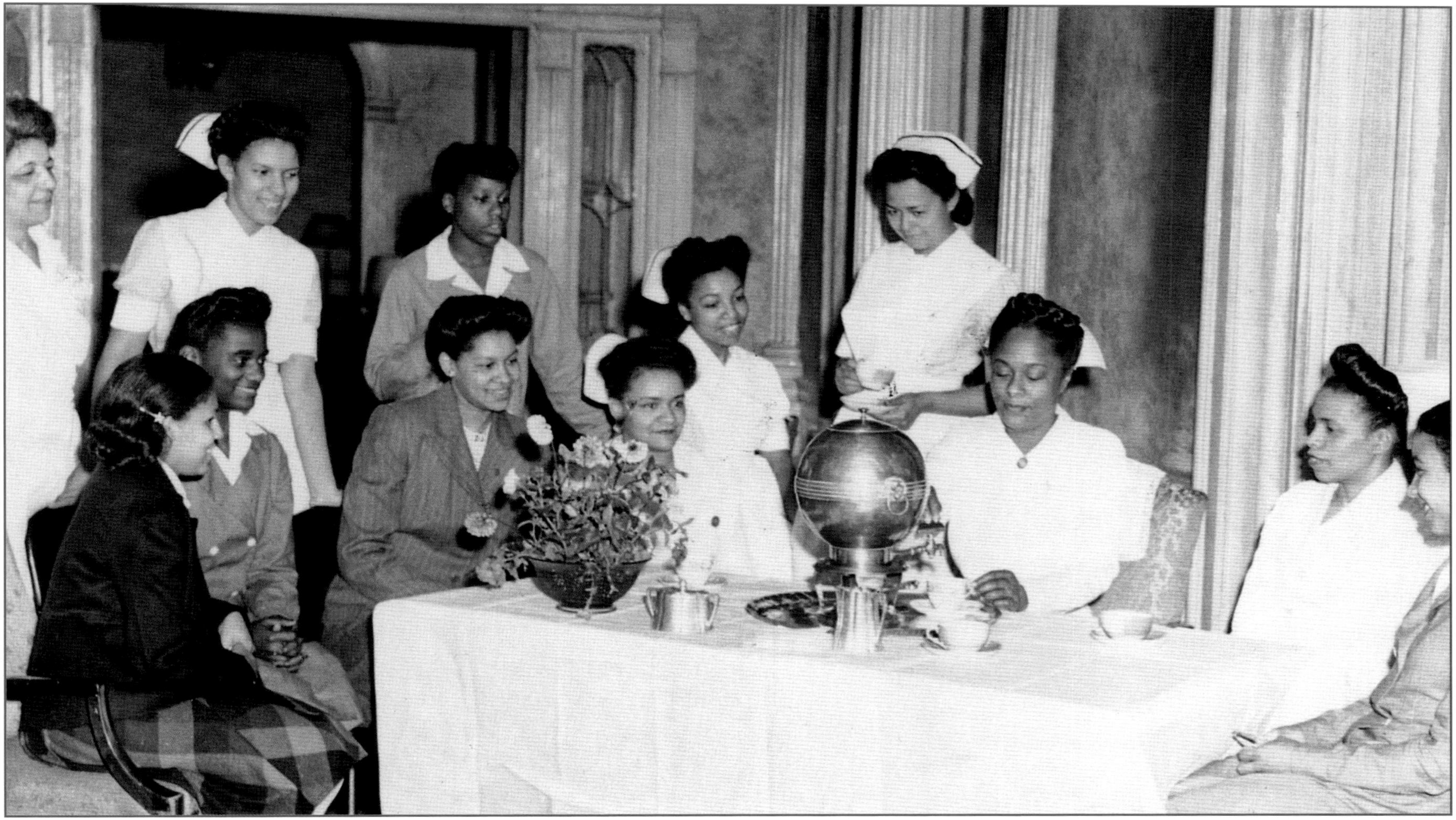

Students and faculty at the Harlem Hospital School of Nursing enjoyed weekly teas.
During World War II, most African-American nurse applicants were turned away by the military.
By the end of the 1940s, many important steps had been taken to fully integrate the profession.
Courtesy the Alumni Association of Harlem Hospital Center School of Nursing.

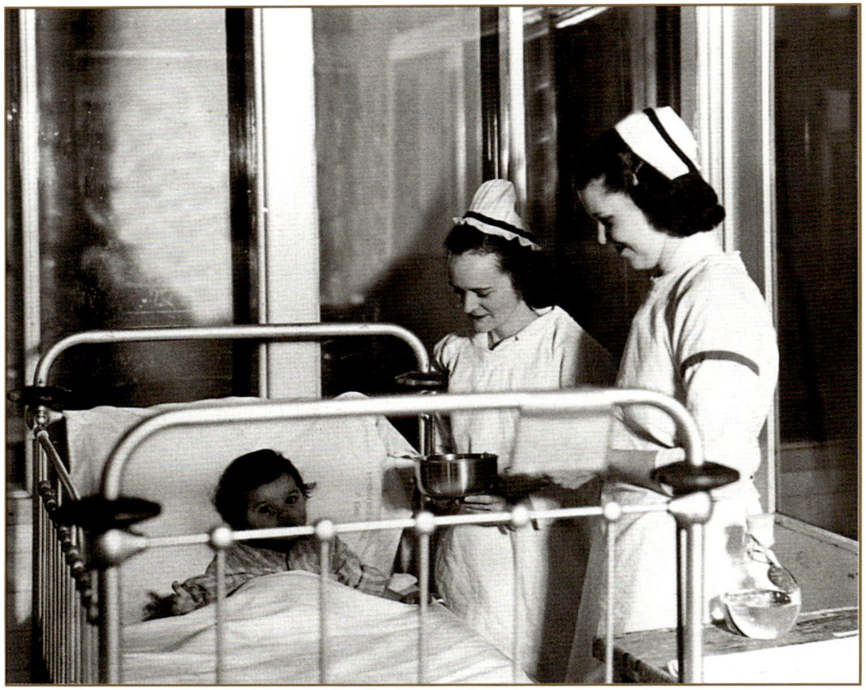

During the 1940s hospital use soared and general duty staff nurses became important providers of patient care. *Courtesy the Archives of the Mount Sinai Medical Center.*

of hours to care for the various kinds of patients, patients ill with various conditions, and that we will have to recommend certain numbers of nurses, so that our nurses will not be overworked in that they carry too much responsibility . . . which perhaps is in excess of what might even be safe from the standpoint of safe nursing care."[51] Delegates voted to develop a comprehensive educational program, use cooperative relationships to achieve improved conditions, and double the dues to "exert every effort and to employ every means" to improve working conditions for the state's nurses. Delegates also rescinded a 1943 resolution designating NYSNA as the bargaining agent for nurses on all matters of employment. This resolution was adopted in response to a request from one of the registries advised by the War Labor Board to designate NYSNA as its representative.[52] "Rather than cast itself in the role of a new labor group, the NYSNA will continue to act for itself in seeking to improve employment conditions for nurses. The House of Delegates, by overwhelming vote, decided to stand behind the ANA's recommendation in fact, although as to form it chose to go along with the New York State Nurses Association's active campaign for the adoption and use of its Personnel Practices."[53]

"How can two general duty nurses,
faced with the entire job of ministering to 20 ill
and uncomfortable patients, be expected to give efficient,
or even adequate nursing care?"

— *Jane Fehr*[6]

Meanwhile, booming hospital construction, advances in medical technology and increased hospital insurance programs contributed to soaring patient census figures. Nurses were struggling to care for an increasing number of patients, and being criticized in the popular press for not doing enough. One nurse lamented, ". . . how can the general duty nurse, who is doing a next-to-impossible job, face the criticisms of the hospital staff as well as the patients for what she had *not* done!"[54]

Growing strain and exhaustion led nurses to wonder whether association efforts were sufficient. In 1947 a Committee to Study the Economic Security Program was formed to determine the status of NYSNA's program, and to study the legality of adopting a collective bargaining program. This committee, too, recommended continuing

NYSNA's current program, which they believed was "every bit as effective as that in states where nurses' associations have become official bargaining agencies."[55] A majority of delegates to the 1947 convention agreed, and the 1948 Advisory Council, following a panel discussion and extensive debate, also voted to reinforce the current program, urging the employment of staff devoted solely to improving employment conditions.[56] Members seemed willing to adopt any and all measures which would improve salaries and working conditions — short of collective bargaining, a term which denoted strikes, industrial practices, and loss of professional status.[57]

The board labored to reconcile conflicting attitudes, and sought the opinion of Albany Law School Professor Robert Jones on the advisability of NYSNA engaging in collective bargaining. Jones believed a simple change in the Articles of Incorporation would allow the association to act legally as a bargaining agent. Shortly after the 1948 meeting, the Board of Directors appointed Jones as legal counsel to "guide a more aggressive program," appointed a Steering Committee for the Economic Security Program to "determine what could be done to enable the New York State Nurses Association to adopt fully the ANA Economic Security Program," and hired Katherine Rehder as assistant executive secretary in charge of the program.[58]

"Don't you think the minds of the public have been matured enough now so that the name 'union' is no longer a stigma? You can be just as professional as a union as you can as any other organization."

— *Mrs. Jasspon*[7]

Jones and Rehder set about preparing for NYSNA's 1949 House of Delegates meeting. They prepared a revision of the Articles of Incorporation and initiated an intense campaign to educate the membership. Three mailings were sent to every member, and Rehder attended district meetings to discuss the issue. President Mabel Detmold opened the convention by noting the continued "dissatisfaction and unrest among nurses . . . We are gathered together at this convention to adopt appropriate measures of grave import to us as nurses, to the profession as a whole, and to the public in whose service we are dedicated." She admonished the group to "deliberate calmly and decide wisely," and reminded delegates to put aside prejudice and consider what would improve the situation for nurses. "If we have achieved legal control of the nursing profession in New York State this is only a first step; we must now find the way to stabilize — to make nursing again a proud profession . . . sheer necessity will compel a change by other means if we are not alert to our responsibility . . . Only you, the delegates here assembled, can provide the framework on which to build a future. If you are good architects, your skill will win recognition and support. A blueprint is offered for your study and action."[59]

The Steering Committee on Economic Security recommended the adoption of ANA's Economic Security Program and amendment of the Articles of Incorporation.[60] Committee chair Yvonne Ward was a strong proponent of adoption of ANA's program in totality, and worked to persuade delegates to include collective bargaining in NYSNA's program. When a motion was formally presented, District 14 President Ethel Prince, closely allied with NYSNA attorney Edward Handelman, immediately rose to speak against the motion. "Our members have been going through this thing for the last several years . . . Do we think that eventually, if we keep on with this kind of deliberation we are going to wear the delegates down?"[61] Handelman was firmly against changing the charter, and believed that NYSNA would "lower its professional status" if the incorporation certificate was changed. Jones agreed with Handelman that the new language could be regarded as permitting collective bargaining, but maintained that the Articles of Incorporation needed to be changed to permit expansion of the Economic Security Program.[62]

Following days of vigorous debate and procedural wrangling, delegates voted to amend the Articles of Incorporation by adding "to assist nurses who are ill, disabled, destitute or otherwise in need; to promote and protect the health and welfare of nurses" to the list of association purposes, but voted down the proposal that NYSNA become a bargaining agent for its members. Thus, NYSNA legally provided for a collective bargaining program, while again resisting the adoption of a full-fledged economic security program. The issue was, however, far from dead. At its closing session, delegates approved a resolution that the board present an estimated budget for an economic security program prior to the next biennial, and conduct a statewide educational program.[63]

RELATIONSHIPS WITH LICENSED PRACTICAL NURSES: Passage of the NYSNA sponsored Nurse Practice Act in 1938 created new problems for the association. In the first year following passage, the association successfully opposed a proposed amendment which provided for nominations to the Board of Nurse Examiners and its Advisory Council from two labor organizations.[64] Severe shortages of nurses for general hospital duty during the summer of 1940 were immediately attributed by hospital administrators to the enactment of the new law, and the association prepared for the introduction of additional amendments by appointing a Nurse Practice Act Committee.[65] In deference to the demands of war, the date of full effectiveness was extended to one year after the cessation of hostilities. Shortages of nurses in the postwar period led to yet another extension to July 1, 1948. In 1947 NYSNA delegates voted to appoint a committee and hire staff to study the nursing shortage in New York and the impact of the law's full enactment. In an attempt to increase the nurse supply, the committee recommended that the Nurse Practice Act be amended to license without examination out-of-state graduates of schools of nursing accredited in any other state, province, or country, and who met all other licensure requirements, and to again postpone the law's effective date to July 1, 1949. Amendments embodying these recommendations were introduced and passed in 1948, and the law finally became fully effective in 1949.[66]

An issue of great importance to many members was the relationship between NYSNA and the practical nurses — now given legal status by the 1938 law. Some districts were so concerned they wanted to call a special meeting of the House of Delegates in early 1939. Instead, the board provided discussion materials so that delegates would be prepared to act at the regular 1939 convention. The central issue was whether practical nurses should become members of NYSNA or form their own organization. Many delegates feared that providing a mechanism for membership of practical nurses within NYSNA would lower standards and jeopardize nursing's tenuous professional status. One member stated, "I think we all feel very keenly that that is one of the most complicated and serious if not one of the most revolutionary questions that most of us have been called upon to face."[67]

The Committee on Practical Nurse Organization recommended amending the bylaws to add practical nurses as a separate class of membership, but because the committee did not submit a written report, the disgruntled assembly voted to re-convene in April to resolve the question. By April "the practical nurses of the state, either oblivious of our work, or impatient with our slowness," had formed the Practical Nurses of New York State, Inc.[68] The committee's recommendation to welcome this group and work together on areas of mutual concern was adopted and a NYSNA member was appointed to serve on the new organization's advisory council. NYSNA members continued to provide guidance and expertise, and when the Board of Regents proposed repealing the law licensing practical nurses, the two associations united in vigorous opposition.[69]

UNPRECEDENTED DEMANDS: The demands of the war years on nursing changed the profession dramatically. Nursing in 1949 was far different than in 1939. Hospital nursing was now the largest field of practice for nurses, and the widespread introduction of practical nurses and nurse's aides had altered the role of the registered professional nurse. The war had highlighted the importance of nursing care and boosted the professional status and expectations of the public, but strained the profession's resources as it tried to keep pace with demand. The turmoil took a toll on NYSNA. Staff turnover, including the resignation of Executive Secretary Hicks in 1944, placed additional strain on the association. The executive secretary position remained vacant until Elizabeth Hall was appointed in 1945, and she resigned just three years later. In 1949 Katherine Rehder was appointed to the position of executive secretary and provided much needed stability. Membership peaked at 21,204 in 1941, then fell steadily. The decline continued throughout the decade, dropping to 13,619 in 1949. In 1941, for the first time in its history, association expenses exceeded income, and reserve funds were expended on defense programs. With falling membership and increased demand for staff and programs, the financial status worsened. As the association approached its fiftieth anniversary, it faced the immense challenges of building its membership, stabilizing its financial status and staffing, and developing an effective program to substantially improve the employment conditions of nurses.

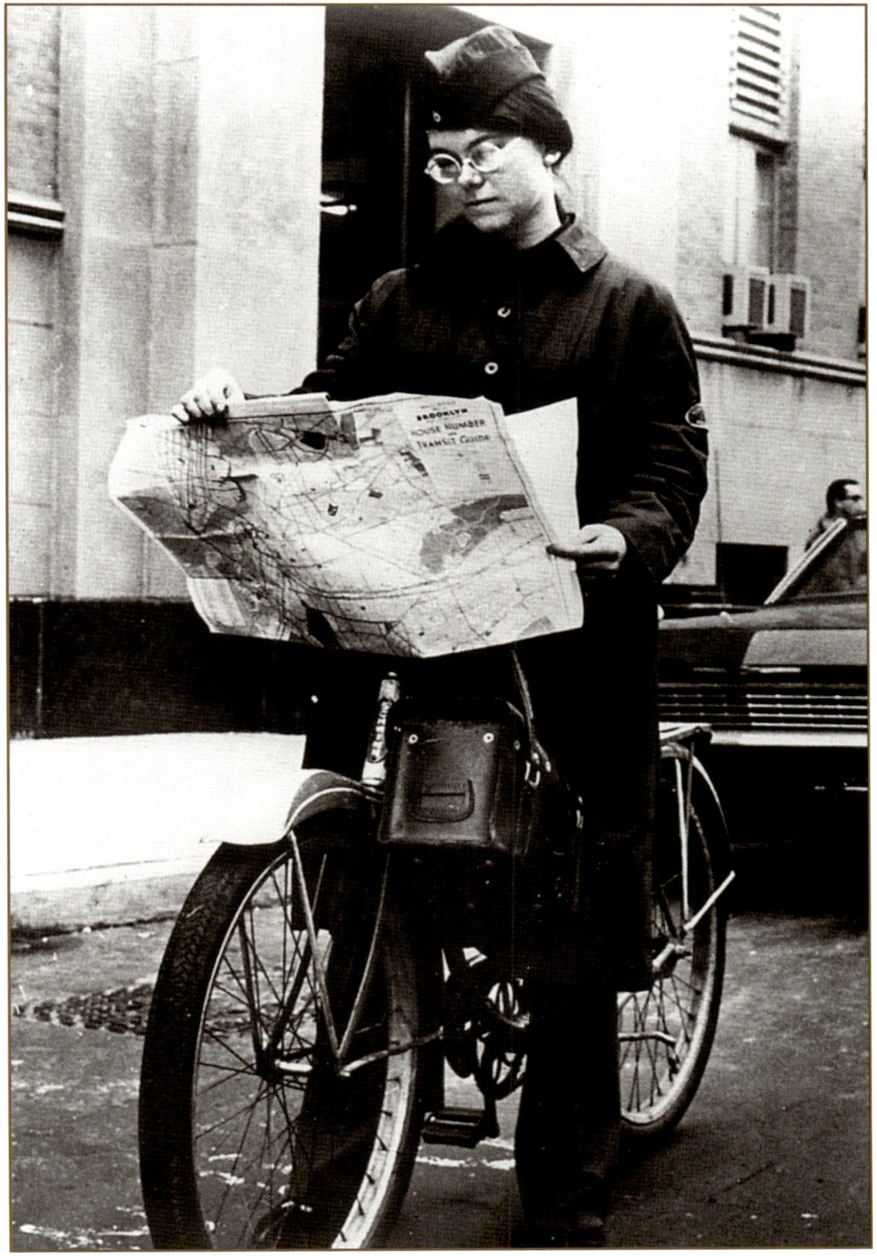

RIGHT: The need for public health nurses grew during World War II. Because of wartime restrictions, many accommodations had to be made, such as using bicycles rather than automobiles to visit patients. *Courtesy the Brooklyn VNA.*

TEXT

1. "The General Staff Nurse," *American Journal of Nursing* 38 (November 1938): 1221–29; and Barbara Melosh, *The Physician's Hand* (Philadelphia: Temple University Press, 1982), 184–91.

2. "The Red Cross and New York State Nurses," *Quarterly News* 12 (January 1940): 21. The Red Cross First Reserve was a pool of nurses theoretically ready to serve when called upon in an emergency. Qualifications for First Reserve nurses were graduation from an approved school connected with a hospital with a daily average of at least fifty patients, state registration, ANA membership, U.S. citizenship, good physical health, 21 to 40 years of age, and single. As the war progressed, and the demand for nurses grew, many of the qualifications were loosened. (Mary Beard and Virginia Dunbar, "Wanted: 10,000 Nurses!" *American Journal of Nursing* 39 [March 1939]: 227–32.)

3. Milton Loomis, "Nursing in Health Defense," *New York State Nurse* 13 (January 1941): 14–15. Loomis was associate commissioner, Department of Education. He went on to maintain that, "The likelihood of attack by foreign powers upon our shores . . . is now diminishing to the vanishing point . . . We have been faithfully promised that we shall not be led into the desperate adventure of a war on foreign soil." A year later Isabel Stewart told NYSNA's 1941 convention delegates that nurses were realists. "There may be a few optimistic souls who still think that the danger is imaginary, and that actual war can be avoided, but I doubt if nurses are among them." ("Proceedings, Second Biennial Meeting, Thirty-Ninth Convention of the New York State Nurses' Association" [Brooklyn, N.Y., 1941, stenotype transcript], 195.)

4. "Second Biennial Meeting," 18. The telegram was sent jointly by the three national nursing organizations, the ANA, the National League of Nursing Education, and the National Organization for Public Health Nursing.

5. Julie M. Pavri, "New York Nurses and the National Nursing Council for War Service" in *Critical Issues in American Nursing in the Twentieth Century: Perspectives and Case Studies,* ed. Darwin H. Stapleton and Cathryne A. Welch (Guilderland, N.Y.: Foundation of NYSNA, 1994), 9.

6. Isabel M. Stewart, "Nursing Preparedness: Some Lessons from World War I," in *Forty-Seventh Annual Report of the National League of Nursing Education* (New York: National League of Nursing Education, 1941), 214.

7. Pavri, "New York Nurses," 6–9. Other organizations represented at the organizing meeting were the ANA, the NLNE, the AJN, the NOPHN, the American Red Cross, and the Association of Collegiate Schools of Nursing. Representatives of other nursing organizations were later included. No other record of Dines' participation in the Nursing Council was found.

8. Hope Newell, *The History of the National Nursing Council* (New York: National Organization for Public Health Nursing, 1951), 6, 108–10. The questionnaire gathered basic identifying information and detailed education and work history. It also asked, "Would you accept assignment to the army or navy service? civilian service? Are you available for full-time duty? part time? volunteer?"

9. Margaret Shetland, "Nursing Participation in Defense Continues, *New York State Nurse* 14 (January 1942): 15–18; and "Nursing Inventory for Defense," *New York State Nurse* 13 (January 1941): 12–13. Executive Secretary Hicks applied to the WPA for additional staff, receiving thirty clerical workers and a full-time supervisor to prepare the mailing. ("New York's Call to Service," *Trained Nurse and Hospital Review* 106 [January 1941]: 52.) In 1943, a re-survey was conducted. NYSNA mailed 82,000 postcard surveys to New York nurses to provide local committees with more recent data on the availability of nurses. ("1943 National Resurvey of Registered Nurses," *New York State Nurse* 15 [October 1943]: 127.)

10. Board of Directors Minutes, NYSNA, 5 July 1941, NYSNA Archives; and Shetland, "Nursing Participation in Defense," 15. At this time, Emergency Departments were rare, and one of the most useful features of the manual was the outline of classes in emergency nursing to prepare nurses for the "demands of modern total warfare." Marriage typically removed nurses from the workplace. However, now they were needed and their skills needed to be updated. Refresher courses for inactive nurses had been organized by the State League of Nursing Education as early as 1941. ("Refresher Courses for Registered Professional Nurses," *New York State Nurse* 13 [January 1941]: 31.)

11. "We See the Face of Danger," *American Journal of Nursing* 42 (January 1942): 62.

12. Janet M. Geister, "A Little Plain Talk," *Trained Nurse and Hospital Review* 107 (January 1942): 38. Geister was now editor of *Trained Nurse and Hospital Review.*

13. Following the entry of the U.S. into the war, the name of the Nursing Council for National Defense was changed to the National Nursing Council for War Service. Both are here referred to as Nursing Council, and the New York State Nursing Council for War Service as the State Nursing Council.

14. "News Alerts: New York State Nursing Council for War Service," *New York State Nurse* 14 (October 1942): 147.

15. New York State Nursing Council for War Service Minutes, March 1943, NACLI Archives; and Financial Statements, NYSNA, 1940–45, NYSNA Archives. NYSNA had also contributed substantially to the Nursing Council in the prewar years. Because of the war effort, most NYSNA committees were disbanded so that energies could be concentrated into the work of the nursing councils.

16. New York State Nursing Council for War Service, "Bulletin No. 2" (2 December 1941, mimeographed).

17. New York State Nursing Council for War Service Meeting Minutes, 1942, NACLI Archives.

18. Procurement and Assignment Division, War Manpower Commission, "Guidelines," NACLI Archives; and "Criteria of Essentiality for Nurses," *American Journal of Nursing* 43 (November 1943): 977–79. Efforts were made to publicize this information in order to reduce the guilt of nurses in essential positions who were barraged with patriotic appeals to enlist, and to reduce disparaging remarks by an unthinking or uninformed public. Private duty nursing was now termed "luxury nursing," and there was little sympathy from anyone for eligible private duty nurses who were not enrolled. Nurses considered available for military service were those under 45 years of age, with no children under 14 years of age. ("State Begins Classification of Nurses," *New York State Nurse* 16 [January 1944]: 17–18.)

19. "Emily C. Creevey," in *Professionalization of Nursing in New York State: Oral History Interview with Six Leaders Who Helped to Advance the Mission of NYSNA,* ed. Elizabeth Carter and Jane Fielding (Guilderland, N.Y.: NYSNA 1988), 37.

20. "State Nursing Council for War Service," *New York State Nurse* 17 (October 1945): 163; and Elmira B. Wickenden, "Nurses United for War Service," *Public Health Nursing* 36 (July 1944): 342.

21. Pavri, "New York Nurses," 20; and Board of Directors Minutes, NYSNA, 15 January 1944, NYSNA Archives.

22. Board of Directors Minutes, NYSNA, 14 May 1943, NYSNA Archives; and Kalisch and Kalisch, *Advance of American Nursing,* 404.

23. Bonnie Bullough, "The Lasting Impact of World War II on Nursing," *American Journal of Nursing* 76 (January 1976): 120.

24. Recruitment materials, 1942, NYSNA Archives; Florence M. Seder to Dorothy Anker, 15 April 15, 1942, NYSNA Archives; and Newell, *History of National Nursing Council,* 26.

25. Committee on Nursing Participation in National Defense Minutes, NYSNA, 31 January 1942, NYSNA Archives; and Board of Directors Minutes, NYSNA, 14 February 1942, NYSNA Archives.

26. New York State Nursing Council for War Service, "Bulletin No. 4," (18 February 1943, mimeographed). Adelphi was established to serve rural Long Island, and Keuka the western New York Finger Lakes region. By May 1943 Hartwick College, the College of Mt. St. Vincent's, Manhattanville College of the Sacred Heart, Wagner College, Alfred University, and Syracuse University were all planning programs. ("Report on Meeting of Local Nursing Council Representatives," 21 May 1943, NACLI Archives.)

27. Kalisch and Kalisch, *Advance of American Nursing,* 341; "Cadet Nurse Corps," *New York State Nurse,* 15 (April 1944): 59.

28. Kalisch and Kalisch, *Advance of American Nursing,* 344–45; and Flanagan, *One Strong Voice,* 117. In late 1944 casualties reached over 1,750 per day. It was later revealed that these Army hospitals were sent without nurses, not because there were none to send, but because it was equipment rather than personnel that these units needed. (Roberts, *American Nursing,* 375–76.)

29. Board of Directors Minutes, NYSNA, 10 April 1942 and 13 February 1943, NYSNA Archives; and Stella Goostray, *Memoirs: Half a Century in Nursing* (Boston: Nursing Archive, 1969), 127. Alta Dines "couldn't visualize" the possibility of a nurse draft, though others stated many private duty nurses were not enlisting because they expected to be drafted.

30. "Chronology of May Bill (Nurse Draft) HR (1284)227," *New York State Nurse* 17 (April 1945): 57; and Clare M. Casey, "A Message from the State President," *New York State Nurse* 17 (April 1945): 57.

31. N.T. Kirk, "Registered Professional Nurses — We Salute You!" *New York State Nurse* 17 (July 1945): 99.

32. Wickenden, "Nurses United for Service," 340–41. In 1942, Alta Dines listed Sheahan, Wickenden, Alma Haupt, Marian Randall, Katharine Faville, Mary Beard, Gertrude Banfield, Dorothy Conrad, Anna Wolf, Adelaide Mayo, Alma Scott, Ruth Haulton, Major Julia Stimson, Mary Roberts, and Isabel Stewart as national leaders who were members of NYSNA. ("Proceedings of the Advisory Council of the New York State Nurses Association," [Poughkeepsie, N.Y., 1942, stenotype transcript], 139).

33. Pavri, "New York Nurses," 25–26.

34. "Proceedings, Forty-First Session and Fourth Biennial Convention of the New York State Nurses Association" (Utica, N.Y., 1945, stenotype transcript), 25.

35. Pavri, "New York Nurses," 20–21.

36. "Bureau to Advise Returning Nurses," *New York Times,* 11 October 1945.

37. "Here's What Your Association Does to Serve You Through Counseling and Placement," *New York State Nurse* 21 (March 1949): 12–13; and History of the NYSNA Counseling and Placement Program, n.d., NYSNA Archives. The state program was adopted only after prolonged debate in both the Advisory Council and the House of Delegates, and was controversial because of its services to non-members and practical nurses. Placement bureaus for nurses had been discussed at both the state and national levels since the studies of the 1920s highlighted problems of distribution. After nine years of comprehensive study, the ANA House of Delegates accepted a proposed national placement program, providing a consultant to assist state nurses' associations in developing state and local programs.

38. Elizabeth Hall, "Twelve Months at State Headquarters," *New York State Nurse* 18 (November 1946): 12–13.

39. "Proceedings, First Biennial Convention of the New York State Nurses Association" (Buffalo, N.Y., 1939, stenotype transcript), 420–21. The spectre of the CIO was raised in many House of Delegates and Advisory Council discussions, including discussions of the Counseling and Placement Program and the question of an organization for practical nurses. A recommendation that practical nurses become members of NYSNA was made primarily because of the threat of an independent practical nurse organization being "taken over" by labor unions.

40. "State Meetings," *Quarterly News* 11 (July 1939): 93. The Joint Committee functioned until 1945, when it became the Coordinating Council on Nursing Problems, and included representatives from MSSNY and the Practical Nurses of New York in addition to HANYS and NYSNA. This council met infrequently to "iron out difficulties which we find in nursing problems." The amiable working relationship with HANYS broke down in 1949, when HANYS representatives refrained from participating when the Coordinating Council voted to oppose any further postponement of the effective date of the Nurse Practice Act, and HANYS sponsored its own bill to postpone the date beyond 1949. The bill was not enacted.

41. "Progress Report," *New York State Nurse* 15 (October 1943): 103–6. It was noted that elementary school teachers' salaries ranged from $2,067–$3,335 for 180 work days per year. ("Editorial," *New York State Nurse* 15 [October 1943]: 102.) Popular practice at the time was to receive a reduced salary plus "maintenance"—room, board, and laundry services. Delegates to the 1943 convention made it clear they preferred a cash salary to cash and maintenance, desiring the same privileges as other groups — to spend their own money as they chose. As one member put it, "responsibility rather than paternalistic supervision."

42. "Convention Adopts Personnel Practices," *New York State Nurse* 16 (January 1944): 14.

43. Board of Directors Minutes, NYSNA, January 1945, NYSNA Archives; Coordinating Committee Meeting Minutes, 3 February 1945; and Elizabeth Hall to Mary Richardson, 5 December 1944, NYSNA Archives.

44. "Wage Increase for Registered Professional Nurses," *New York State Nurse* 17 (July 1945): 125.

45. "Fourth Biennial Convention," 96.

46. Ibid., 329–30; and Emily J. Hicks Memo, 30 August 1946 and 31 August 1946, NYSNA Archives.

47. Clare M. Casey, "$50.00 for 40 Hours!" *New York State Nurse* 18 (July 1946): 107–8. In fact, additional factors contributed to the failure of nurse veterans to flock to hospital nursing. They wanted time to rest, to get back into the life of family and friends, and satisfy longings for "luxuries." Many nurses took advantage of the GI bill to obtain additional education, and others married and started raising a family. (Mary Walker Randolph, "What Army Nurses Expect from the Profession," *American Journal of Nursing,* 46 [February 1946]: 95–97.)

48. "Hospital Official McCormack Favors Levels Rise for Nurses," *New York State Nurse* 18 (July 1946): 108.

49. Clare Casey to ANA, 11 October 1946, NYSNA Archives. Casey also stressed the formation of state and district personnel practices committees, the appointment of Seyffer to work full-time on the promotion of improved employment conditions, and a comprehensive public relations program. Florence Smith Vincent had been hired to coordinate NYSNA's public relations efforts. Standards were first completed for general duty staff nurses in 1945, and nearly every state had requested copies.

50. "Proceedings of the Advisory Council and the Special Meeting of the New York State Nurses Association" (Albany, N.Y., 1946, stenotype transcript), 45–68.

51. Ibid.,134.

52. Clare M. Casey, "Our Hand to the Plow!" *New York State Nurse* 18 (December 1946); and "Proceedings, Fortieth Session and Third Biennial Convention of the New York State Nurses Association," (Rochester, N.Y., 1943, stenotype transcript), 331. At the 1943 meeting, Ethel Prince, later a vocal opponent of collective bargaining, stated, "Madam chairman, I cannot understand why anyone would object to having the New York State Nurses Association be the collective bargaining agency if we have to have one. The New York State Nurses Association should be the group to represent us in any policy." Handelman, believing the resolution illegal, advised the board to rescind the resolution, but no action was taken until the 1945 meeting. There is evidence that delegates expected the dues increase to pay for full-time staff for the program. However, there was a great deal of staff turnover during this period, and there was no staff member consistently designated for the program.

53. Clare M. Casey, "Faithfully Yours, NYSNA," *New York State Nurse* 19 (January 1947): 5.

54. "Relief Proposed for General Duty Nurses," *New York State Nurse* 21 (February 1949): 7. At the same time, the association was promoting its economic security activities. In a March article in the *New York State Nurse,* it was noted that "Proof of the program's effectiveness lies in the fact that while in 1942, hospitals reported a maximum salary of $120 (for a 44–60 hour week), a 1948 survey shows that salaries for nurses now range from $165 to $215 (for a 40–44 hour week)." The article reviewed the history of the personnel practices program. ("Here's What Your Association Does to Improve Your Economic Security," *New York State Nurse* 21 [March 1949]: 8–9.)

55. Committee to Study the Economic Security Program Minutes, NYSNA, 15 March 1948, NYSNA Archives; and Florence Smith Vincent, "Success Crowns Genessee Valley Nurses Spring Institute," *New York State Nurse* 20 (May 1948): 12.

56. "Proceedings, Advisory Council of the New York State Nurses Association" (Lake Placid, N.Y., 1948, stenotype transcript), 154–55.

57. Roberts, *American Nursing,* 570. "Collective bargaining" was seen as nearly synonymous with "trade unions" which were perceived by many to be allied with communism. As the Cold War intensified, the suggested connection between unions and communism became even more troubling.

58. "Here's What Your Association Does," 9; and Board of Directors Minutes, NYSNA, 15 December 1948 and 1 March 1949, NYSNA Archives. The Personnel Practices Committee was made inactive at the 15 February 1949 Board of Directors meeting.

59. "Proceedings, Forty-Fourth Meeting and Sixth Biennial Convention of the New York State Nurses Association" (Buffalo, N.Y., 1949, stenotype transcript), 4–7.

60. Ibid., 136–37.

61. Ibid., 209–11. Discouraged with the House of Delegates action, Ward became an ANA staff member soon after the meeting.

62. Ibid., 222–24. Edward Handleman had been NYSNA's legal counsel for many years, as well as counsel for District 14, Nurses House, and several other nursing organizations. Jones was retained in December 1948 specifically to handle economic security matters, while Handleman continued to provide legal services for all other NYSNA matters. Handleman was not invited to participate in the 1949 convention until a spokesperson for District 14 requested his participation. A motion to this effect was carried, and Handelman was called to Buffalo for the remainder of the meeting. (Ethel Mockler and Robert Smith, "Report on the Biennial," *New York State Nurse* 21 [November 1949]: 5.)

63. Mockler and Smith, "Report on Biennial," 6.

64. "Legislature Proposes Nursing Bills," *Quarterly News* 12 (April 1940): 71; and Board of Directors Minutes, NYSNA, 26 April 1940, NYSNA Archives.

65. Board of Directors Minutes, NYSNA, 13 September 1940, NYSNA Archives.

66. "Proceedings, Advisory Council," 1942, 103; Survey Study Committee Report on Nursing Situation in New York State, NYSNA, 1947, NYSNA Archives.

67. Board of Directors Minutes, NYSNA, 11 March 1939, NYSNA Archives; and "First Biennial Convention," 230.

68. "First Biennial Convention," 234–36; and "Proceedings, Adjourned Meeting, House of Delegates of the New York State Nurses Association" (Syracuse, N.Y., 1940, stenotype transcript), 4.

69. "Special Meeting," 298. By November 1942 membership had reached one thousand and the practical nurse group had established an office and hired an executive secretary.

FEATURE

Mabel Keaton Staupers

1. Darlene Clark Hine, *Black Women in White: Racial Conflict and Cooperation in the Nursing Profession 1890–1950* (Bloomington, In.: Indiana University Press, 1989), 179.

2. Ibid., 163; and American Nurses Association Hall of Fame Nomination Form, 1995, NYSNA Archives.

EXCERPTS

1. "Second Biennial Meeting," 14.
2. Wickenden, "Nurses United," 340.
3. "Fourth Biennial Convention," 168.
4. Leah Bryan, "Committee on Personnel Practices," *New York State Nurse* 18 (July 1946): 129.
5. "Fourth Biennial Convention," 157–58.
6. "Letters," *New York State Nurse* 21 (April 1949): 4–5.
7. "Sixth Biennial Convention,"166.

CHAPTER SIX

Nursing in 1950

BY 1950 THERE WERE NEARLY EIGHTY-FOUR THOUSAND REGISTERED nurses in New York State, and half of the active professional nurses were employed by hospitals and other health institutions. The number of registered nurses engaged in private duty had dropped to approximately 20 percent of the total, many of whom restricted their practice to special duty service in hospitals. The "average nurse" was now a hospital staff nurse, working an eight-hour shift. The average nurse no longer lived within the confines of the hospital complex, and more than likely was married.[1]

As technology and medicine advanced, nursing care became more and more complex. During World War II, bold and risky surgery for war injuries had led to new and accepted surgical procedures. The use of blood transfusions, intravenous therapy, and innovative rehabilitation techniques increased enormously. Physicians ordered earlier post-operative ambulation, and hospital stays were shortened. These reduced periods of bed rest altered traditional nursing care practices. Perhaps most significantly, new drugs were developed to fight infections. Sulfonamides and antibiotics radically changed the patterns of hospital care, reducing admissions of patients with infectious diseases, and dramatically shortening the length of hospitalization. Nurses were increasingly called on to make judgments regarding physiological processes and the emotional and psychological needs of the patient.[2] The nurse began to plan for the patient following discharge, making referrals and providing health teaching to the patient and family members.

Many hospitals were beginning to organize staff into teams, with a professional nurse as team leader who determined nursing needs of the patients, and worked with other team members —

graduate nurses, students, practical nurses, and attendants — to develop comprehensive plans of nursing care. The registered nurse had become an essential member of the hospital staff, and the nurse's unique patient-centered skills in assessing, planning, and delivering care were beginning to be realized. Unfortunately, severe understaffing in many hospitals prevented the full realization of this role. Time to assess and plan was too often an unheard of luxury, and in-service training to upgrade skills was a rare benefit. Increasing division of labor added administrative duties while it took registered nurses away from the bedside — the very thing they cherished most about their profession. Too often, instead of providing hands-on care or teaching patients, the nurse's time was spent in "non-nursing" tasks such as folding linen, delivering meals, and transporting patients. Too many patients, too few staff, and demeaning salaries created growing anger and frustration, and nurses began to explore new ways to improve patient care through an improvement in employment conditions.[3]

RIGHT: *Courtesy Ellis Hospital School of Nursing Collection, Foundation of NYSNA Archives.*

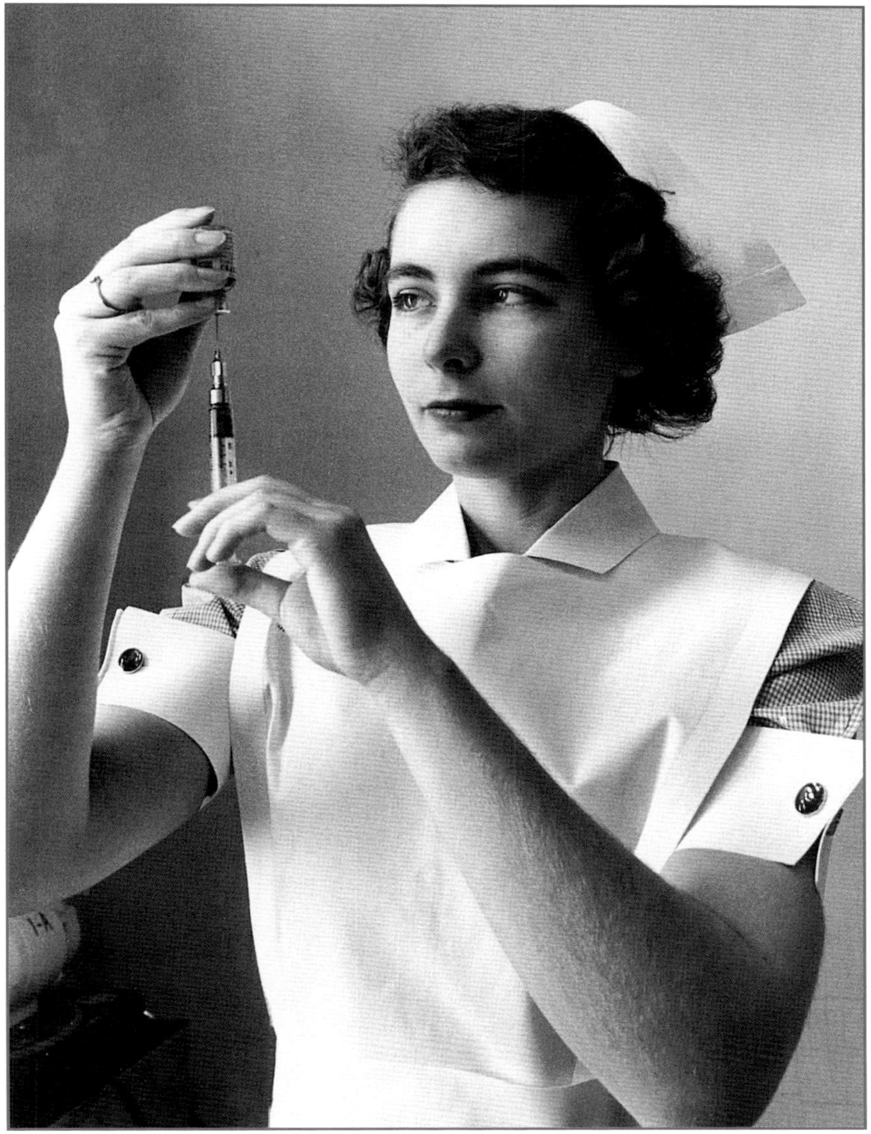

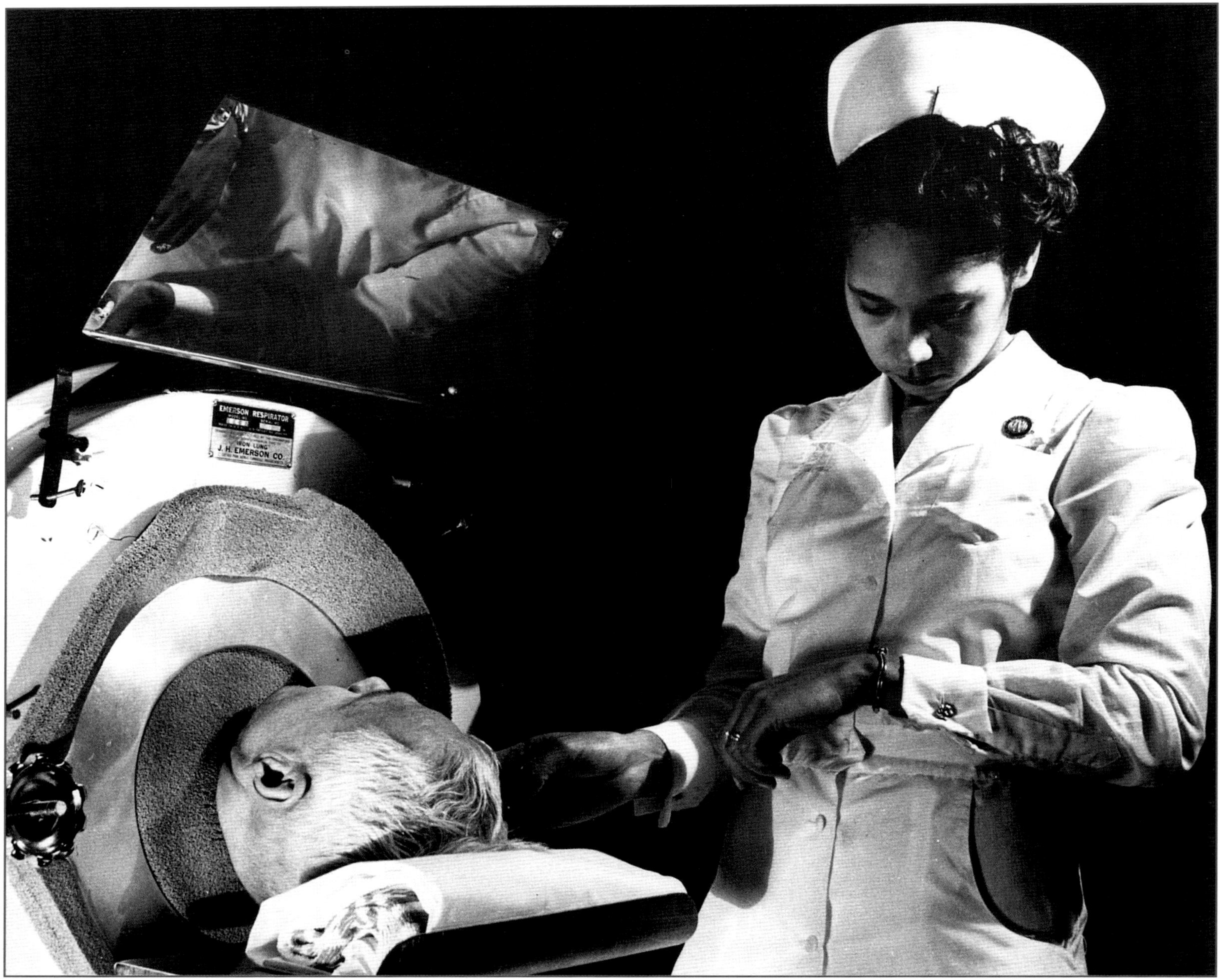
EMERSON RESPIRATOR
IRON LUNG
J. H. EMERSON CO

POSTWAR TRANSITION 1950~1960

The long-standing problems of supply and distribution of nurses, poor salaries and working conditions, and the utilization of auxiliary personnel continued to plague nursing, and the severe shortage of nurses continued to be the central issue around which nursing's energy was focused. An article in the *New York Times* in the summer of 1950 attributed the shortage to recent implementation of the 1938 Nurse Practice Act, but NYSNA leaders blamed the proliferation of new and expanded hospitals which required unprecedented numbers of registered nurses. Since 1943 the nurse population had increased — often spectacularly — in all but three of the state's counties. Enrollment in New York's schools of nursing was the highest in any peacetime period, but many graduates were lost to the workplace when they married young, and chose home and family over career. At the same time, the birth rate soared, life expectancy lengthened, and the demand for nursing services skyrocketed.[4]

FACING PAGE: Polio epidemics were a common health problem during the 1950s. Patients treated in an iron lung required a great deal of nursing care. *Courtesy Westchester Medical Center.*

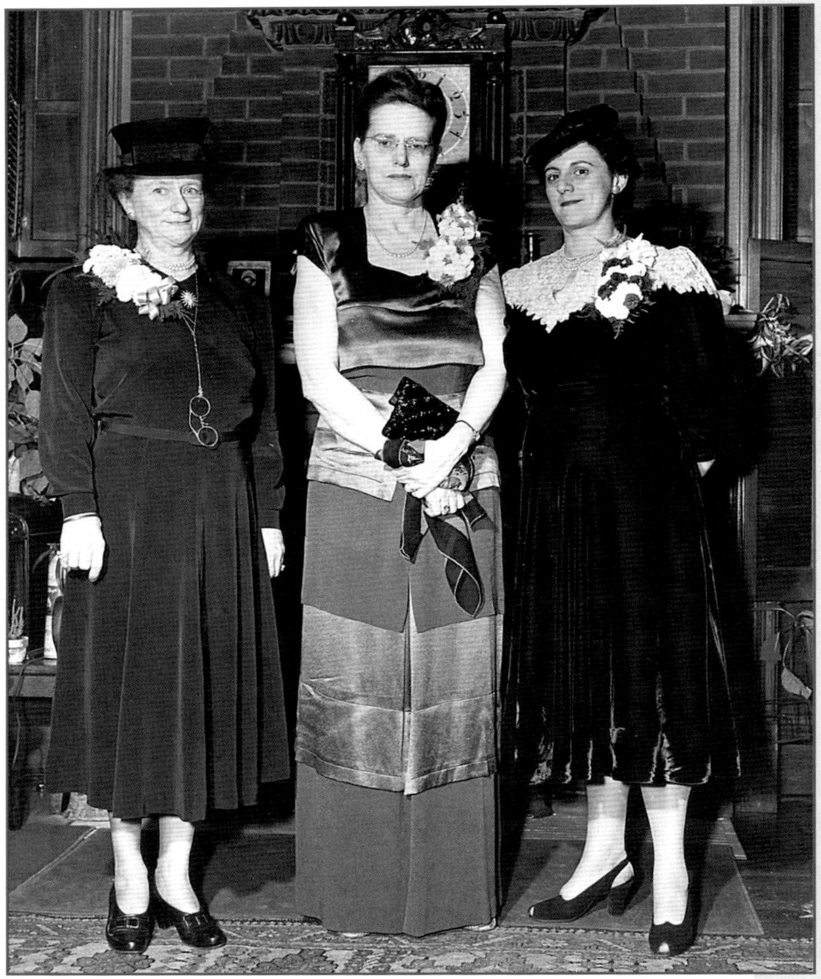

Mabel Detmold, center, is shown here with Laura Fineholt at left and Ruth Brooks at right in 1948. *Photograph by Casey.*

Mabel Detmold
1880 - 1964

Mabel Detmold, a graduate of St. Luke's Hospital School of Nursing in New York City, worked as a private duty nurse and as an office nurse. After 1935 she served as manager of the Turtle Bay Holding Company, a real estate firm primarily devoted to the management of a group of brownstone houses surrounding the Turtle Bay Gardens on Manhattan's east side. Despite this obligation and her role as a devoted wife and mother, Detmold worked to advance the nursing profession through her participation in nursing organizations. As president of District 13's registry, she introduced the resolution authorizing NYSNA to represent nurses in all matters of salaries and conditions of employment. The resolution was passed in 1943, but was later rescinded. As NYSNA president from 1947 through 1951, she continued to work for the adoption of a full-scale Economic Security Program, and was bitterly disappointed when delegates repeatedly rejected collective bargaining as an association responsibility. Following her presidency, she served the profession as chairman of NYSNA's Committee on Legislation and as president and director of Nurses House, Inc. An author of a history of Nurses House and of the Turtle Bay Gardens community, Mrs. Detmold is described as having an unforgettable personality, intelligent, warm, witty, and honest.[1]

At NYSNA's Golden Anniversary convention in 1951, President Mabel Detmold assessed the challenges ahead. "Standing today on the threshold of our next half-century, it requires courage to face the tasks that loom before us . . . All around us we see more hospitals being built, and realize, sometimes with despair, that if we did not have enough nurses to care for patients before the hospital expansion plans were considered, we certainly can't fill future demands without drastic changes... We must vigorously pursue the program to conserve nurses for nursing; to consign the thousand odd jobs to less skilled but well trained personnel. We must also guard against the assignment of tasks which belong to nurses to those inadequately trained to perform such tasks. We must increase our efforts to secure adequate compensation for services rendered. This is not a selfish desire. Without a just wage we are promoting a condition which is depriving patients of the care they have a right to demand."[5] In addition to these challenges, widespread epidemics of polio and the spectre of war placed ever greater demands on the profession.

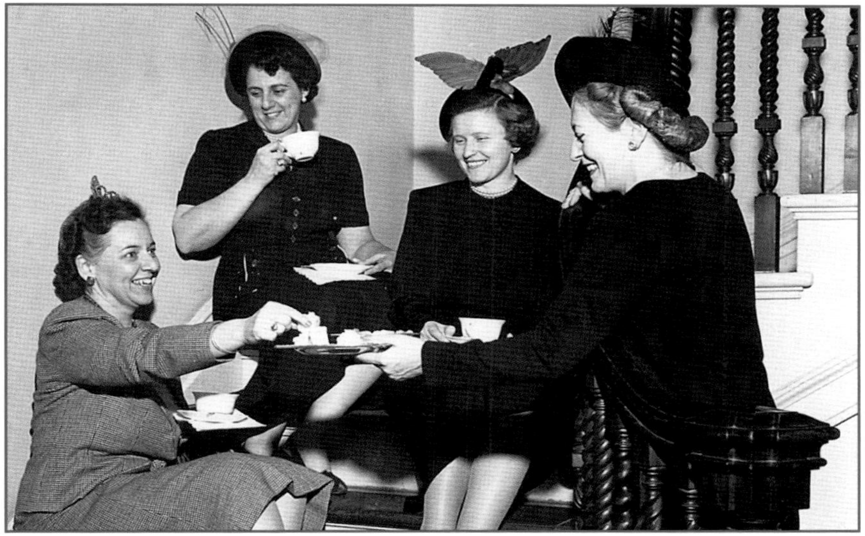

When NYSNA purchased its own headquarters at 385 State Street in Albany, a tea was given to welcome nursing leaders from across the state. Shown here are, from left to right, Dorothy Clark, Ruth Brooks, Teresa Yarwood, and Assistant Executive Secretary Anne Harrington. *Photograph by Floyd Adams.*

CIVIL DEFENSE : The 1945 bombing of Hiroshima ushered in the atomic era and the Soviet Union exploded its own atomic bomb a few years afterward. Communism was spreading worldwide, and the possibility of atomic warfare during these Cold War years was frightening and a very real threat. In 1950, with memories of World War II painfully fresh, the United States entered the Korean Conflict. The Army Nurse Corps assured nursing leaders that it was not experiencing a shortage of nurses, and had a well-organized reserve to draw from if needed.[6] NYSNA leaders were alarmed despite these assurances. In August 1950 NYSNA's board appointed a Committee on Nursing in the Defense Program to work with the State Civilian Defense Commission to define nursing duties in a disaster or emergency and plan for the allocation of nurses in all phases of "any war emergency." The board directed each district to send a representative to an official course on nursing care and atomic warfare, and cancelled all programs not concerned with defense.[7]

Fearful that global warfare on a scale never before seen was close at hand, the 1950 Advisory Council meeting focused on the nurse's role in civilian defense. Civil Defense Committee chairman Mary Parker warned, "It isn't if it [war] comes, it is when it comes, and nobody knows exactly when that is going to be . . . there won't be hospitals enough . . . there probably won't be enough nurses . . . we will have many, many more casualties than has ever been experienced before."[8] Statewide institutes trained nearly two hundred nurses to respond to atomic

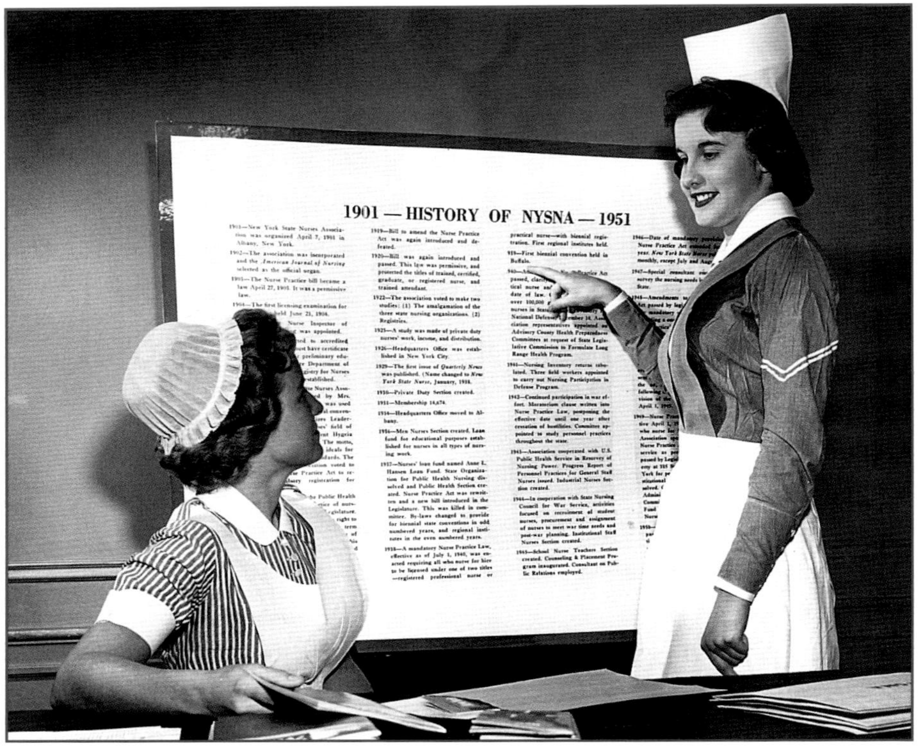

Student nurses assisted with NYSNA's 1951 convention, which celebrated the association's fiftieth anniversary. Early in 1951 students from over fifty New York State schools of nursing met to form a state association of student nurses. The newly formed organization met during the convention and adopted a constitution. NYSNA provided an advisor to the student organization. *Photograph by Paul Parker.*

disaster, and to set up and teach local workshops.[9]

Only months after the outbreak of the Korean War, casualties mounted, and the Army issued an urgent request for additional nurses. NYSNA emphasized accepting male nurses into the military, relieving nurses of non-nursing duties, and facilitating employment of inactive nurses as means of insuring an adequate supply of nurses.[10] The association continued to participate in the state civil defense program, but by late 1952 the sense of urgency had dissipated. ". . . civil defense is not an emergency. It is something that we are going to live with the rest of our lives. It is just as much a part of our public health services as measles or tuberculosis or any of the other diseases which we feel we have conquered — as long as we have the atom bomb and as long as we have no better way of solving the problems which cause war."[11] By 1954 the committee had shifted its focus to planning disaster programs, including disaster nursing in school curricula, and promoting disaster education programs for graduate nurses.[12] While the threat of atomic warfare was never realized, it was through nursing's response to these defense initiatives that emergency nursing and disaster planning were developed.

INTRAVENOUS THERAPY: In planning and preparing for large-scale disaster, it became evident that additional trained persons were needed to administer blood and intravenous medications. "Certainly in any large size bombing there is going to be a great deal of blood to be given, so much that the physicians won't be able to give it . . . nurses are one of the groups who have had experience at least in dealing with patients . . ."[13] The NYSNA board directed legal counsel to obtain a reinterpretation of the 1942 attorney general's opinion which placed intravenous therapy within the realm of medical practice, and barred nurses from giving intravenous medication except in extreme emergency, and then only with special training and under physician supervision.[14]

Despite the 1942 ruling, there was a growing trend in schools of nursing to teach intravenous therapy, and many nurses and even non-nurses were administering IV therapy in some institutions.[15] In 1953 the Department of Health announced a plan to train nurses in IV therapy skills in preparation for atomic attack, but opinions rendered by the Office of the Attorney General, the State Civil Defense Commission, and the Education Department demonstrated a lack of consensus on the legality of such training, and delegates to the 1955 convention voted to again request an opinion from the attorney general. Issued in 1961, the new opinion concluded that registered nurses could lawfully administer intravenous therapy under the specific order of a physician. NYSNA published the opinion with an introduction and interpretation by President Lucille Notter. The pamphlet was widely distributed, and marked the beginning of NYSNA's continuing practice of clarifying and publicizing scope of nursing practice issues.[16]

> "The General Duty Section is a new group . . . We are the young people, the leaders of tomorrow, and if we don't make an effort to get and to develop the young talents we have, then certainly the faces we see here won't be here maybe 20 years from today."
>
> — *Elois Holt*[1]

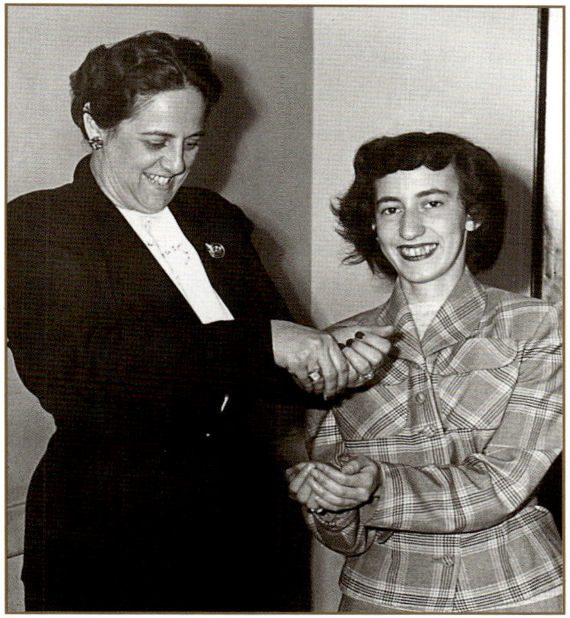

Mary Perrone, on the right, chairperson of NYSNA's General Duty Unit, urged association members to adopt collective bargaining as a component of the Economic Security Program. Miss Perrone is shown here with Ruth Brooks, chairperson of the Private Duty Section.

STRENGTHENING ECONOMIC SECURITY: The 1949 House of Delegates' rejection of a program of collective bargaining was demoralizing to many NYSNA members. At the 1950 Advisory Council meeting, President Detmold stated, "I do not think we have faced this issue fairly and squarely. I believe we are letting nurses down . . . Two years ago we recommended the employment of a person to implement the program but no one to date has defined 'the program,' except in the haziest of terms. A year ago we vigorously decided what we did *not* want—a negative step . . . One cannot be optimistic about the economic security program of the New York State Nurses Association. It is crippled by indecision, by a failure to face facts, by a neglect of the realization that only when all nurses work together for the common good can improvement be achieved."[17]

In 1951 NYSNA announced a three-point program to ease the shortage of nurses. Hailed by the *New York Times* as deserving national attention, the program was aimed at making the profession desirable enough to draw inactive nurses back into practice and stimulate enrollment in schools of nursing through improving salaries and other conditions of employment.[18] Meanwhile, hospitals were severely understaffed and the morale of the staff nurse plummeted. Mary Perrone, chair of the General Duty Nurses Section, wrote to NYSNA President Detmold that nurses at Bellevue Hospital were being "asked to carry double loads by covering two wards instead of one . . . When the nurses attempted to protest this double-ward routine, they were told that this is a situation they would have to learn to handle in

Prototype Local Unit at Nathan Littauer Hospital

In 1955 staff nurses at Nathan Littauer Hospital in Gloversville banded together to form a General Duty Unit, one of several local units formed in the 1950s under the guidance of the Economic Security Program. These units were the cornerstone of the program in its early years, and provided groups of nurses both voice and vote in matters of employment. NYSNA provided assistance in identifying issues to bring to employers, supplied supporting information, and participated in meetings with management to discuss proposals. Discussions continued until agreement was reached on all issues by all parties, after which the agreed upon proposals were put into effect.[1]

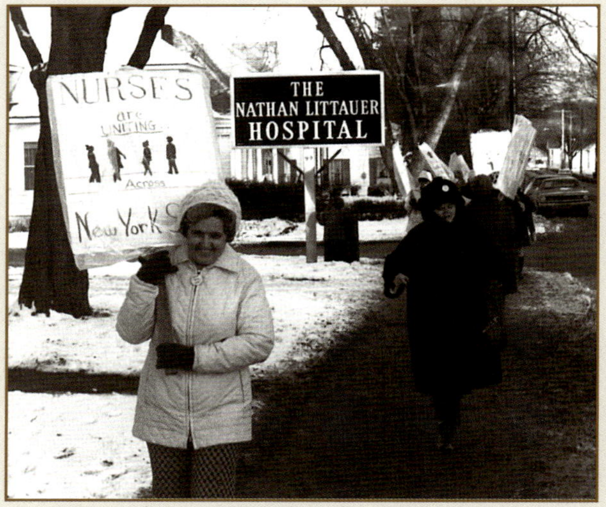

Nathan Littauer's General Duty Unit became the first unit represented by the Economic Security Program when it requested assistance from NYSNA in 1957.[2] Association representatives met with the unit to discuss needed improvements in personnel policies and participated in meetings with hospital administration. Under the leadership of Selma Gifford and Mrs. Arden Crouches, the nurses requested a raise in starting salaries, from $55 to $60 per week, increased sick and vacation time, and provisions for leave of absence, physical examination, and annual review of personnel policies. Following several months of discussions, hospital management and the nurses agreed to a compromise that included a beginning salary of $57.75, no change in sick and vacation leave, and acceptance of the remaining proposals. NYSNA celebrated this "excellent demonstration of what professional nurses, acting in a professional manner, can accomplish for themselves . . . The basic principle of recognition of nurses' right to have a voice in determining policies that affect them was clearly recognized by the administration . . ."[3]

NYSNA continued this informal representation of the nurses at Nathan Littauer until 1976, when a concerted effort was initiated to formalize the relationship. Designation cards were signed, and NYSNA requested voluntary recognition as collective bargaining agent for the nurses, but the hospital declined and a petition was filed with the NLRB. Local 200, SEIU, also attempted representation of the nurses, but in a March 1976 election, NYSNA received over 91 percent of the votes.[4] Negotiations commenced in April 1976. When contract talks stalled, the nurses brought their case to the public through a community rally and informational picketing.[5] Finally, in March 1977 the first contract between Nathan Littauer Hospital and NYSNA was fully executed. As NYSNA's program evolved, Nathan Littauer's local unit became a Council of Nursing Practitioners. Today, nearly forty-five years after the unit was first formed, nurses at Nathan Littauer continue to be represented by NYSNA.

preparation for the descent of the atom bomb . . . It really is a new wrinkle when I think of the flattering given our egos during the last war. The continual praise didn't lessen the fact that we were overworked nor did it raise our salaries but we felt a lot more necessary, insincere praise and all."[19] Perrone urged staff nurses to form district general duty sections to consider and discuss whether NYSNA should be authorized to represent nurses for collective bargaining. Apparently referring to past votes on the issue, she noted that ". . . minority opposition has often been able to block the adoption of programs designed to meet the needs of the majority within the profession."[20] On behalf of the General Duty Section, Perrone introduced a resolution at the 1951 convention authorizing NYSNA to represent registered nurses as their collective bargaining agent in all matters affecting salaries, hours, and working conditions. Discussion mirrored the debate at the 1949 convention, and the resolution was defeated two to one. Instead, delegates adopted a program proposed by the Committee on Employment Conditions to develop a pilot project on local staff organizations.[21]

"It seems to me that one of the greatest inducements that you can offer to any potential member is economic security."

— *Joseph L. Julien*[2]

Local staff units were organizations formed by nurses within a hospital or other employing agency which used group discussion, negotiation with the employer, and mutual agreement to improve employment conditions. Delegates voted to initiate a pilot project to develop local units in one of the smaller districts. District 7, surrounding the upstate city of Utica, was an area where hospital personnel policies were among the worst in the state, and was chosen as the site of the pilot project. NYSNA staff worked with district representatives and general duty staff nurses to establish local units in five hospitals. The units enjoyed modest successes, and the following year, the project was expanded.[22] With the assistance of NYSNA staff, some improvements were achieved, but the units were not sustained and by 1960 most had dissolved.[23]

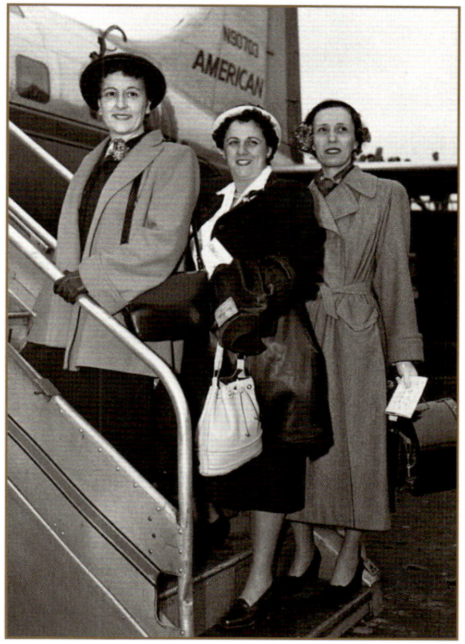

RIGHT: Katherine E. Rehder, far right, an experienced private duty and public health nurse, was appointed assistant executive secretary in charge of the Economic Security Program in 1949. Later that year, she became executive secretary. When ill health forced her to retire in 1963, members adopted a resolution noting that Miss Rehder's "untiring efforts have won for her the lasting affection of the members of this association." Rehder is shown here with Mary Benedict, on the left, and Ruth Brooks, center, departing for ANA's 1950 convention.

Recommended standards of employment, the centerpiece of the Personnel Practices Program in the 1940s, continued to be an important component of the employment conditions program. Sections were charged with setting functions, standards, qualifications, and employment standards for their own occupational groups. Following board approval, the recommended minimum standards of employment were printed and distributed to nurses and employers. Again, some improvements were realized, but progress was painfully slow.[24] A dynamic program geared to enlighten the traditional attitudes of both nurses and hospital administrators was needed, but the poor financial status of the association seriously impeded progress. Dues had not been increased since 1946, and with markedly increased costs, the association had in effect less money with which to work. Delegates to NYSNA conventions defeated proposed dues increases for five consecutive years, and directed the board to cut programs as necessary to keep expenses from exceeding income.[25] Meanwhile, more and more requests for assistance on matters of employment came into headquarters from across the state.

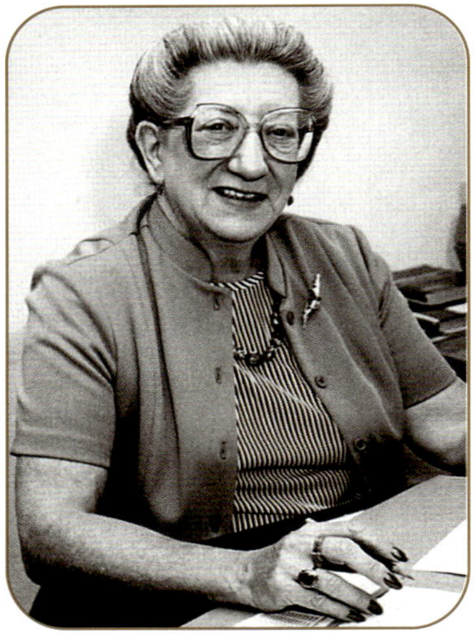

LEFT: Ruth Harper held the position of executive director of District 14 for twenty-six years (1957–1983). She was an active participant in NYSNA's Advisory Council and Bylaws Committee, and received NYSNA's Honorary Recognition and Membership Awards. Through her work with District 14 members employed by New York City's Department of Hospitals, she played a major role in forming the first bargaining unit.

REPRESENTING THE CITY NURSES: When New York City Mayor Robert Wagner developed a labor relations program for city employees, NYSNA carefully studied how the association could best ensure city-employed nurses a strong voice in workplace issues. In 1955 the city's newly adopted Career and Salary Plan reclassified nurses, and in effect downgraded instructors and many supervisors. After nurses requested assistance through Districts 13 and 14, NYSNA filed appeals on their behalf.[26]

This assistance to the more than three thousand Department of Hospitals nurses no doubt influenced NYSNA's board when it conducted a three-day workshop to develop association goals. The board spent a significant amount of time discussing implementation of a better employment conditions program, and the proposed goals included a strengthened Economic Security Program. The goals were adopted at a 1956 special meeting of the House of Delegates, along with a dues increase to finance the proposed programs. With this financial support, the board authorized employment of additional staff and special legal counsel to assist the New York City employed nurses.[27]

In 1957 a New York City report proposed an executive order to allow city employees to designate an exclusive representative in matters of employment.[28] At the 1957 convention, members again discussed the employment conditions program, and directed the board to outline specific steps to strengthen the program. In the wee hours of the following morning, board members prepared and adopted a statement which included a section on the purpose of the association's Economic Security Program and a list of specific steps to strengthen the program. While avoiding the inflammatory term "collective bargaining," the statement clearly provided for a "full-scale active economic security program," and directed "maximum support on all organizational levels to the New York City pilot program."[29] Following presentation of the statement to the House of Delegates, "President

"This is the same collective bargaining motion that we have had before us year after year, time after time . . . I thought we were going to wait until next year before we went into that fight again."

— *Anne Goodrich*[3]

Thompson stepped to the microphone and advised delegates that it was the proper time to debate the issue — and called for speakers. The silence was deadening. The President — an expression of wonderment on her face — repeated 'the time for debate is now.'" Following a single brief comment from the floor, the statement was unanimously adopted.[30]

The 1957 House of Delegates action, together with the 1949 change in the association's charter, allowed the association to expand its Economic Security Program and pursue formal representation of the New York City employed nurses. A three-day workshop, co-sponsored with the New York State School of Industrial and Labor Relations at Cornell University, was held to teach key concepts of labor relations to members and staff. The development of local units increased, and Associate Executive Secretary Marion Klappmeier joined four of the units in negotiation sessions with employers. In early 1958 NYSNA filed appeals and re-appeals to raise the salaries of New York City employed nurses by four grades, and a public relations campaign was conducted to build consumer support. Meetings were held with Mayor Wagner and other city officials, and in November 1959 an additional two-grade increase was approved. Though only 75 percent of the goal, the increase was celebrated. "All of this did not just happen. It came through intensive and prolonged activities . . . It is the professional way for professional nurses to achieve economic betterment."[31]

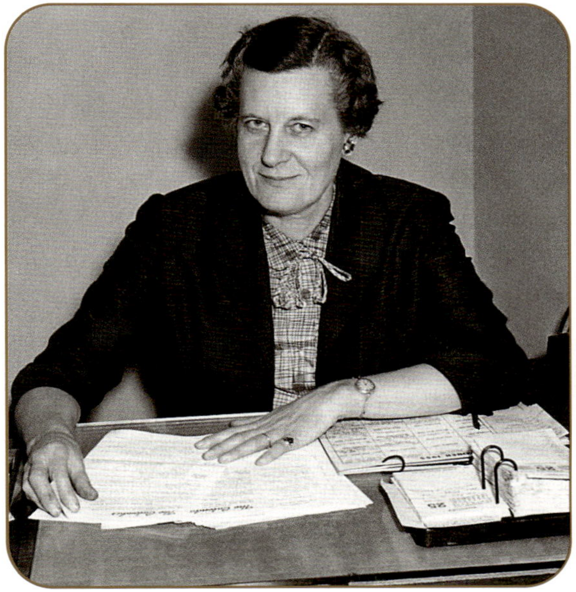

Olga Fessenden served as executive secretary of District 13 from 1955 to 1973. During her tenure, she participated in the early efforts of nurses employed by New York City's Department of Hospitals to be represented by NYSNA. *Photograph by Thomas Leigh Wood.*

In August 1958 NYSNA filed applications requesting that the association be named exclusive bargaining representative for staff nurses and supervisory nurses at the Department of Hospitals.[32] The applications were disputed by District Council No. 37, Department of Hospitals Employees of the American Federation of State, County and Municipal Employees, who charged that NYSNA was not a labor organization, and not "empowered by its internal regulations to negotiate collectively." A decision, however, cited the 1957 House of Delegates action and NYSNA's ongoing salary appeals on behalf of Department of Hospitals nurses, and ruled the objections without merit. Finally, in May 1960 NYSNA was officially designated as the exclusive bargaining representative for registered nurses employed by New York City's Department of Hospitals, the first time a U.S. governmental jurisdiction recognized a professional organization as a collective bargaining representative of nurses.[33] Executive Director Klappmeier paid tribute to all who contributed to the effort. "This recognition climaxed over three years of intensive, and often discouraging, work on the part of many people . . . a herculean job was done by districts 13 and 14. Innumerable meetings, conferences and telephone calls were only a part of the task. Getting designation cards to and from over 3000 nurses was a truly laborious job. But this is now all in the past, and the real challenge is the future."[34] The association had finally taken the momentous final step into the realm of collective bargaining. As the association moved forward, Klappmeier admitted to trepidation. "As I have said before, this whole New York City business scares me to death when I think of the time, personnel and wisdom it demands."[35] Nonetheless, she vowed that the association would meet the challenges ahead as best it could.

REORGANIZATION AND EXPERIMENTATION: LEGACIES OF THE NATIONAL NURSING COUNCIL: The successful cooperation of the national nursing organizations in the National Nursing Council during the war led to further study of the functions and structure of the six national nursing organizations. Raymond Rich Associates reported on their study of the organizations and offered recommendations for a restructured profession at ANA's 1946 convention.[36] NYSNA's Committee on the Structure Study discussed the report, and recommended the amalgamation of all the national organizations into one professional organization on a district-state-national basis. NYSNA's House of Delegates adopted the recommendation, but ANA's 1950 House of Delegates adopted a two-organization plan. This plan provided for the ANA, which accepted only nurses as members, and the National League for Nursing, composed of nurses, lay persons, and agency members. Staffing plans and bylaws were developed, and the new structure was adopted at ANA's 1952 convention.[37] NYSNA continued to favor a single organization on the state level, and formed a joint committee with the New York State League for Nursing to promote cooperation and work toward the goal of one professional state organization.[38] Throughout the decade, the New York State League for Nursing declined, and NYSNA became increasingly involved in nursing education issues. By 1960 the association was poised to assume leadership in nursing education in New York State.

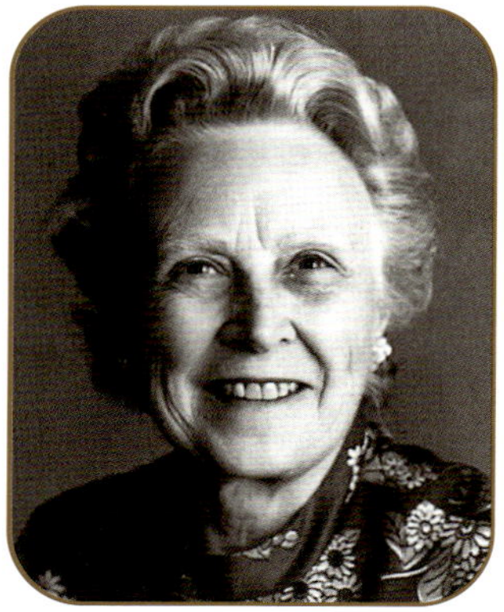

Mildred Montag initiated the nursing program at Adelphi College in 1943, and later served as a professor of nursing education at Teachers College, Columbia University, for over twenty years. Her prototype educational program accelerated nursing education into a two-year program which was markedly different from existing hospital and baccalaureate programs.

Another National Nursing Council project was a study on the nursing needs of society as reported in *Nursing for the Future* by Esther Lucile Brown. The study advocated that preparation of professional nurses belonged in institutions of higher learning, and called for a system of accreditation for schools of nursing. The Brown report spearheaded a movement for educational reform and support of the baccalaureate degree as the basic educational preparation for registered nurses began to build.

The joint boards of the six national nursing organizations formed the National Committee on the Improvement of Nursing Services (NCINS), directed by New York's own Marion Sheahan, to implement the Brown report. NCINS called for better preparation for faculty, administrative, and supervisory positions, more effective in-service education, additional practical nurses, and experimentation in nursing curricula, particularly in the development of two-year programs.[39] New York provided national leadership in developing experimental two-year programs. R. Louise McManus, head of the Department of Nursing at Teachers College, Columbia University, addressed NYSNA's 1950 Advisory Council and presented an experimental patient-centered curriculum based on a prototype educational program developed by Mildred Montag. The Advisory Council approved the proposed program, and urged discussion at the district level.[40]

Esther M. Thompson

1902 - 1990

Esther Thompson came to Rochester in 1943 as director of the nursing program in the Education Department of the University of Rochester. In the early 1950s Miss Thompson became involved in the activities of NYSNA as chair of the Conference Committee for the Improvement of Nursing Care for the People of New York State, where she utilized skills she had developed in research on the functions of nurses in the Rochester region.

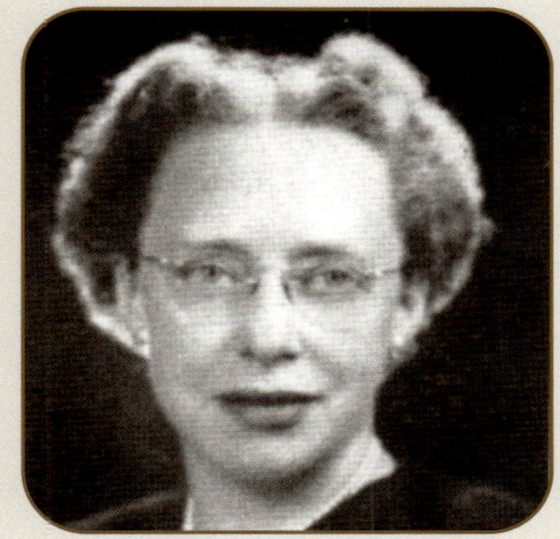

In the late 1940s, Miss Thompson attended the first National Training Laboratory Conference on Group Dynamics, and participated in subsequent intensive training experiences in group techniques. She put her group dynamics skills to good use when she was elected NYSNA president in 1955. She was responsible for initiating a three-day conference to identify association goals, and board minutes reported on "buzz sessions" and other small group activities. She led a successful campaign to raise association dues for the first time in ten years, and guided board members in developing the historic economic security proposal that was adopted at the 1957 convention.

Miss Thompson continued her involvement in NYSNA after the end of her presidency in 1959. As the association grappled with issues of nursing education in the 1960s, her commitment to baccalaureate nursing education and her skills in group dynamics were ongoing assets to the professional association.[1]

"It will only be another 49 years when we can have a centennial party."

— *Mary Delehanty*[4]

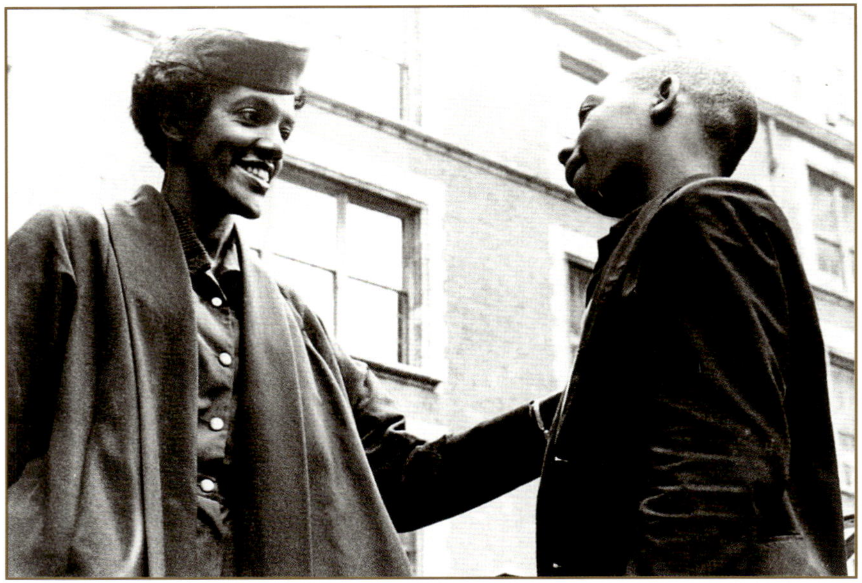

ABOVE: Public health nurses provided a wide spectrum of nursing services, including counseling. *Courtesy the Alumni Association of Harlem Hospital Center School of Nursing.*

The Board of Regents' Advisory Committee on Experimental Programs in Nursing also recommended experimentation in nursing curricula. In 1952 Orange County Community College inaugurated the state's first associate degree nursing program based on Montag's curriculum, one of seven nationwide. After five years of development, Orange County's curriculum was fully approved by the Department of Education, and by mid-1957, ninety-four New York associate degree graduates had passed the licensing examination, 65 percent with scores above the national average. All found immediate employment.[41] The associate degree system of nursing education proliferated nationwide, and by the end of the decade was accepted as a legitimate method of educational preparation for nurses.

BELOW: NYSNA's Men's Section advocated for full participation of men in the military nurse corps for many years. Edward Lyon of Kings Park, N.Y., shown here with ANA President Agnes Ohlson on the left and NLN President Ruth Freeman on the right, was the first male nurse ever commissioned in the U.S. Army Nurse Corps Reserve. *U.S. Army Photograph.*

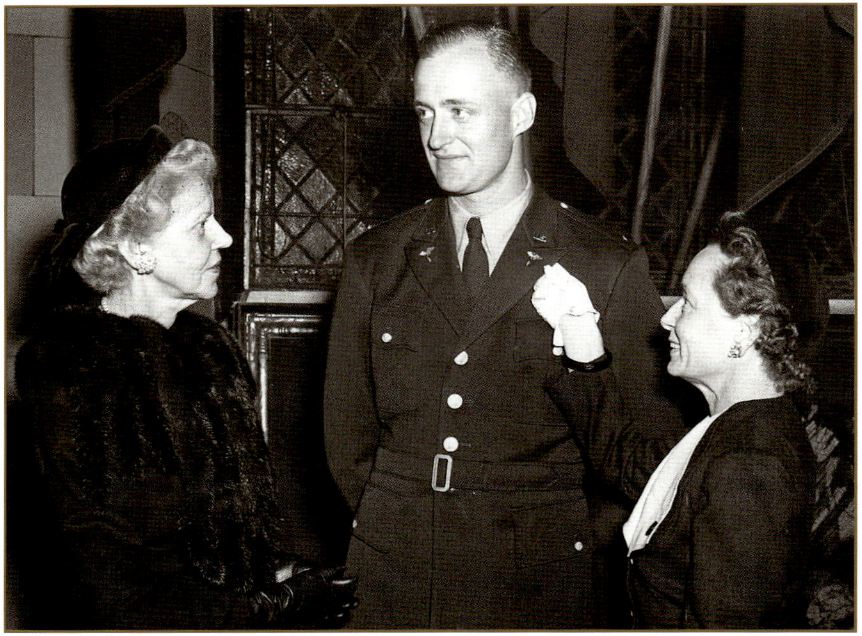

"Today as never before Membership in one's professional organization is important. Nurses have been silent and placid about their Profession for too long."

— *Ruth M. Brooks*[5]

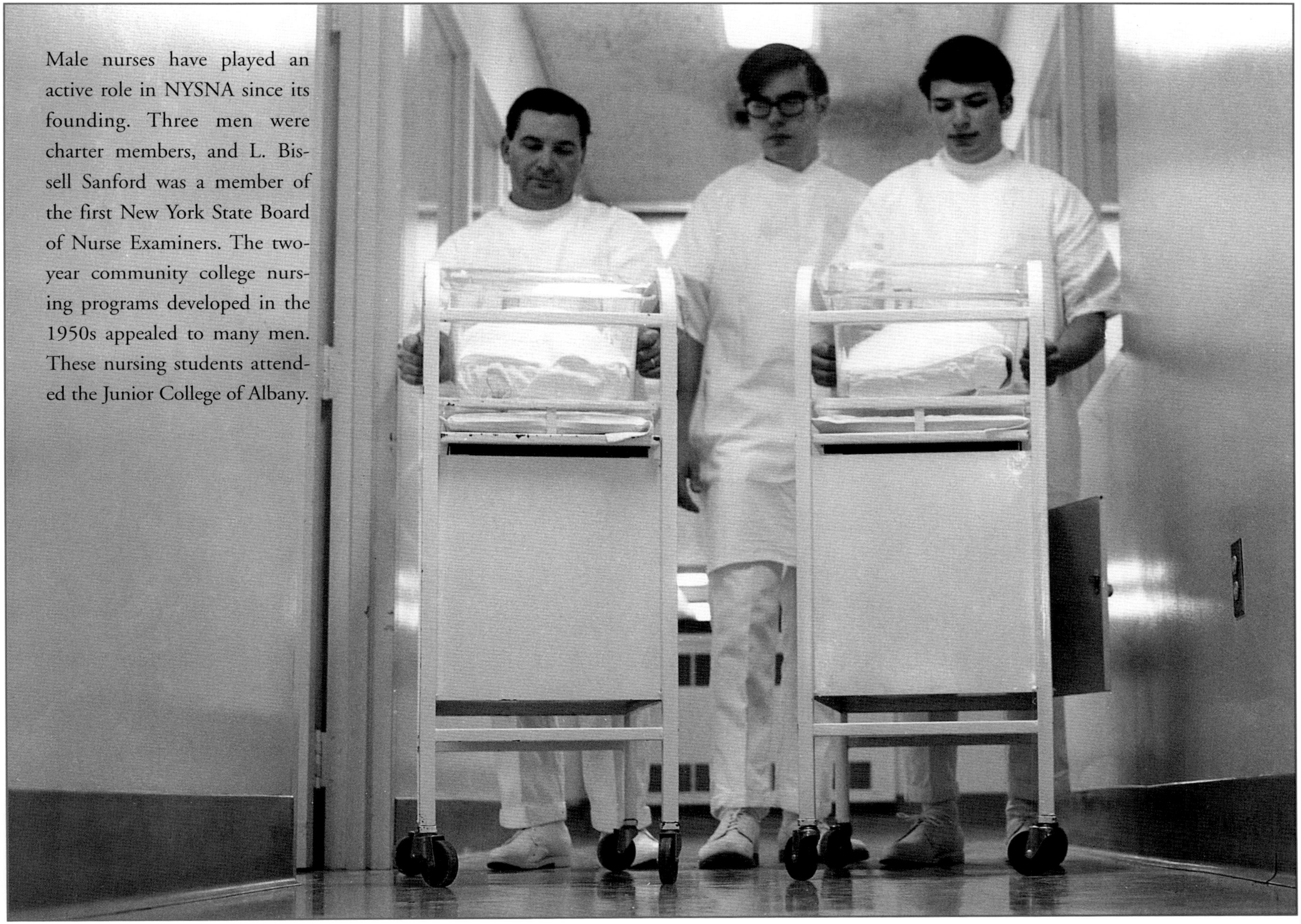

Male nurses have played an active role in NYSNA since its founding. Three men were charter members, and L. Bissell Sanford was a member of the first New York State Board of Nurse Examiners. The two-year community college nursing programs developed in the 1950s appealed to many men. These nursing students attended the Junior College of Albany.

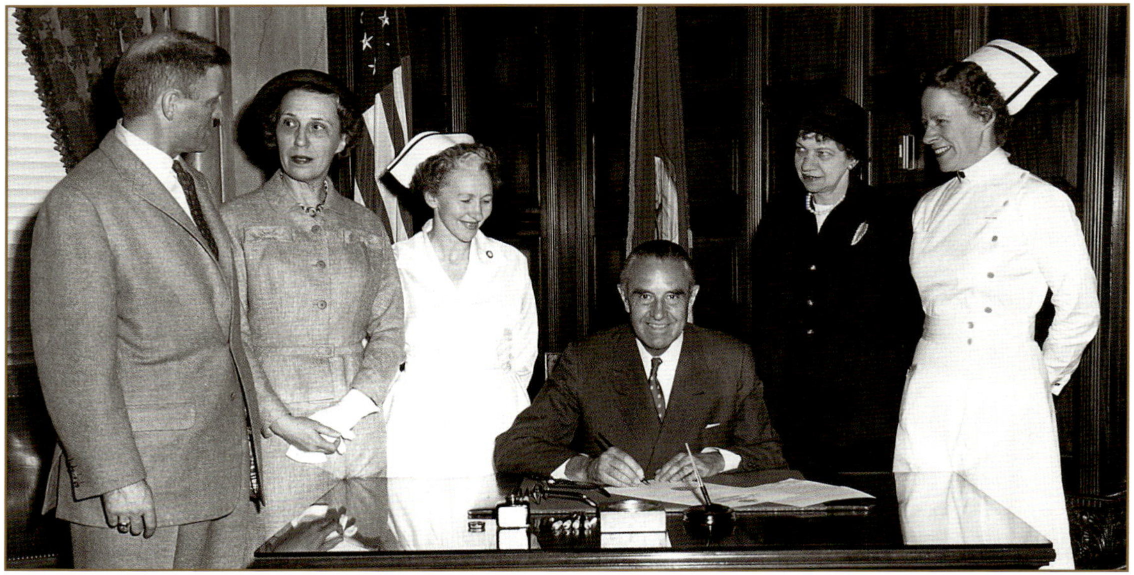

NYSNA sponsored legislation providing scholarships for nursing education beginning in 1951. In 1955 and 1956 Governor Harriman signed into law bills providing scholarships for basic and advanced nurse education. Harriman is shown here with, from left to right, NYSNA legal counsel Robert Jones, Executive Secretary Katherine Rehder, Legislative Committee member Mrs. Martin P. Cassidy, Secretary of the Board of Nurse Examiners Mary Ellen Manly, and Legislative Committee Chairperson Ruth Ogden.

A TIME OF TRANSITION: Declining membership and an unstable financial base stalled many NYSNA activities during the early 1950s. The association found itself in a vicious circle. Morale among nurses was poor, and no doubt contributed to declining membership. ". . . our hospitals are inadequately staffed and the nurses who remain are spread too thinly for the workload. Someone said recently, 'Young nurses won't take it; the older ones can't.' Even when we worked a 12-hour day we did not find our nurses so exhausted, so discouraged."[42] Yet, without a strong membership base financial resources were diminished and association activities designed to improve employment conditions and the morale and status of the staff nurse had to be curtailed. The Counseling and Placement Program, newly consolidated with the Registry Committee, continued with a reduction in staff and services. No fieldwork was done, referrals dropped, and a fee was imposed for some services.[43]

With the 1956 increase in dues, the association was able to once again build up its programs. Legal counsel Robert Jones monitored legislative issues, and the association successfully opposed many bills, supported minor modifications to the Nurse Practice Act, and sponsored scholarship legislation. There were a growing number of educational institutes and workshops sponsored by the sections to meet the increasing interest of nurses in continuing education, and the association participated in many multi-disciplinary groups studying the shortage of nurses and analyzing nursing functions.

The decade was, in fact, marked by experimentation and reflection on the state of the profession in a new postwar world. The movement toward baccalaureate and associate degree nursing education, the entry into collective bargaining, and the changes in nurses' scope of practice continued to be the focus of the association's work. During this transition period, association activities prepared NYSNA for new initiatives in the turbulent years ahead.

TEXT

1. Kalisch and Kalisch, *Advance of American Nursing,* 370; and Roberts, *American Nursing,* 488.

2. Wanda C. Hiestand, Eleanor K. Herrmann, and Elizabeth A. Shields, "Nursing Practice — Home, Hospital, and Battlefield," in *Prologue to Professionalism: A History of Nursing,* ed. M. Louise Fitzpatrick (Bowie, Md.: Brady Communications, 1983), 30.

3. Roberts, *American Nursing,* 495; Ruth Sleeper, "Nursing Care Throughout Fifty Years," *American Journal of Nursing* 50 (October 1950): 587–9.

4. Mabel Detmold, "We Set Our Sights," *New York State Nurse* 22 (October 1950): 2–3; and "Proceedings, Advisory Council of the New York State Nurses Association" (Albany, N.Y., 1950, stenotype transcript), 8.

5. "Proceedings, 46th Session and the Seventh Biennial Convention of the New York State Nurses Association" (New York, N.Y., 1951, stenotype transcript), 16–17.

6. Mary G. Phillips to Ellen Best, 11 July 1950, NYSNA Archives.

7. Board of Directors Minutes, NYSNA, 1 August 1950, NYSNA Archives.

8. "Advisory Council," 1950, 129.

9. "NYSNA Members Attend Four Defense Institutes," *New York State Nurse* 22 (December 1950): 5.

10. "NYSNA Asks That Nurses Respond to Army Appeal," *New York State Nurse* 23 (January 1951): 10.

11. "Proceedings, 47th Session of the New York State Nurses Association" (New York, N.Y., 1952, stenotype transcript), 120–21.

12. "Biennial Reports" (Albany, N.Y., 1959, mimeographed).

13. "Advisory Council," 1950, 128.

14. Robert H. Jones to Katherine E. Rehder, 11 May 1951, NYSNA Archives; and Board of Directors Minutes, NYSNA, 7 December 1950, NYSNA Archives.

15. "Seventh Biennial Convention," 24–25.

16. Robert H. Jones, "The Intravenous Therapy Problem," *New York State Nurse* 25 (January 1953): 11–14; Lillian Howell, "The Need of Nurse Training in Intravenous Therapy for Civil Defense," *New York State Nurse* 25 (January 1953): 9; and *The Professional Nurse — And Intravenous Procedures: The 1961 Opinion of New York State Attorney General* (Albany, N.Y.: NYSNA, 1961).

17. "Advisory Council," 1950, 72–74.

18. Ethel Mockler, "New York State Association Attacks Nursing Shortage with Progressive Plan," *Nursing World* 125 (April 1951): 145, 162–63.

19. Mary Perrone to Mabel Detmold, n.d., NYSNA Archives.

20. Mary Perrone, "General Duty Section, NYSNA," 1951, NYSNA Archives, 3.

21. "The NYSNA Golden Anniversary Convention," *Nursing World* 125 (December 1951): 564; and Lucille Notter, "The New York State Nurses Association Employment Conditions Program, 1942–55," *New York State Nurse* 27 (May 1955): 8–9.

22. "Seventh Biennial Convention," 199–201; Notter, "Employment Conditions Program," 9–10; and Ed Graham, "Convention Highlights," *New York State Nurse* 24 (November 1952): 3.

23. Minutes of Meeting of Special Committee on Economic Security, NYSNA, 13 May 1960, NYSNA Archives.

24. "Some Things Every Member Should Know: Executive Secretary Reports," *New York State Nurse* 27 (September 1955): 3; and Notter, "Employment Conditions Program," 6. Efforts were also successful in increasing private duty nursing fees through a "very fine publicity campaign. The New York City Hospitals — the largest and best-organized group in the country — had attempted to deny the nurses their rights in the matter of salaries. The complete defeat of the hospitals in the battle they chose to make will undoubtedly serve as a warning to other employing groups across the country." ("Annual Reports, 1951–1952" [Albany, N.Y., 1952, mimeographed].)

25. "How Would You Vote?" *New York State Nurse* 28 (September 1956): 10–11; and Notter, "Employment Conditions Program," 10. NYSNA membership fluctuated throughout the decade. It increased in 1958 to 14,594, then dropped. By 1960 membership was 13,079, lower than it was in 1950, despite various membership promotion activities. In 1955 NYSNA dues were lower than those of forty-two other states, and other state nurses' associations of comparable size had staff of eight to eighteen, while NYSNA employed only four full-time professional staff.

26. Marion M. Klappmeier, The New York State Nurses Association Acts, 7 July 1960, NYSNA Archives.

27. "NYSNA Immediate Long-Term Goals," *New York State Nurse* 29 (March 1957): 3; Board of Directors Minutes, 6–7 March 1957, NYSNA Archives; and "Let's Measure Intangibles," *New York State Nurse* 29 (September 1957): 4. The two day workshop was held at Grasslands Hospital in Westchester County, and appears to be the first instance of long range planning in a retreat-like format. (Board of Directors Minutes, 13–15 June 1956, NYSNA Archives.) Dues were increased from $7 to $10 per capita. ANA and district dues were in addition to this amount. ("A Happy Compromise," *New York State Nurse* 28 [November 1956]: 1.)

28. Klappmeier, The Association Acts; and Special Committee on Economic Security.

29. "Statement from Board of Directors to House of Delegates," *New York State Nurse* 29 (November 1957): 5.

30. "A Professional Experience," *New York State Nurse* 29 (November 1957): 4; and "Proceedings, 49th Session of the New York State Nurses Association" (Syracuse, N.Y. 1957, stenotype transcript), 50.

31. Katherine E. Rehder. "An Eventful Biennium," *New York State Nurse* 31 (September 1959): 13–14; "Major Victory Scored by NYSNA Economic Security Program," *New York State Nurse* 32 (January 1960): 2; and Special Committee on Economic Security.

32. The association also filed applications to represent staff and supervisory public health nurses at the Department of Health. However, certification for these units was not granted. (Special Committee on Economic Security.)

33. "Nurses Choose NYSNA . . . As Exclusive Bargaining Representative," *New York State Nurse* 32 (September 1960): 5–6; and Olga C. Fessenden and Ruth W. Harper, "Operation: Pilot Project," *New York State Nurse* 33 (March 1961): 6–7.

34. Klappmeier, The Association Acts.

35. Marion M. Klappmeier to Ruth W. Harper and Olga C. Fessenden, 19 October 1959, NYSNA Archives.

36. Roberts, *American Nursing,* 578. The six organizations were the ANA, the NLNE, the NOPHN, the National Association of Colored Graduate Nurses, the American Association of Industrial Nurses, and the Association of Collegiate Schools of Nursing.

37. "Structure Program in 1950," *American Journal of Nursing* 50 (April 1950): 230–31; and Donahue, *Nursing, The Finest Art,* 329. ANA's 1948 House of Delegates agreed it preferred one national nursing organization, to include non-nurse members, as did the NLNE and the NOPHN. The inclusion of non-nurse members, however, jeopardized ANA's membership in the International Council of Nurses. ("Structure Committee," *New York State Nurse* 20 [August–September 1948]: 25.)

38. "Convention Summary," *New York State Nurse* 25 (November 1953): 5. This discussion was far from new. In 1922, NYSNA had studied the amalgamation of the three state nursing organizations. ("Seventh Biennial Convention," 15.)

39. Roberts, *American Nursing,* 473–4, 503–5. Ninety percent of nursing programs, however, were still apprentice programs owned and operated by hospitals. Kalisch and Kalisch, *Advance of American Nursing,* 412.

40. "Advisory Council," 1950, 112–26; Board of Directors Minutes, 12 October 1950, NYSNA Archives; and "Idea + Experiment = New Program," *New York State Nurse* 29 (September 1957): 7. New York State's university system, established in 1948, provided for the development of two-year community technical colleges. Many educators felt that nurses could be adequately prepared in less than the traditional thirty-six months, and believed the growing demand for nursing services justified experimentation. The five-year research project developed and evaluated two-year nursing programs in seven community colleges. (Kalisch and Kalisch, *Advance of American Nursing,* 411–12.)

41. "Idea + Experiment," 7–8.

42. "Seventh Biennial Convention," 17.

43. "Headquarters Report," *New York State Nurse* 25 (September 1953): 25; and "NYSNA Board," *New York State Nurse* 31 (September 1959): 16. In 1959 new policies were adopted that restricted counseling and placement services to members, new graduates, and instances of "critical need."

FEATURES

MABEL DETMOLD

1. Mabel Detmold, *The Brownstones of Turtle Bay Gardens* (New York, N.Y.: The East 49th Street Association, 1964).

PROTOTYPE LOCAL UNIT AT NATHAN LITTAUER HOSPITAL

1. Mary D. Burr, "Strength Through Unity," *New York State Nurse* 33 (March 1961): 14; and "The Local Unit-Key to Your Economic Security," *New York State Nurse* 33 (March 1961): 8-9.

2. Margaret Rooney to Registered Professional Nurses Employed by Nathan Littauer Hospital, Memo, 13 February 1976, NYSNA Archives. Rooney was the director of the Economic Security Program.

3. "A General Duty Unit Acts," *New York State Nurse* 30 (September 1958): 10–11. The agreed upon annual salary was $3,003. NYSNA employment standards recommended minimum starting salaries of $4,000–$4,400. ("Employment Standards for General Duty and Head Nurses of New York State" [Albany, N.Y., 1957, mimeographed].)

4. Margaret Rooney to Nursing Practitioners, Nathan Littauer Hospital, Memo, 9 January 1976 and 3 March 1976, NYSNA Archives.

5. Nathan Littauer/Extended Care Facility Summary of Negotiations, 8 June 1976, NYSNA Archives; and Littauer Hospital Nurses to Hold Public Rally Friday, Press Release, 3 November 1976, NYSNA Archives.

ESTHER M. THOMPSON

1. "Esther M. Thompson," in *Professionalization of Nursing in New York State: Oral History Interviews with Six Leaders Who Helped to Advance the Mission of NYSNA,* ed. Elizabeth Carter and Jane Fielding (Guilderland, N.Y.: NYSNA, 1988), 50-55.

EXCERPTS

1. "47th Session," 174.

2. Ibid.

3. Ibid., 178.

4. Ibid., 45.

5. "Ruth M. Brooks," in *Professionalization of Nursing in New York State: Oral History Interviews with Six Leaders Who Helped to Advance the Mission of NYSNA,* ed. Elizabeth Carter and Jane Fielding (Guilderland, N.Y.: NYSNA, 1988), 98.

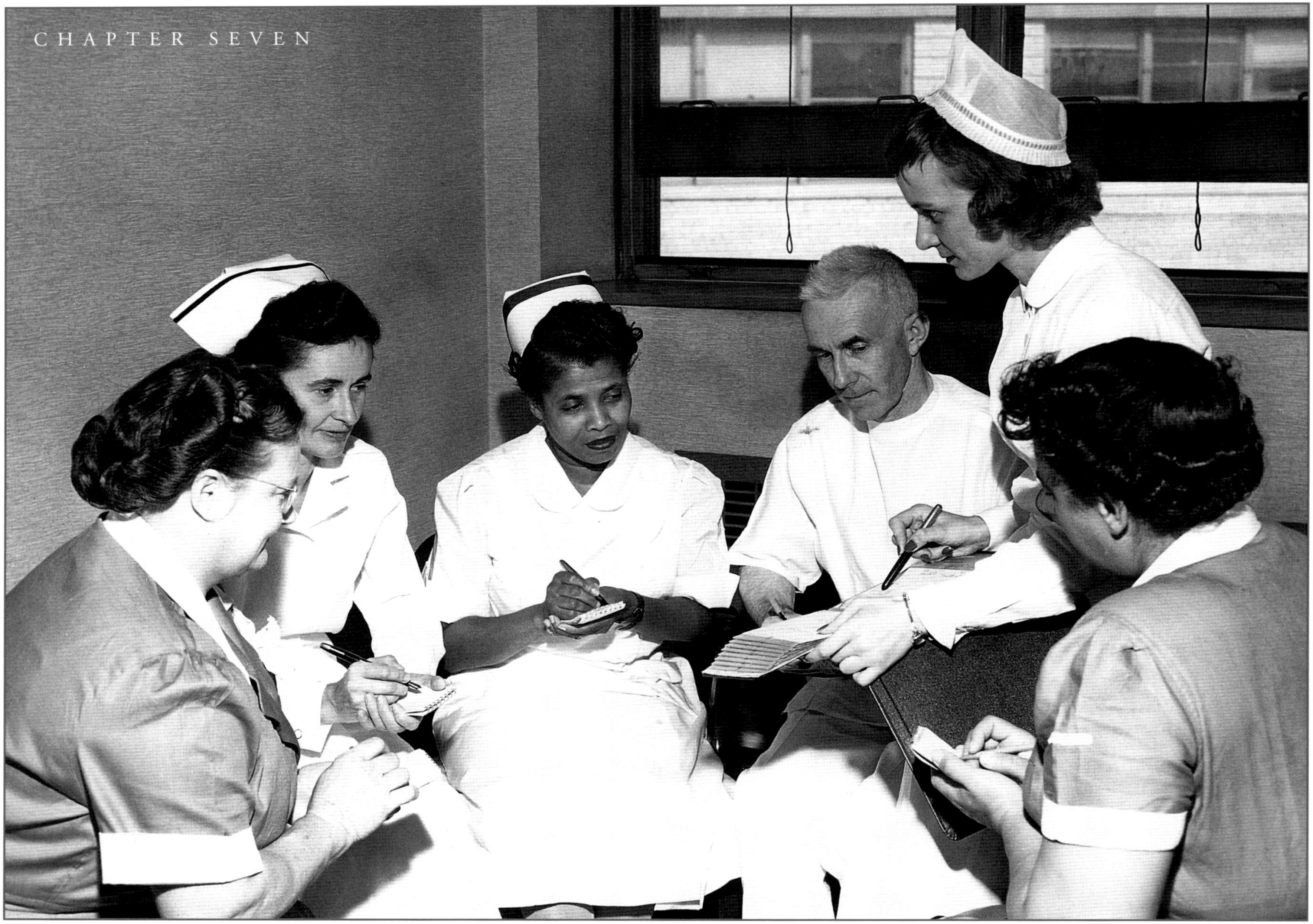

CHAPTER SEVEN

CHANGE AND CONTROVERSY
COURAGE AND CONVICTION
1960 ~ 1969

The association entered the 1960s facing many challenges, as the postwar nursing shortage continued unabated. Changing nursing functions required new ways of assisting nurses to maintain their clinical competence and close examination of the educational system that was preparing nurses. "Professional nurses now are expected to do and understand many things that their counterparts of 25 years ago either never heard of (because nobody had) or considered the physician's prerogative. Yet the new technical skills are easy to acquire compared with the ability to exercise judgments incident to use of these skills. A nurse must have psychological and physiological insights of considerable depth to observe and report patient reactions adequately to the doctor who so seldom now can stay long by the bedside, or to take emergency action as required."[1] The time had again come for the profession to confront critical issues: nursing education, new trends in health care, the continuing shortage, the role of subsidiary workers, staffing patterns, and "What is meant by 'nurse'?"[2] These were the old questions the association had faced time and again, now shaped by the unique forces of the new decade.

FACING PAGE: Members of the nursing team planned patient care during ward conferences. *Courtesy Lambertsen Collection, Foundation of NYSNA Archives.*

PLANNING FOR THE FUTURE: LET THE NURSE NURSE: A societal focus on planning — urban planning, planning for expanded highway systems, and planning for adequate educational resources for "baby boomers" — affected the nursing community, and the decade of the 1960s was marked by intensive study and planning. The growth of graduate nursing education programs in the 1950s created highly educated leaders who brought new skills and methods of study, evaluation, and planning to the work of the association.

The first of many NYSNA-sponsored conferences during the 1960s was held in March 1960 at Arden House in Harriman, New York, to study the nursing situation and plan for the future. President Notter noted that "today's plans must be for a future shaped by rapid change in the immediate past, and by even more rapid change to come."[3] Leaders urged conference participants to speculate about the future, and the kind of nurses that would be needed in 1970. Recommendations served as the basis of a comprehensive program adopted by the Board of Directors, which included promoting in-service and continuing education programs, implementing ANA's Functions, Standards, and Qualifications, encouraging research, developing a mechanism to recognize clinical excellence, improving the general welfare of nurses through the Economic Security Program, strengthening diploma schools, establishing new associate and baccalaureate schools, and eliminating non-nursing functions to "let the nurse nurse."[4] This first Arden House Conference set an ambitious agenda for both the state and district associations.[5]

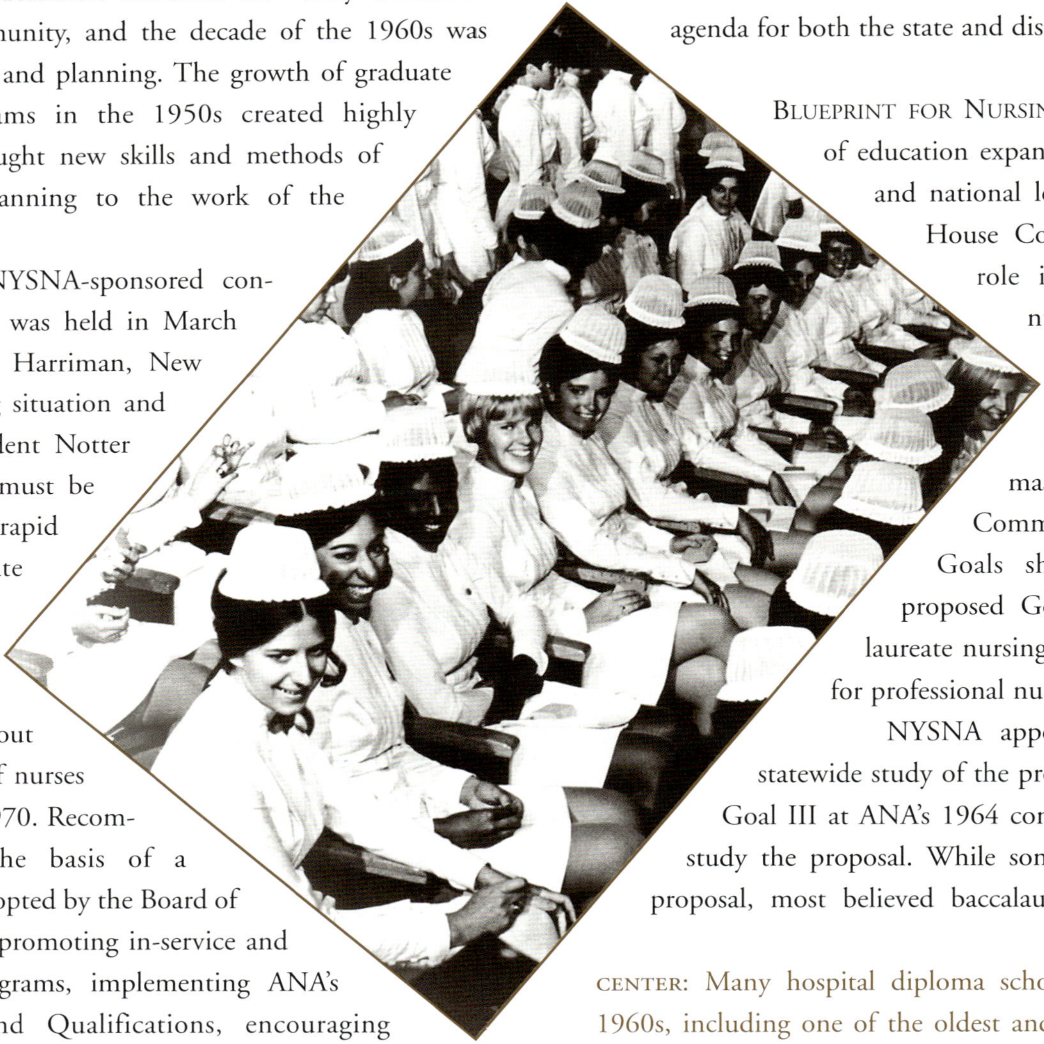

BLUEPRINT FOR NURSING EDUCATION: Nursing's scrutiny of education expanded dramatically at both the state and national levels in the 1960s and the Arden House Conference focused NYSNA on its role in nursing education. Trends in nursing education were changing, with diploma schools in decline, and an increasing number of associate degree, baccalaureate, and master's programs. Nonetheless, ANA's Committee on Current and Long-Term Goals shocked the profession when it proposed Goal III, the promotion of baccalaureate nursing education as the basic foundation for professional nursing.[6]

NYSNA appointed a committee to plan for statewide study of the proposal in preparation for action on Goal III at ANA's 1964 convention, and held a conference to study the proposal. While some participants disagreed with the proposal, most believed baccalaureate education was necessary to

CENTER: Many hospital diploma schools of nursing closed during the 1960s, including one of the oldest and most revered. Bellevue School of Nursing's last class, the class of 1969, is shown here. *Courtesy Bellevue Alumnae Association.*

"We believe that planning for nursing is one of the most important tasks facing the profession today. The work being done at the local level is crucial to the development of an overall plan at the State level."

— *Mildred Schmidt*[1]

prepare nurses for increasingly complex and demanding functions, and to "keep in step" with current societal trends toward collegiate education. Following the conference, district nurses' association representatives promoted discussions in the districts.[7]

Goal III raised many emotionally charged questions and generated a great deal of controversy, resulting in postponement of further action by ANA's Board of Directors. A large majority of practicing nurses were diploma graduates concerned about the impact of the proposal on their own careers, and there were questions about the fate of diploma schools and associate degree programs.[8] Nonetheless, in a surprise move, delegates to ANA's 1964 convention approved a recommendation to "work toward baccalaureate education for future practitioners . . ." Shortly thereafter, ANA's board adopted a Position Paper on Nursing Education which embodied the recommendations in Goal III. This was ANA's first definitive statement on nursing education.[9]

"There is a practical place for a marriage between education and service. The teaching should be more realistic, and there should be more hands and bridges across to the work situation."

— *Frances Purdy*[2]

NYSNA moved swiftly to act on the position paper's recommendations. A Committee on Education was formed to establish the association's leadership role "during this great transitional period in nursing education."[10] The committee sponsored another Arden House Conference where representatives of nursing education and nursing service discussed the transition to baccalaureate education and recommended that immediate steps be taken to implement ANA's position paper.[11]

NYSNA's board and Committee on Education agreed that studies had adequately appraised the current status of nursing, and action was now needed. The board directed the committee to prepare a "blueprint" — "a concise and definitive plan of action" — for orderly transition from the current nursing education system to that outlined in the position paper. The blueprint, developed under the leadership of Associate Director Veronica Driscoll, outlined a plan designed to meet the nursing needs of the people of New York by educating nurses in institutions of higher learning. It called for a plan to be completed by 1972 for the transfer of all nursing education programs in New York to institutions of higher learning, and an immediate halt to the establishment of new diploma and practical nurse programs. Associate degree education was proposed as the minimum preparation for "beginning generalized nursing practice," and baccalaureate education as minimum preparation for "professional nursing practice." The plan vested primary responsibility for implementation in community planning groups, although NYSNA and the districts were also assigned vital roles.[12]

The blueprint was widely distributed and, as expected, received mixed reactions. President Notter predicted the difficulties ahead. "New York State nurses are taking responsible action in shaping the future of nursing. They are doing this despite the problems involved because they believe that this action is appropriate and necessary to meet the future nursing needs of the people of New York State . . . Those who do not understand will be fearful, and we must do all we can to help them understand; but we cannot wait

Eleanor C. Lambertsen . . . Speaking for Nursing

Eleanor Lambertsen was the primary spokesperson for NYSNA's positions during the 1960s. Dr. Lambertsen was a member of ANA's Committee on Education when the 1965 position paper was prepared, and consultant to NYSNA's Committee on Education which developed the "Blueprint." She was a frequent speaker at NYSNA meetings and provided expert testimony at the 1966 fact-finding sessions regarding NYSNA's efforts to secure an appropriate contract for nurses employed in New York City's Department of Hospitals. She subsequently served as consultant to NYSNA's Special Committee to Study the Nurse Practice Act, and was chairperson of NYSNA's first Council on Nursing Research. She received NYSNA's Honorary Recognition Award in 1982. In 1965 she delivered an address at NYSNA's convention on the controversial subject of the future of nursing education.

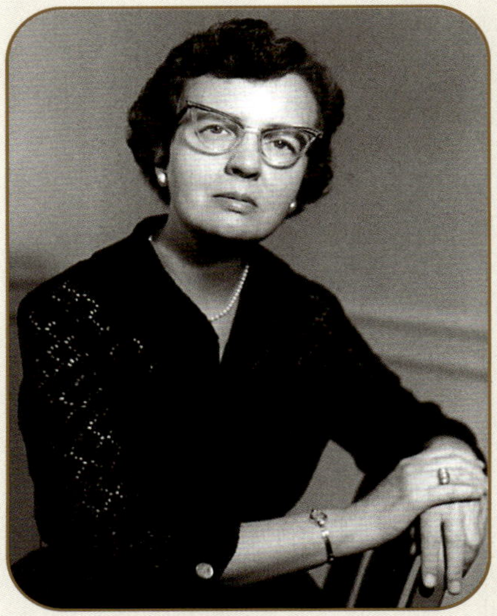

ABOVE: *Courtesy the Lambertsen Collection, Foundation of NYSNA Archives.*

"Is one of our problems that of reinforcing our already well established beliefs about these systems? . . . Emotional overtones cloud objective appraisal . . . Major changes are essential. But an inescapable element is an attitude favorable to change . . . The role of nursing in the changing social order places increasing responsibility on nurses in case finding, prevention, rehabilitation, and supportive services as well as therapeutic services . . . our desperate need is for nurses who are more broadly prepared than narrowly prepared — nurses who can move effectively in nursing services from situation to situation and not be bound by the routines, mores and traditions of one particular employment situation. Nurses who can establish precedent rather than conform to the immediacy of the situation . . . How much longer are we going to continue to debate the virtues of the various systems of nursing education in isolation? Our greatest single responsibility is to recognize that change is not only imperative but inevitable."[1]

until everyone understands or agrees with us, pleasant as this would be. We are not in a popularity contest; we are committed to a difficult but reasonable goal — the proper preparation of the nurses of the future — and we must move toward this goal by making use of the most effective means available.

"We may sometimes have been hesitant to use our leadership, but we have a social responsibility to do so where the health and welfare of the people are concerned. With faith in ourselves and the courage of our convictions we will take the steps needed to insure that the public will have the quality of nursing care it will require in the years to come."[13]

Although a large majority of participants in NYSNA's conferences and meetings had endorsed the move to baccalaureate education, the blueprint's concrete plan for implementation, which included target dates, alarmed many nurses. Opponents of the plan believed implementation of the blueprint would immediately exacerbate the existing nursing shortage and necessitate changes in licensing requirements. Furthermore, they charged that the costs of baccalaureate education would affect not only nursing students, but patients and taxpayers as well, and they were concerned about the morale of diploma and associate degree graduates if these programs were eliminated or viewed as non-professional.[14] The Hospital Association of New York State (HANYS), too, expressed its displeasure with the blueprint, charging it was "completely unrealistic and unsound," "centered on the personal status and educational prestige of the nurse," and "not related to the bedside care of the patient." Although the NYSNA membership remained divided in its response to the blueprint, it united in a vigorous response to HANYS' assertions, particularly denouncing the contention that nursing faculty need not have even baccalaureate education.[15]

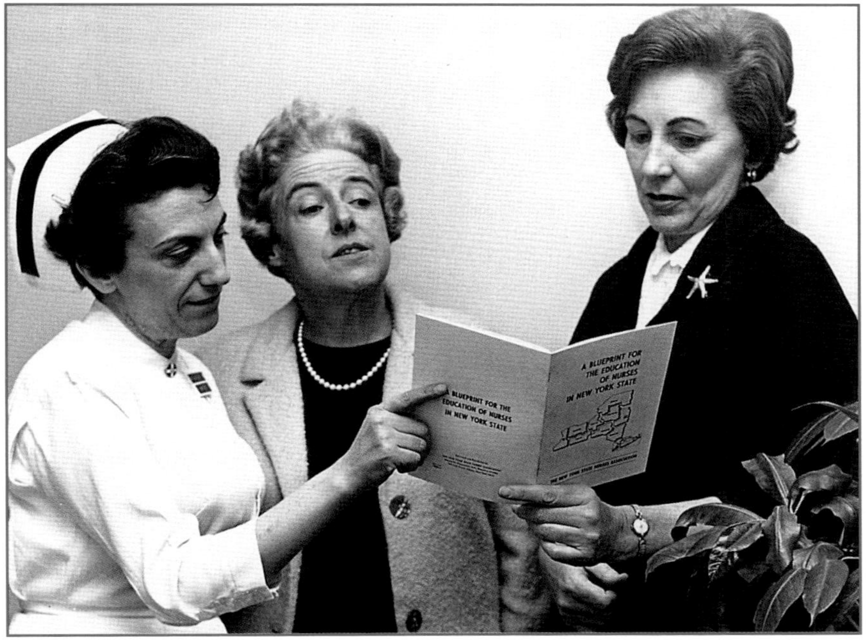

NYSNA members studied and discussed NYSNA's plan for nursing education in New York State known as the "Blueprint." *Courtesy the District 14 Collection, Foundation of NYSNA Archives.*

NYSNA moved forward to complete its responsibilities as assigned by the blueprint, developing a plan for assistance to practical nurses, associate degree graduates, and diploma graduates in seeking advanced preparation, and compiling lists of schools and available scholarships. Districts were challenged to secure both professional and public understanding, and to establish community planning groups. By October 1969, however, only five such groups had been formed, and the development of a statewide planning council was delayed. Already, implementation was behind schedule.[16] Despite several years of discussion, the proposed change in nursing education was considered radical, and the blueprint was pushing it to happen all too quickly. Many nurses were just not ready to abandon so rapidly the old, traditional pattern of nursing education.

A New Era for Economic Security: The 1960 certification to represent over three thousand New York City employed nurses marked a shift in focus of the Economic Security Program. Instead of concentrating on developing local units, the program poured its resources into representing the nurses employed by the city's Department of Hospitals, and sought representation of large numbers of nurses employed by the Veterans Administration (VA) hospitals.

Scarcely a week following certification to represent nurses employed by the Department of Hospitals, a Special Committee on Economic Security

> "It is difficult for the city hospitals
> to hold their nurses in the competitive market . . .
> It is a vicious cycle.
> The less nurses you have, the less you can attract."
>
> — *Mary Mullen*[3]

met to consider the implications for the total Economic Security Program. Aware that labor unions were eager to take over representation, and recognizing the potential effect of the New York City program on other cities around the state, the committee recommended an all-out commitment of substantial amounts of time, money, and effort to effectively represent the "city nurses." The committee reaffirmed the value and focus of the Economic Security Program, and raised questions about the possibilities of forming alliances with labor unions and using tactics such as "token strikes" and mass resignations — questions that would remain relevant and controversial for decades.[17]

The association acted quickly to organize representation of the city nurses. Staff planned intensive educational programs, hired consultants to assist with organization and membership promotion, developed and implemented an organizational structure, published a monthly newsletter, *The Spotlight,* and instituted an experimental payroll deduction system.[18] On May 9, 1961 — a full year after certification — the first negotiation session with New York City representatives was held. The nurses were represented by NYSNA Associate Director Marion Klappmeier, attorney Robert Jones, and NYSNA's newly hired consultant on civil service.[19] After four sessions, all parties agreed on a contract that provided salary upgrades and increases in shift differentials.[20]

By NYSNA's convention in 1961, most of the New York City public hospitals had formed staff nurse units and supervisory nurse units, the Executive Council was formed, and President Notter reported that "The economic security program has grown by leaps and bounds and could easily keep several additional staff busy."[21] The association secured office space at 31 Union Square West and in 1962 hired Emma Torchia to work exclusively with the city nurses. Torchia instituted classes for unit representatives on the handling of grievances, and grew increasingly busy providing information and representing nurses — both members and non-members — at grievance hearings.[22]

While the program was flourishing in New York City, the eighteen active upstate local units were in decline, although during 1960–1961 Marion Klappmeier and Veronica Driscoll traveled over twenty thousand miles organizing local units and negotiating with employers on their behalf.[23] Many of these local units encountered tremendous resistance from employers. A provision of the New York State Labor Relations Act which exempted non-profit voluntary hospitals from the mandate to engage in collective bargaining constituted a major barrier to early program growth. At its meeting during the 1961 convention, NYSNA's General Duty Section urged the association to continue to pursue an amendment to the law which would remove the exemption.[24] In 1963 a NYSNA supported bill was

LUCILLE E. NOTTER

1907 - 1993

Lucille Notter was NYSNA's first doctorally prepared president. Although most well known for her interest in and promotion of nursing research as the editor of *Nursing Research,* she was also an educator and public health nursing administrator. She was an extremely active member of District 13, serving as its president from 1952 to 1956, and in other capacities too numerous to mention. Elected president of NYSNA in 1959, she subsequently served eight additional years on the Board of Directors.

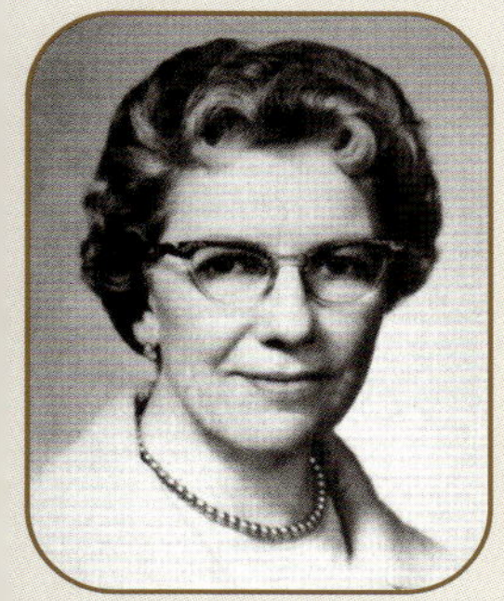

Dr. Notter was committed to collegiate education and career mobility for nurses, and used her role as NYSNA president to promote the advancement of nursing education. She guided the association in planning for the future in the historic 1960 Arden House Conference, contributed to the development and implementation of the "Blueprint," and was a strong supporter of association activities to improve conditions of employment. An eloquent speaker and prolific writer, Dr. Notter motivated and inspired. "The next ten years are going to be ten of the most exciting, most challenging, and most crucial ones for nursing. We cannot be content to be the victims of the winds of change and the resulting demands for services; we must assume responsible leadership, in cooperation with other health professions, for determining the proper direction of nursing action for the good of society."[1]

During an oral history interview in 1988, Dr. Notter advised nurses. "You need to be a professional person, secure in your knowledge, secure in your values, secure in knowing what is right and wrong and getting up and saying so . . . "[2] In 1980 NYSNA conferred upon Lucille Notter its highest award, Honorary Recognition, for the vision, inspiration, and courage she provided to professional nurses everywhere.[3]

ABOVE RIGHT: *Photograph by the Frumkin Studio.*

MARION M. KLAPPMEIER

Marion Klappmeier was hired as NYSNA's assistant executive secretary in 1955. In that position she provided assistance to NYSNA's sections, and led the Economic Security Program. When Katherine Rehder resigned in 1963, Ms. Klappmeier assumed the position of executive director, and served in that capacity until her retirement in 1969.

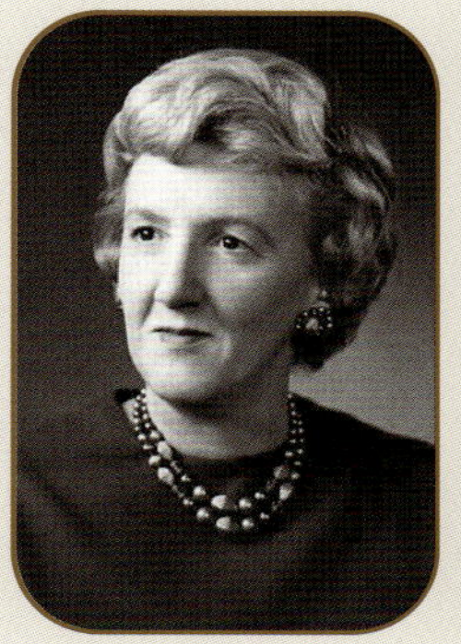

Marion Klappmeier was a graduate of the Russell Sage College School of Nursing, and held a master's degree in nursing service administration from Columbia University. She served on many boards of directors and committees connected with the health professions. She provided national leadership by serving on ANA's Board of Directors and Economic and General Welfare Committee. Ms. Klappmeier was commended for her wisdom, perseverance, and foresight. Under her leadership NYSNA focused on the development of an Economic Security Program "designed both for the present and for the changes and challenges of the future."[1] Other noteworthy accomplishments during her tenure included the establishment of a Council on Nursing Practice, the establishment and strengthening of liaison activities with allied organizations, and the development of educational offerings. Her first report to the membership expressed the heart of her directorship. "Many major issues face both the nursing profession and the association which is the spokesman for the profession. These must be recognized and faced up to with courage and wisdom. Most important, nurses must be strong enough to make their own decisions and take their proper place in today's society . . . Today, and tomorrow, and the day after tomorrow, do indeed need to be a time of reappraisal, both for the professional association and for each individual nurse. Only as we re-appraise and re-evaluate can we be prepared to make decisions with the wisdom required of us . . . What can be accomplished in the future depends, in the last analysis, upon the relative value nurses place on their profession and their professional association."[2]

passed that extended collective bargaining rights to employees of non-profit institutions in cities with populations over one million, and in 1965 the exemption was removed for all non-profit hospitals in the state.[25] Meanwhile, some nurses were fired for trying to form units, while others encountered refusals to bargain, delay tactics, and broken promises.[26] One hospital refused to meet with nurses and NYSNA representatives, then raised salaries 2¢ per hour, stating that salary increases were more desirable than other fringe benefits. "This is a fine example of the outmoded paternalistic attitude . . . which is an insult to the intelligence and dignity of employees . . . Decisions as these have a shattering effect on the morale of nurses, who on one hand have the responsibility of life and death, but on the other, are not even given the courtesy of expressing an opinion on matters which personally affect them."[27] Refused the right to negotiate, staff and unit members often turned to publicity to develop community support. Some units suffered from a lack of leadership because of the time and effort involved, local politics, and "personal abuse."[28] Discouraged, local units weakened, and many disbanded.

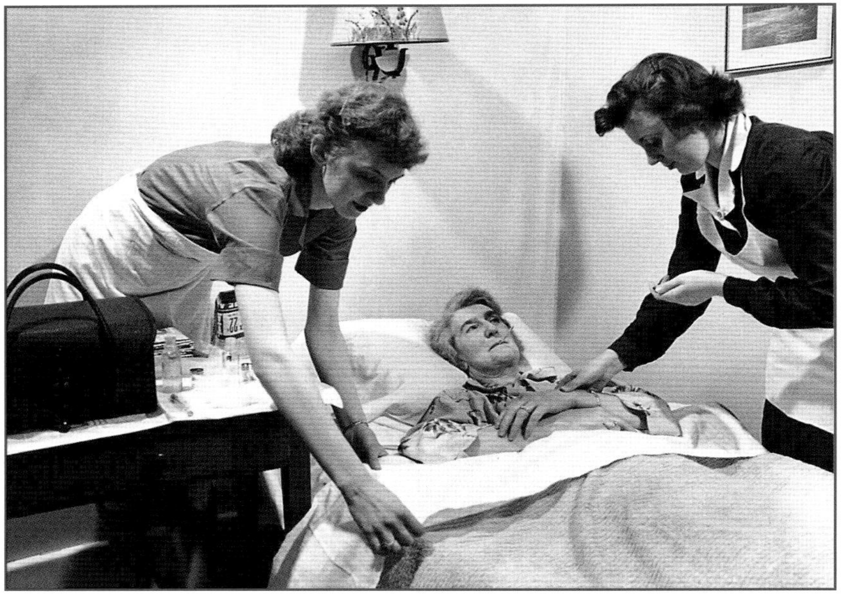

As medicine advanced and the population aged, more elderly required nursing care and constituted a significant proportion of the case loads of public health nurses. *Courtesy Ellis Hospital School of Nursing Collection, Foundation of NYSNA Archives.*

In 1962 President John F. Kennedy issued an executive order which created an employee relations program for federal employees. The association initiated a membership drive targeted at federally employed nurses, and staff visited all thirteen VA hospitals in New York to provide information and distribute designation cards. NYSNA received signed cards from a majority of nurses at both the Brooklyn and Bronx VA hospitals, becoming the first state nurses' association to request exclusive recognition for VA employed nurses.

Action on the request was delayed when the VA raised questions regarding ANA's status as a professional organization versus an employee organization, and whether there was a conflict of interest if nurses in VA management also served as ANA officers. Months of discussions between ANA and the VA followed, but the VA held to its restrictive interpretation of the conflict of interest provision. Because of the limitations the VA policy would impose on represented VA nurses' participation in association leadership positions, ANA advised NYSNA to withdraw its requests for recognition. Although gravely concerned about the affect of withdrawal on VA nurses who had expressed interest in representation by NYSNA, and on program growth and membership efforts, the association believed it had no other recourse than to comply with ANA's directive.[29]

ANA continued discussions with the VA, and over the next few years the VA modified its conflict of interest interpretation. By 1968 several states had been granted exclusive recognition to represent nurses at VA hospitals.

The Nurses at Westchester Square Hospital

The story of the nurses at Westchester Square Hospital is in some ways typical of local unit development. Precedent-setting elements of the story, however, make it truly extraordinary. The unit developed much like other early local units. In September 1961 nurses at Westchester Square Hospital in the Bronx sent a letter to NYSNA requesting representation of thirty-three of the thirty-six registered nurses employed by the hospital, becoming the first request for a local unit in District 13. The nurses were "greatly disturbed," and identified the standard two-week vacation, few holidays, and the absence of sick leave, standardization of pay, retirement plan, and regular increments as the most urgent problems. NYSNA staff met with the nurses, after which the nurses formed and organized a local unit, elected officers, and signed cards designating NYSNA as their chosen representative for purposes of collective bargaining. The unit's first officers were H. Lucile Crossen, Ona Morrison, Josephine Ryan, and Eileen Torpey. The Westchester Square unit was the first NYSNA unit of nurses employed by a private proprietary hospital, and thus the first unit that came under the scope of the New York State Labor Relations Act.[1]

When the hospital refused to recognize NYSNA as the nurses' representative, the association petitioned the New York State Labor Relations Board, requesting designation. Following two informal conferences, the hospital demanded a formal hearing on the petition. Hospital administration contended that NYSNA was not a "labor organization" as defined by law, and maintained that the only appropriate bargaining unit was one composed of the entire nursing staff, including practical nurses and nurse's aides. "Five long grueling days" of testimony in the spring of 1962 produced 643 pages of transcript, which, together with documents submitted as evidence, were examined and considered by the Labor Relations Board.

The decision rendered by the Labor Relations Board in November 1962 represented a major victory for the nurses at Westchester Square and for the association. The board agreed that NYSNA was a labor organization, and determined that the unit, consisting solely of registered nurses, was appropriate for the purposes of collective bargaining within the meaning of the law. "We find that the registered professional nurses do not have sufficient common interests with the licensed practical nurses and the nurses' aides to warrant placing them all in the same unit."[2]

The nurses at Westchester Square were commended by Marion Klappmeier and Veronica Driscoll. "Without your belief in the principle that nurses must speak for nurses, and without your confidence in the New York State Nurses Association as the only spokesman for professional nurses in this state, and without your persistence, despite the frustrating obstacles of time and undue pressure, the achievement of this victory would never have been possible."[3]

Following an election, official certification designating NYSNA as the nurses' exclusive representative, and negotiations, a written contract covering all terms and conditions of employment was achieved, and nurses immediately began receiving some of the benefits gained. The contract, signed in September 1964, was the association's first contract with a proprietary institution. Thanks to the courage and conviction of the Westchester Square nurses, particularly the "unusual ability and dedication" of unit chair Lucile Crossen, the rights of the professional association to speak for professional nurses was affirmed in legal precedent.[4]

Nurses at Canandaigua Veterans Administration Hospital requested assistance from NYSNA and in 1968 became the first VA nurses represented by the association.[30]

During the first half of the decade, improvements in employment conditions by the Economic Security Program were slow and gradual. Many agreements represented only token gestures by the employer, and the program was hampered by staff shortages. The nursing shortage continued, with 40 percent of all staff nursing positions in the New York City metropolitan area vacant, and the situation in the nineteen municipal hospitals was reaching crisis proportions.[31]

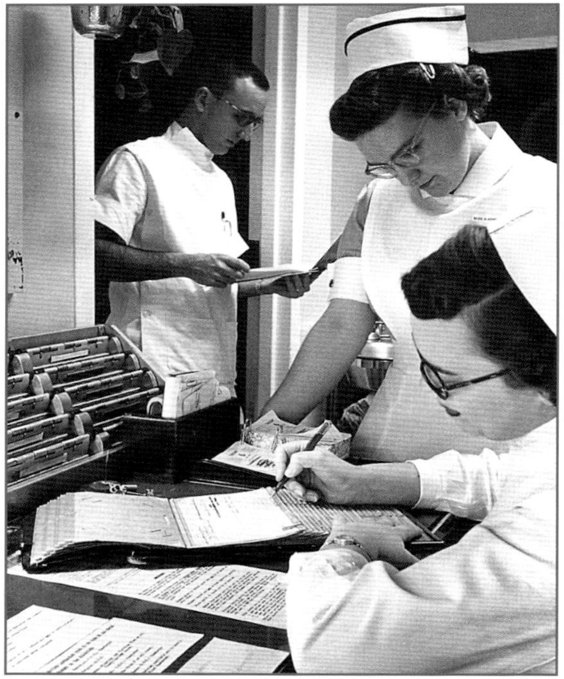

As the health care bureaucracy grew, so did nurses' paperwork responsibilities. *Courtesy Ellis Hospital School of Nursing Collection, Foundation of NYSNA Archives.*

City Hospital Crisis: New York City's municipal hospitals had undergone years of neglect. Buildings were deteriorating, supplies were deficient, and equipment was antiquated and unsafe. Nurses were saddled with a host of non-nursing functions — from distributing linen to substituting for pharmacists—and the situation was worsening. The hospitals were severely understaffed, with only thirty-four hundred of eight thousand professional nursing positions filled. Receiving an annual starting salary of $5,150 for a forty-hour week, nurses were paid less than city garbage collectors. Nurses were leaving daily for jobs in New York's voluntary hospitals where salaries were better, supplies and equipment were more plentiful, and staffing levels averaged 80 percent.[32] An article in the *Daily News* described what a new graduate nurse could expect in a city hospital. "After three years of hard work and dedicated study . . . She will work a 40-hour week, not including the half-hour allowed for meals. The half-hour meal period will become academic because she will usually be so busy she won't have a chance to eat. The new nurse will find that she is responsible for multiple wards, sometimes 70 or 80 patients. If there isn't enough time in her eight-hour shift to do all her work (as is too often the case), and she is required to stay overtime, she will receive no extra pay. How long will the nurse stay in the city hospital?"[33]

When John Lindsay campaigned for mayor of New York in 1965, he published a White Paper on conditions in the city hospitals. His proposal to "restore the status of nurses and to attract nurses of high caliber, to bring our hospitals back up to the standard of excellence which they should set," secured the votes of countless nurses and raised their hopes for better days ahead. Proposals developed by the bargaining units and presented to the city in October 1965 closely reflected the Mayor-elect's recommendations.[34] These proposals included salary increases to make the city hospital salaries "in any way competitive with the local voluntary hospital for a dwindling supply of registered professional nurses." Premium compensation for overtime, holiday, and weekend work was proposed to remedy the practice of giving nurses only equivalent time off for overtime and holiday work. Veronica Driscoll explained, "they don't usually even get that, because there would literally be no professional nurses left to cover wards and floors if they took

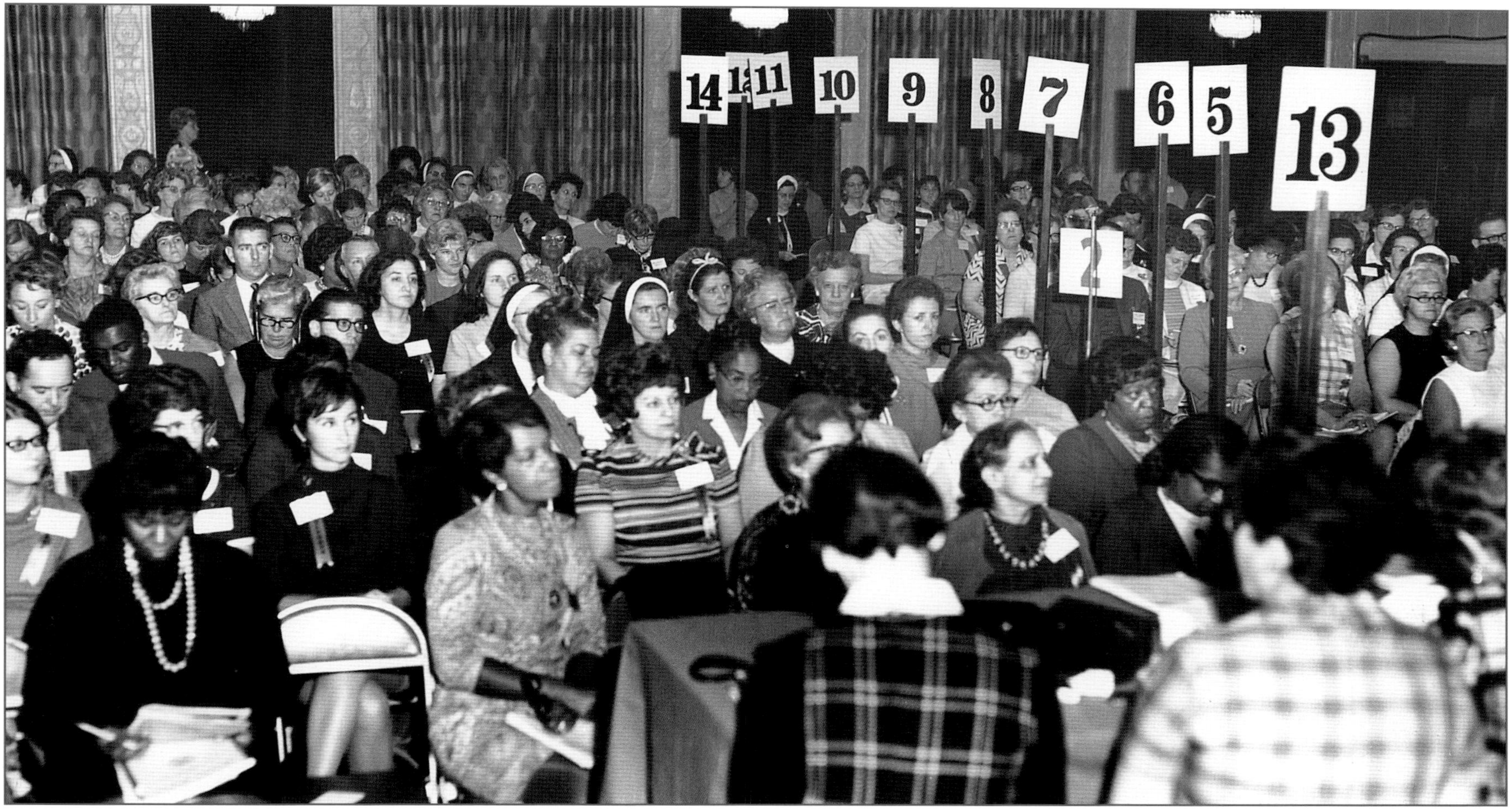

ABOVE: NYSNA conventions have been an important time for members to thoughtfully consider the work of the association. President Cora Pike commented on this in 1965, "To provide the finest care for our patients, we need to keep our profession actively alive and that in one important sense is why we are here today. And that is why we shall return." *Photograph by Empire Photography.*

the time off later." Other proposals included additional pay for prior experience and education, fully paid health insurance, and a shortened work week. City officials, however, were reluctant to enter into negotiations before the Lindsay administration took office, and the contract expired with no agreement in place.[35]

Early in 1966 representatives of the nurses sent Mayor Lindsay a congratulatory letter reminding him of his campaign promises, but the nurses were bitterly disappointed when the city offered only a one-grade salary increase and rejected all other proposals. The bargaining team, composed of unit representatives Beatrice Schorr, Ruth Wasserman, and Marguerite Thibodeau, NYSNA staff members Mary Finnin and Veronica Driscoll, and NYSNA attorney Robert Jones, refused the city's counterproposal, and negotiations quickly reached an impasse. In February 1966 NYSNA requested mediation and fact-finding arbitration proceedings.[36]

Discouraged by delays and a lack of progress, it was a difficult period for both NYSNA staff and the represented nurses. Bargaining units began to meet more frequently to keep members informed and meetings grew increasingly intense as unit leaders struggled to hold the groups together. Discussion turned to "what do we have to fight with."[37] Bellevue unit chairman Mary Tomaselli recalled raising the issue of mass resignation. "I remember standing up and giving this speech, my knees knocking, and I said, 'people are resigning from here every week. The impact is not dramatic . . . suppose two hundred of us went at the same time.' "[38] The decision to resign was not an easy one, and discussion continued for several weeks. Nurses who resigned would lose pensions and vacation time, and many were graduates of the hospital's school of nursing, and intensely loyal to the hospital. "Bellevue had been good to me . . . there was that kind of internal fight while you're standing up trying to convince other people to do this, saying to yourself, 'when push comes to shove am I going to do it? Am I going to have the guts to do it?' "[39]

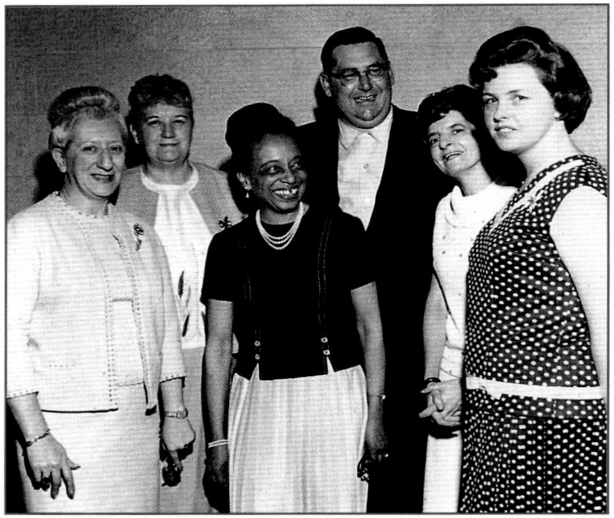

District 14 members including, from left to right, Ruth Harper, Dorothy McLaughlin, Janice Phillips, and Robert Sprecht, met frequently with Economic Security Program staff Veronica Driscoll and Mary Finnin. *Courtesy the District 14 Collection, Foundation of NYSNA Archives.*

As the bargaining units struggled to plan their next steps, mediation sessions were held. Assistant Executive Secretary Mary Finnin described the sessions. "We presented our proposals; the city presented its refusals."[40] Extensive newspaper, radio, and television coverage on the plight of the nurses and conditions in the hospitals raised public awareness. "The nurses in city hospitals have always put the welfare of their patients first. There has never been a threat to strike the hospitals by the nurses. But our members throughout the city are threatening to resign en masse if steps are not taken to alleviate the critical nurses' situation."[41] The frustration of the nurses was vividly described. "The care given is inadequate and substandard, not because the nurses are not trying or don't care, but simply because it is physically impossible for them to do the work assigned . . . Day after day, I'm required to violate my principles and the principles of my profession. I would rather resign than see this continue."[42]

On April 14, 1966, the nurses' frustration reached a climax. Forty-one nurses in the Bronx Hospital Center bargaining unit, chaired by Margot Hahn, spontaneously submitted their resignations. Veronica Driscoll reported to the Board of Directors, "The nurses believe they can no longer condone conditions which are legally, professionally, ethically and physically indefensible."[43] The day following the Bronx resignations, Mary Tomaselli and other nurses at Bellevue resigned. ". . . it was a very stressful time, it was a very uncertain time for us, because it was new ground, it was something that, we just never thought we would be doing. You know, you just didn't do things like this."[44] Nurses at other hospitals quickly followed suit. In all, 1,480 nurses — nearly half of all the nurses employed by the Department of Hospitals — submitted resignations effective May 23, 1966.[45]

After eight mediation sessions, the city finally agreed to submit the dispute to fact-finding. NYSNA brought in expert nursing witnesses, nurses holding various positions in city hospitals, schools of nursing board members, and physicians to support the nurses' demands, while the hospitals braced for the impending resignations by reducing admissions and preparing patients for discharge. The fact-finder terminated proceedings on May 17 because of the impending crisis. Late the following night, the city and the nurses agreed to accept the fact-finder's report. The agreement raised salaries, bringing the minimum staff nurse salary to $6,400 by January 1967. Shift differentials were increased, education and experience were taken into consideration, and tuition assistance was established. Neither overtime pay nor the shorter work week were included, but the fact-finder's report called for joint study on non-nursing duties. "Perhaps more than anything else, this assured the nurses that their right to function as professional persons at long last was recognized."[46] The fact finder summed up the decision, "The overriding consideration here is the forthwith resolution of this dispute so that essential nursing services in the City hospitals will not further be disrupted nor the morale of this highly-skilled, dedicated and loyal professional group be permitted to deteriorate."[47]

Jubilant nurses, relieved that the ordeal was finally over, rejoiced in the results of professionals joining together to improve their working conditions. An editorial in the *American Journal of Nursing* noted, "The remarkable outcome of this story is that the administration of the largest city in this country had to bow to a fantastically effective combination of forces. There was the grim determination of half the city hospital nurses to seek work elsewhere if the administration failed to come through with a settlement which could attract other nurses. There was a sophisticated professional nursing organization representing them, using impeccable and skillful political, negotiating, and public relations techniques. And, cheering from the sidelines was an enlightened and sympathetic public." Professional nursing had proved it could succeed in the "big game of labor disputes."[48]

The settlement had both local and national impact. Within twenty-four hours, New York City voluntary hospitals were considering raising salaries to compete with the municipal hospitals, and Mayor Lindsay lifted a job freeze on nonprofessional positions, thus relieving nurses of some non-nursing duties.[49] A national salary goal of $6,500 was adopted at ANA's 1966 convention, and the city nurses received special commendation. "To a degree more apparent than in many years, [NYSNA's] efforts were successful in improving the economic and professional status of many nurses directly, of all nurses by precedent and through inspiration. The very success of the New York nurses represented by NYSNA was credited at the San Francisco ANA Convention with providing the impetus for adoption of ANA's first

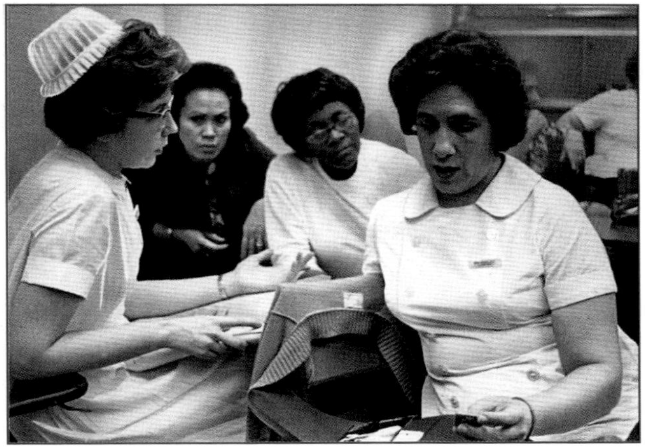

Mary Tomaselli of Bellevue Hospital, at left, and Lucille Frank of Coney Island Hospital, at right, waited anxiously for the outcome of contract talks with New York City's Department of Hospitals. *Courtesy* New York Post; *photograph by Ensel.*

National Salary Goal. This in turn strengthens the real economic security of every career nurse now and for the future."[50]

Widely publicized in the public and professional press, the New York City contract initiated an unprecedented increase in requests for NYSNA to assist nurses. The focus of the Economic Security Program again shifted — this time to simply responding to a flood of inquiries. By January 1967, for the first time, there was a backlog of requests. ". . . suddenly nurses are aware of their plight, and have raised their voices across the state."[51] Pleas poured in, contracts were negotiated, and petitions were filed before the New York State Labor Relations Board on behalf of nurses at five hospitals. In rapid succession, Jewish Hospital of Brooklyn became the first voluntary hospital in the city of New York to recognize NYSNA as a bargaining agent, NYSNA negotiated its first multi-employer contract for directors of nursing employed in member nursing homes of the Metropolitan New York Nursing Home Association, and passage of the Taylor Law opened even more opportunities.[52]

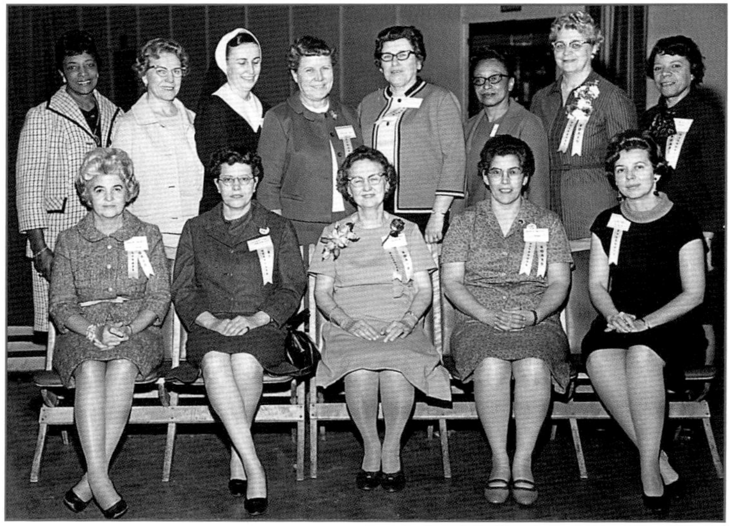

This photograph of the Board of Directors elected in 1967 is the earliest existing photograph of an NYSNA board. Shown, seated from left to right, are Mrs. Laura M. Loring, Evelyn M. Peck, Katherine M. Disosway, Maude B. Miller, and Eileen M. Bonner. Standing are Mrs. Leota P. Brown, Lucille E. Notter, Sister Marie Michael, Catherine Lynch, Mrs. Hazel Harvey, Janice R. Phillips, Mrs. Margaret Sydow, and Mrs. Iris Brice. Not shown are Alberta Bowes, Beatrice Latremore, Anne Lee, Esther M. Thompson, Rita Clarke, and Celia Heffron. *Courtesy the District 14 Collection, Foundation of NYSNA Archives.*

The Taylor Law, passed in 1967, provided for the organization of all state, county, city, and village employees for purposes of collective bargaining. NYSNA immediately became embroiled in controversy when, despite its history of representing publicly employed nurses, Governor Rockefeller recognized the Civil Service Employees Association (CSEA), and refused the association's appeal to represent state employed nurses. NYSNA petitioned the Public Employment Relations Board (PERB) to decertify CSEA and to certify NYSNA as the representative of state employed nurses. PERB declined, and placed nurses in a bargaining unit with other professional and technical employees.[53]

The Board of Directors authorized staff to take any necessary measures, including the formation of a coalition with other groups, to protect the interests of the state employed nurses. NYSNA staff held meetings with representatives of other professional groups and the AFL/CIO to form a coalition. Meanwhile, CSEA attacked the association's efforts by publicizing that NYSNA was forming a relationship "with this very evil group known as the AFL/CIO," and NYSNA failed to get adequate support from the state employed nurses to authorize such a coalition.[54] Delegates to the 1969 convention raised the issue and Veronica Driscoll responded, "I wonder if we're at the point of sophistication where we are still looking upon unions as some horrible thing. I think we have to realize in this day and age, we have a new ball game and we have to use new strategies. The fact that we tried to have this relationship with the union was in no way lessening our interest to protect the nurses.

In fact, it was the only way in which we could protect the nurses."[55] A motion to require approval of the House of Delegates before entering into any coalition with outside groups was defeated.

The nursing shortage continued in crisis proportions. NYSNA cited the economic exploitation of nurses, the poor use of nursing skills, and the lack of respect for the profession as the major contributing factors, and believed that "Only a bold, massive and costly program of action can halt the nursing crisis."[56] Associate Director Mary Finnin blamed the continuing crisis in New York City's municipal hospitals on "failure by the city to implement in good faith the terms of the 1966 contract," noting that it took thousands of telephone calls to Mayor Lindsay before nurses received their differential checks for summer duty.[57] Early in 1968 two of New York's voluntary hospitals raised beginning salaries to $7,200, and NYSNA appealed to the Department of Hospitals to raise salaries to meet the increase. In an attempt to ease the nursing shortage, Mayor Lindsay granted an unprecedented "emergency raise" which increased starting salaries to $7,000.[58]

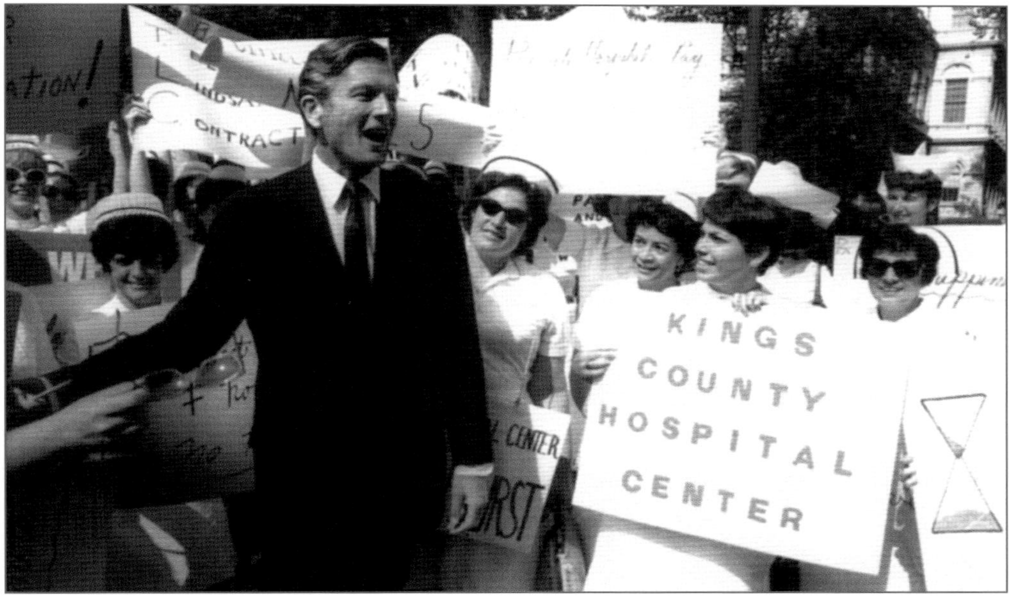

In 1968 nurses employed at New York City's Department of Hospitals rallied at City Hall to emphasize to Mayor John Lindsay the gravity of their concerns. *Courtesy* DAILY NEWS *L.P. Photo.*

In 1968 the nurses' contract again expired before agreement was reached, and the city nurses again took drastic action. At Coney Island and Fordham hospitals, nurses called a one-day walkout to protest the stalled negotiations. Coney Island unit chair Patricia Barry reported that except for "emergency coverage if requested, nurses will not be at work."[59] Nurses at Elmhurst Hospital demonstrated their displeasure in a sidewalk demonstration, nurses at Bronx Municipal Hospital Center again threatened mass resignation, and nearly five hundred uniformed off-duty nurses demonstrated in front of City Hall. An agreement, reached ten days later, raised starting salaries to $7,900, increased differentials, and established a welfare fund to administer insurance benefits. It also provided for the establishment of an unprecedented "parity formula" to keep Department of Hospitals salaries comparable to those of voluntary hospitals.[60]

During the second half of the sixties, the Economic Security Program experienced dramatic growth precipitated by the 1966 New York City contract and passage of the Taylor Law. Despite the failure of NYSNA to achieve representation of state employed nurses, there was a marked increase in representation of city and county employed nurses. By 1969 the association represented 7,539 registered nurses in seventy-seven bargaining units in voluntary, proprietary, federal, and municipal hospitals and agencies across the state, and the program conducted special projects in sixteen of the eighteen district associations. The Board of Directors approved centralization of program activities in the New York City office, now at 11 West 42nd Street, and six staff positions were assigned to the Economic Security Program.[61]

In the early 1960s there was concern that "The program has not been totally accepted by all those affected by it nor has it been allowed to become part of the professional nurse's life," and basic information on the program was provided in the *New York State Nurse* to "clear away some of the confusion."[62] By the close of the decade, members had become both knowledgeable and opinionated. At the 1969 convention delegates entered into lively debate about the "no strike" policy. ANA had recently voted to grant nurses the right to use the strike when necessary, and Janet Sollenberger, who charged that NYSNA's policy restricted the program to function "under out-dated and out-moded methods of bargaining," introduced a similar motion at NYSNA's 1969 convention. Although the Taylor Law prohibited publicly employed nurses from striking, and the Labor Relations Act prohibited strikes by employees of non-profit hospitals and agencies, Sollenberger maintained that the strike should be available as a bargaining tool for those who were not legally prohibited. Following lengthy debate, the motion was defeated.[63] During this decade of social protest, nurses courageously protested poor working conditions — not only for their own professional dignity, but for the well-being of their patients. When bargaining and negotiation failed, they used demonstrations, mass resignation, and walkouts, but as a body, the association was not ready to embrace the strike as a collective bargaining tool.

"We preface everything with the good of the patient.
Do we mean it, or don't we?
If we are going to walk out on our patients,
I don't want to be any part of it."

— *Anne Goodrich*[4]

"With modern trends — rapid change —
it is possible we could be submerged in these changes."

— *Frances Reiter*[5]

CHANGES IN NURSING PRACTICE: The association had always been concerned with nursing practice, but never before had NYSNA addressed nursing practice so broadly as it did in the 1960s. Nursing functions were altered by new systems of care, such as "progressive patient care," the health team, intensive care units, home care plans, and changes in the treatment of mental illness, and by new technology, such as the heart-lung machine, pacemaker, artificial kidney, and the "constant discovery of new drugs."[64] These changes raised concerns regarding the ethics and legality of nursing practice, the recognition of clinical excellence, growth of "gray areas" of practice, keeping pace with new medical advances, and coping with an increasing number of subsidiary workers.

In 1959 NYSNA formed a Committee on Professional Nursing Practice to address the legal control of nursing practice through the monitoring of appropriate legislation and enforcing the Nurse Practice Act. Emphasizing that the law was only good if it was enforced, members were encouraged to report violations.[65] Ethical issues were also of concern, and the committee investigated both legal and ethical complaints, including medication administration by nurse's aides, practicing nursing without a license, and television advertising by nurses. The committee contacted the offender or referred the problem to the State Education Department Division of Professional Conduct, the Secretary of the Board of Nurse Examiners, or the state medical society.[66] In 1965 the committee developed guidelines on the discipline of members found in violation of the code of ethics, and NYSNA passed bylaws amendments providing for reprimand, censure, suspension, or expulsion of members found in violation of the code.[67]

During the 1961-1963 biennium, there was an association-wide focus on the improvement of nursing care, and the scope of the committee's work broadened to include defining standards of practice.[68] A Committee to Clarify Nursing Roles was formed to study problems "created by different levels of nursing," and a statement was published on the registered nurse's responsibility for directing and supervising nursing care provided by Licensed Practical Nurses and auxiliary workers. These concerns only increased throughout the decade, when federal legislation funded training programs for nonprofessional health workers. A variety of new programs of concern to the association trained "baby aides," geriatric aides, and medical assistants.[69]

During these years of tremendous medical advancement, traditional medical and nursing practices were being rapidly altered, and nurses were often asked to perform tasks that appeared to be medical functions.[70] President Cora Pike commented to delegates at the 1963 convention, "One area that is of vital concern to all of us is supporting the nurse practitioner in the area of dependent nursing function. More and more often we are being called upon to perform functions within this dependent area. A few of these are closed chest cardiac resuscitation, administration of investigative drugs, vena puncture, intratrachael [*sic*] suction, administration of anesthesia during labor and vaginal examinations."[71] Meetings were held with representatives of the state medical society to explore areas of questionable practice, and joint statements were developed. The statements recommended the establishment of Medical-Nursing Practice Committees in institutions, and provided guidelines on the nurse's role in closed chest cardiac resuscitation, administration of investigational drugs, administration of anesthesia during labor, insertion of intravenous catheters, and the care of patients with cardiovascular disease in coronary care or intensive care units. All six statements were published in 1968 and widely distributed.[72]

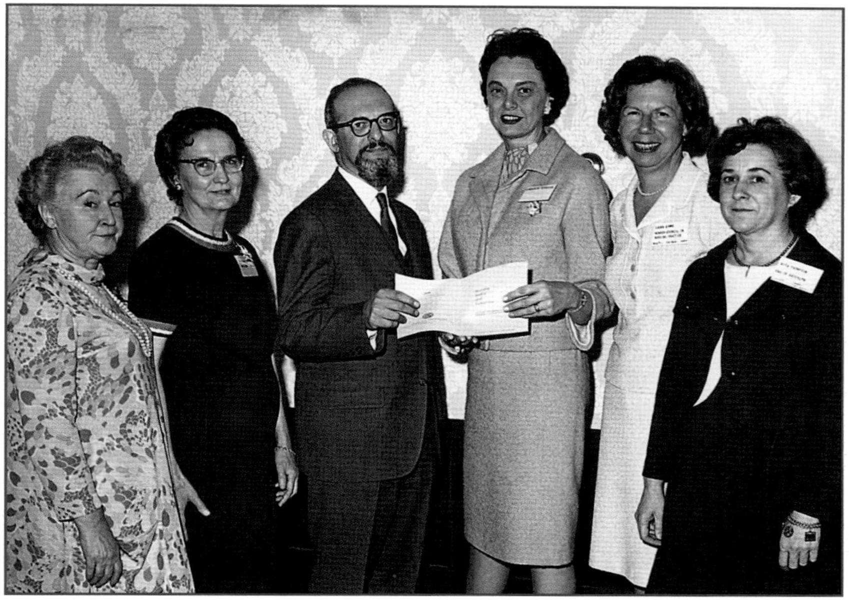

NYSNA sponsored a growing number of conferences and educational programs for nurses. This group attended the "Nursing: Today and Tomorrow" conference in 1968. From left to right are Lydia Hall, Katherine M. Disosway, Mr. Fox, Cynthia R. Kinsella, Laura L. Simms, and Rita Thompson.

As the nursing shortage led to increased recruitment and hiring of foreign nurses, the committee considered the ramifications of this practice. The 1963 House of Delegates voted to reconsider the association's position supporting citizenship as a requirement for licensure, which hampered the employment of foreign nurses in New York State. The association successfully sponsored legislation to remove citizenship requirements, and recommended that prospective employers investigate qualifications, immigration status, and licensure status of foreign nurses prior to hiring.[73]

Throughout the sixties, there was rapid growth in the number of educational programs offered by the association. Typically these offerings focused on emerging technology and health-care trends. Topics included communication skills, home care, radiation therapy, alcoholism, illness in the aging population, and nursing diagnosis ("the first time the term had been discussed publicly in New York State").[74] In 1967 the committee became the Council on Nursing Practice. The council planned workshops for nursing service administrators and educators to discuss and identify clinical nursing competencies expected of the new practitioner, and to set up guidelines defining specific responsibilities of nurses in the face of a revolution in technology. 1968 programs on the theme "Coping with Change" included sessions on computerization and electronic monitoring of patients.[75] Such foresightedness reflects the association's consistent leadership in nursing practice, as well as in the legislative and health policy arenas.

THE TURBULENT SIXTIES: During the sixties nurses faced tremendous change and controversy with courage and conviction. The acute nursing shortage in 1960 worsened as medicine advanced, hospital admissions continued to rise, and the advent of Medicare and Medicaid added new demands for health-care personnel. NYSNA attacked the problem through its Economic Security Program and through legislative efforts. State legislators, though they expressed concern over the nursing shortage, failed to pass legislation designed to ease the crisis.[76] However, in a major national effort to ease the critical shortage, the Nurse Training Act of 1964 provided financial assistance to nursing students and to schools of nursing. The legislation authorized over $287 million for construction of facilities for diploma, associate degree, and collegiate programs, student loans, traineeship programs to increase graduate students preparing for positions as administrators, supervisors, clinical specialists, and faculty, and special projects. NYSNA's Committee on Legislation described the law as "the most important piece of federal nursing legislation ever to be enacted."[77]

"Our collective voices are strong, if we will but use them. If each of us fulfills her responsibilities as a citizen and as a nurse, by giving active support to legislation, we can have . . . the most successful legislative program ever."

— *Ruth Ogden*[6]

During the decade, the association met growing needs with increased activity and growth. The number of professional staff grew from five in 1959 to fifteen authorized positions ten years later. The Counseling and Placement Service declined, while other program areas expanded dramatically. By the end of the decade, staff were hired for the specific program areas of membership, organizational units, legislation, nursing education, nursing practice, or economic security, and the headquarters had again moved to larger offices.

Following a decline in membership in the late 1950s, NYSNA experienced strong growth in 1961, and received a membership promotion award from ANA. The pattern did not continue, however, and the association launched several promotional activities, including an experimental payroll deduction system for state employed members, a flexible membership year, campaigns in state institutions and agencies, and an "unprecedented" statewide membership drive aimed at increasing district and state membership by 20 percent. While falling short of its goal, membership rose 15.5 percent, bringing association membership in 1966 to the highest level in twenty years.[78]

The tremendous changes in the profession of nursing faced by the association during the sixties were more than matched by sweeping social changes. Americans faced assassinations, escalating involvement in the war in Vietnam, civil strife, and an emphasis on improving the status of women. Many New York nurses served in Vietnam, caring for soldiers with massive multiple injuries. On the home front, nurses grieved over the violent loss of national leaders and celebrated man's first walk on the moon. Many nurses were active in the civil rights movement, and some protested American involvement in Vietnam while others supported the war effort. As a profession, however, nursing was embroiled in its own problems, and association records are silent on many of these social issues.[79] In 1967 President Katherine Disosway made some general comments on the changing society, and the unchanging need for nursing to be in control of its own destiny. "Change has never been more sweeping than it is today. We have seen men walk in space, the atom harnessed to produce electric power and fight disease, and travelers jetted across the continent and oceans in a matter of hours. We are in a period of scientific change, social complexity and rapid evolution in new ways of organizing services. And nursing is affected all the way along . . . Nurses must speak for Nurses and Nursing."[80]

"We ask again, who is the professional nurse? . . .
I think she is the person at the patient's bedside
who should be prepared in all depths and skills."

— *Grace Nugent*[7]

CHAPTER NOTES

TEXT

1. R. Louise McManus, *An Open Letter* (Albany, N.Y.: NYSNA, 1960), 5.

2. *Nurses and Nursing 1960–1970: A Report of a Conference, Sponsored by the New York State Nurses Association, Held March 21–23, 1960, at Arden House, Harriman, N.Y.* (Albany, N.Y.: NYSNA, 1960), 7.

3. Ibid., 2. Each of the eighteen districts was invited to send three participants — one engaged in nursing education, one in nursing service, and one in bedside nursing.

4. Ibid., 30–32. The ANA, through its sections and the sections of the state associations, had been striving to develop statements on the functions, standards, and qualifications for each of the various groups of nurses (general duty, office nurses, school nurses, public health, etc.) since the 1950s. Statements were developed and published throughout the 1950s and into the 1960s, but there was concern that the information was not getting out to employers and to nurses themselves, and that even for those familiar with the standards, no practical use was being made of the information.

5. A second Arden House conference was held jointly with the Hospital Association of New York State in December 1961. Following a format similar to the first conference, the focus was on "Our Mutual Interest — The Patient." Recommendations from this conference again highlighted the need for improved educational opportunities, in-service education programs, stable staffing patterns, and effective utilization of nurses. (*Our Mutual Interest — The Patient: A Report of the Conference held jointly by the Hospital Association of New York State and the New York State Nurses Association, Arden House — Harriman, New York, December 13–15, 1961* [Albany, N.Y.: NYSNA, n.d.], 34.)

6. "Proceedings, 52nd Meeting of the New York State Nurses Association" (New York, N.Y., 1963, stenotype transcript), 74–75; and Flanagan, *One Strong Voice,* 184–85. In 1962 ANA had added the enunciation and implementation of standards of nursing education to its list of functions, and appointed a Committee on Education. (Esther M. Thompson, "Meeting NYSNA Responsibilities Toward Nursing Education in Transition," *New York State Nurse* 38 [May 1966]: 4.) It is often overlooked that Goal III proposed that this shift in educational preparation for nurses was to be completed over a twenty to thirty-year period.

7. "NYSNA's Sagamore Conference on ANA's Proposed Goal III," *New York State Nurse* 35 (November 1963): 6; and Reports from Conference Discussion Groups, 25 October 1963, NYSNA Archives. A follow-up conference was held in March 1964.

8. "What is Happening to Proposed Goal III?" *American Journal of Nursing* 64 (March 1964): 95.

9. Barbara G. Schutt, "The Recent Past," *American Journal of Nursing* 71 (September 1971): 1790; and Flanagan, *One Strong Voice,* 242.

10. Thompson, "Meeting NYSNA Responsibilities," 4.

11. "Arden House: Education for Nursing Practice," *New York State Nurse* 38 (May 1966): 2–3.

12. "A Blueprint for the Education of Nurses in New York State," *New York State Nurse* 39 (January 1967): 11–13; "Board Action," *New York State Nurse* 38 (September 1966): 18; and "Biennial Reports of the New York State Nurses Association 1965–1967" (Albany, N.Y., 1967, mimeographed), 23–24. It was

recommended that community planning groups appraise the nursing needs of the community and identify the educational and clinical resources available for nursing education. The concept was remarkably similar to the central registries and community nursing centers proposed in the 1920s.

13. Lucille E. Notter, "The Profession's Commitment," *New York State Nurse* 39 (March 1967): 6, 10.

14. Klappmeier to Participants in Sagamore Conference.

15. "Transition in Nursing Education: One State Nurses Association's Proposal," *American Journal of Nursing* 67 (June 1967): 1212–14.

16. "The Tripartite Link to Successful Transition . . ." *New York State Nurse* 39 (January 1967): 14; "Biennial Reports of the New York State Nurses Association 1967–1969" (Albany, N.Y., 1969, mimeographed), 4–7; and "The 'Blueprint' and the Registered Nurse Contemplating Baccalaureate Education," *New York State Nurse* 40 (September 1968): 19–22. All five of the community planning groups were formed in upstate regions.

17. Special Committee on Economic Security. Members of the committee were Mary Burr, Olga Fessenden, Ruth Harper, Adeline Krowinski, Gloria Stewart, Gracemary Dunna, and Amelia Saunders. The committee discussed the need to use contracts, but believed it prudent to wait until units were more well established.

18. Fessenden and Harper, "Operation: Pilot Project," 7. At this time, association membership was voluntary for represented nurses. ANA approved the payroll deduction system of dues collection on an experimental basis. Approval was also secured from the boards of NYSNA and Districts 13 and 14. The first dues checks began arriving in February 1961. (Report of Headquarters Staff to the Board of Directors, NYSNA, 12 June 1961, NYSNA Archives.)

19. Report of Headquarters, 12 June 1961. Already there were threats from other unions. Teamsters Local 237 was actively campaigning to organize nurses in New York City, and held a meeting at Kings County Hospital in April 1961. Their aim was the "sole collective bargaining right for professional nurses employed by the Department of Hospitals."

20. "State and District News," *American Journal of Nursing* 61 (September 1961): 112; and Report of Headquarters Staff to the Board of Directors, 7 October 1961, NYSNA Archives. Only the director of nursing and assistant directors were exempt from the bargaining units. While NYSNA could not negotiate for these nurses, it did submit salary appeals on their behalf.

21. Report of Headquarters Staff to the Board of Directors, NYSNA, 4 December 1961, NYSNA Archives; and "Proceedings, House of Delegates, 51st Meeting of the New York State Nurses Association" (Buffalo, N.Y., 1961, stenotype transcript), 11. The first Executive Council was announced in September 1961. Each hospital formed bargaining units and elected officers and representatives to the district units. The Executive Council was made up of representatives of the Staff Nurses Unit Councils of Districts 13 and 14 and the Supervisory Nurses Unit Councils of Districts 13 and 14, and representatives of Districts 13, 14, and NYSNA. Members of the first Executive Council were Edamay Bialko, Gladys-Marie Costelloe, Dorothy Breznyak, Shirley Hyman, Olga Fessenden, Ruth Harper, and Marion Klappmeier. Executive directors of Districts 13 and 14 were members of the Executive Council, and Klappmeier, as NYSNA staff, was chairman. (Marion M. Klappmeier to Ruth W. Harper, 8 September 1961, NACLI Archives.) In 1969 all sections voted not to adopt employment standards for the forthcoming biennium, believing the standards were no longer effective in improving the economic status of nurses. ("NYSNA's 55th Convention 'Now!' " *New York State Nurse* 41 [November 1969]: 4.)

22. Board of Directors Minutes, NYSNA, 5 December 1961, NYSNA Archives; Report of Headquarters Staff to Board, 4 June 1962, NYSNA Archives; and Economic Security Program Report to Board, NYSNA, 1 October 1962, NYSNA Archives. Because NYSNA was the exclusive bargaining representative for all registered nurses employed by the Department of Hospitals, it was obliged to provide services to both members and non-members.

23. Katherine E. Rehder, "60 Years — A Long Way," *New York State Nurse* 33 (September 1961):11. Driscoll and Klappmeier were solely responsible for staffing the Economic Security Program until early 1962.

24. "Sixty Years of Nursing Progress," *New York State Nurse* 33 (November 1961), 5.

25. Marion M. Klappmeier, "Two Years of Purpose/Practice/Progress," *New York State Nurse* 37 (September 1965): 5. In hearings on the proposed amendment, NYSNA attorney Robert Jones presented a statement articulating NYSNA's position that registered nurses constitute a separate bargaining unit, and should not be included with other professionals or with non-professional health care employees. (Report of Headquarters Staff to Board of Directors, 6 October 1963, NYSNA Archives.)

26. Katherine E. Rehder, Report to the Board of Directors, NYSNA, 12 December 1960, NYSNA Archives. Rehder reported one such instance to the board. "It was the opinion of all of the nurses that the dismissal was a direct result of the formation of a unit and they felt it was unfair to the individual nurses and stated they were willing to support her all the way, even if it meant resigning from their jobs." Following unsuccessful meetings with administration, "The nurse then requested a meeting with the hospital board and permission to have a NYSNA representative attend also. The board agreed to hear her case but not with the NYSNA [representative] present. We accompanied the nurse to the meeting but were refused entry. After sitting in the hall for over an hour, we were called into the meeting. The nurse's case was argued, but to no avail." The following morning, the nurse was reinstated by a nursing administrator who was appalled by the manner in which NYSNA staff were treated by the Board of Directors, and work began on requests for improved working conditions.

27. "Economic Security Briefs," *New York State Nurse* 34 (November 1962): 10.

28. Economic Security Program Report, 1 October 1962.

29. "No. 10988 . . . A New Era . . . A New Challenge," *New York State Nurse* 35 (May 1963): 3–4; Committee on Economic and General Welfare Minutes, NYSNA, 25 June 1963, NYSNA Archives; "52nd Meeting," 4; and "Representation by Professional Organization Denied VA Nurses," *New York State Nurse* 36 (May 1964): 14.

30. Report on Status of NYSNA Request for Recognition on Behalf of Nurses at Canandaigua Veterans Administration Hospital, 22 November 1968, NYSNA Archives; and Economic Security Program Report for the Board of Directors, NYSNA, 5 December 1969, NYSNA Archives.

31. "The Status of Nursing in New York State Hospitals," *New York State Nurse* 38 (March 1966): 3; and Marion M. Klappmeier, "Executive Director's Report," *New York State Nurse* 35 (September 1963): 2. In early 1963, Florence Manly, in charge of the Counseling and Placement Program resigned, and Executive Secretary Katherine Rehder resigned in March. Marion Klappmeier was appointed executive secretary, and Veronica Driscoll was promoted to associate executive secretary, leaving two professional staff positions unfilled. This lack of staff and a period of "very minimal assistance" from Jones created a delay in follow-through on many economic security issues. (Report of the Executive Secretary to the Board of Directors, NYSNA, 27 May 1963, NYSNA Archives.)

32. Edith P. Lewis, "The New York City Hospital Story," *American Journal of Nursing* 66 (July 1966): 1527; and Hope MacLeod, "The Nurses' Fight With the City," *New York Post,* 21 February 1966.

33. Peter McLaughlin, "City Hospital Crisis: Nurses Feel the Mayor Has Let Them Down," *Daily News*, 9 April 1966.

34. McLaughlin, "City Hospital Crisis," 9 April 1966.

35. NYSNA Tells City: To Improve Nursing Service, Improve Salaries, Press Release, 8 November 1966, NYSNA Archives. The city's subway workers' contract also expired, and their strike in early 1966 created havoc with New York City's transportation system. Nurses continued to work without a contract *and* had to arrange for alternate transportation. ("New York City's Hospital Crisis," *RN* 29 [July 1966]: 67.)

36. "New York City's Hospital Crisis," 68–69; Veronica M. Driscoll to Board of Directors, Memo, 18 April 1966, NYSNA Archives; and Lewis, "New York City Hospital Story," 1529. The city's first counterproposal was not presented until the third negotiating session.

37. NYSNA endorsed ANA's 1950 no strike policy, believing such a tactic to be unprofessional, and because of this voluntary relinquishment of the strike, nurses believed employers had an increased moral obligation to deal justly with nurses through their authorized representative. However, nurses in the public sector were prohibited by law from striking. ("Misconceptions and Misinformation Concerning the Economic Security Program" *New York State Nurse* 34 [March 1962]: 8.)

38. Interview with Mary Tomaselli, New York City, 14 August 1997.

39. Ibid.

40. Lewis, "New York City Hospital Story," 1529.

41. McLaughlin, "City Hospital Crisis," 9 April 1966. The speaker is Mary Finnin.

42. Peter McLaughlin, "City Hospital Crisis: Overworked Nurses, Little Equipment — & Crowding," *Daily News,* 8 April 1966.

43. Driscoll Memo, 18 April 1966.

44. Tomaselli Interview.

45. The mass resignations were not unprecedented in New York. In late 1963 nurses employed by the Sullivan County Home and Infirmary, hopeless and discouraged over the lack of progress in bettering their employment conditions, unanimously decided "that they should all resign rather than to continue working under the present sub-standard conditions." NYSNA staff reported to the board that, "In view of all circumstances involved, we felt we could not justifiably persuade the nurses to rescind their decision." (Report of the Executive Staff, NYSNA, 9 December 1963, NYSNA Archives.) After it was informed of the nurses' decision, the Board of Supervisors authorized more nurses and raised salaries, and the nurses rescinded their resignations. ("Economic Security Briefs," *New York State Nurse* 36 [March 1964]: 4.)

46. Lewis, "New York City Hospital Story," 1531–33.

47. "A Lesson In Professional Commitment," *New York State Nurse* 38 (September 1966): 4.

48. Barbara G. Schutt, "You Can Fight 'City Hall,'" *American Journal of Nursing* 66 (July 1966): 1523.

49. "Lesson in Professional Commitment," 2; and "Nurses, Patients and Paychecks," *New York Times,* 28 May 1966.

50. "Lesson in Professional Commitment," 2; and "Belonging is Doing Something About It," *New York State Nurse* 38 (November 1966): 8.

51. "Economic Security Briefs," *New York State Nurse* 39 (January 1967): 2.

52. "Voluntary Hospital Recognizes NYSNA as Bargaining Agent," *American Journal of Nursing* 67 (July 1967): 1373; and "Biennial Report — Economic Security Program" *New York State Nurse* 39 (August 1967): 6.

53. "Economic Security and the Public Employed Nurse," *New York State Nurse* 40 (March 1968): 3–4.

54. "Proceedings, 55th Meeting of the New York State Nurses Association" (New York, N.Y., 1969, stenotype transcript), 99–100.

55. Ibid., 101.

56. "Fourteen Recommendations Aimed at Overcoming Nurse Shortage In Preliminary Report of Joint Legislative Committee," *New York State Nurse* 39 (January 1967): 6.

57. "Nurse Blames Low Salaries on Hospital Collusion," *American Journal of Nursing* 68 (February 1968): 240–41.

58. "New York City: Salaries Raised, Precedents Broken," *New York State Nurse* 40 (May 1968): 14; "NYC Nurses March for $8500 Contract," *American Journal of Nursing* 68 (September 1968): 1837; and "Voluntary Hospital Contract Starts Nurses at $7,200," *American Journal of Nursing* 68 (March 1968): 450.

59. Stephen Brown, "Nurses Defy Leaders; 1-Day Coney Tieup Set," *Daily News,* 2 August 1968.

60. Arthur Mulligan, "Hospital Braces for Nurses' Strike," *Daily News,* 21 August 1968; and "New York City Nurses: 'Gorgeous,' 'Responsible' — and Now Better Paid, Too," *New York State Nurse* 40 (November 1968): 16. Mayor Lindsay came out to talk with the demonstrators, saying, "For three years we've had demonstrations around City Hall, but never have we had such gorgeous girls."

61. "16 Out of 18," *Report* 1 (December 1969): 2; Report of Executive Director to Board of Directors, NYSNA, 11 December 1968, NYSNA Archives; and "The Taylor Act and the Nurse," *New York State Nurse* 40 (November 1968): 3–11.

62. "Misconceptions and Misinformation Concerning the Economic Security Program," *New York State Nurse* 34 (January 1962): 7. Already the association was seen as a "single purpose" organization by some. One of the questions posed in the article was, "Is this all the NYSNA is concerned about: improving the economic status of nurses? Answer — No, but unfortunately this is what many people choose to believe." The response then goes on to describe other NYSNA programs.

63. "55th Meeting," 143–58.

64. Progressive patient care was a system of organization of facilities, services, and staff around the medical and nursing needs of the patients. The program organized patient care in five units: intensive care, intermediate care, self care, long-term care, and home care. (Faye G. Abdellah and E. Josephine Strachan, "Progressive Patient Care," *American Journal of Nursing* 59 [May 1959]: 649–50.)

65. Robert H. Jones, III, "Professional Control of Standards of Nursing Practice," *New York State Nurse* 32 (March 1960): 4–6; "NYSNA Special Committee Active on Professional Nursing Practice," *New York State Nurse* 32 (May 1960): 6; and "Legislation '61," *New York State Nurse* 33 (May 1961): 8. The committee also recommended legislation to require the State Education Department to publish rosters of duly registered nurses.

66. "Biennial Reports of the New York State Nurses Association 1961–1963" (Albany, N.Y., 1963, mimeographed), 12.

67. "Proceedings, 53rd Meeting of The New York State Nurses Association" (Rochester, N.Y., 1965, stenotype transcript), 44.

68. Klappmeier, "Executive Director's Report," 3. Sections held institutes throughout the period on various clinical and ethical topics.

69. "51st Meeting," 10; "Responsibilities To Be Assigned To Different Groups of Nursing Personnel," *New York State Nurse* 34 (November 1962): 3; and "Biennial Reports 1965–1967," 11–13, 20. The committee updated statements on the Licensed Practical Nurses in 1965, and a special committee to study the roles of various nursing service personnel was authorized by the board in 1966 in response to requests for guidelines to be used in assigning personnel, especially practical nurses. When the work of the committee was completed with publication of "The Appropriate Functions of the Licensed Practical Nurse in Nursing Service," it was felt there should be a continuing committee to deal with problems of allied nursing personnel.

70. Board of Directors Minutes, NYSNA, 12 March 1963, NYSNA Archives; and Joint Position Statements of the Medical Society of the State of New York, New York State Nurses Association, Hospital Association of New York State, [1968], NYSNA Archives.

71. "52nd Meeting," 49–50. Dependent nursing functions were defined as administration of medications and treatments prescribed by physicians or dentists. (Edythe L. Alexander, "Are Your Eyes on Professional Nursing Practice?" *New York State Nurse* 36 [November 1964]: 3.)

72. "Biennial Reports of the New York State Nurses Association 1963–1965" (Albany, N.Y., 1965 mimeographed), 15–16; and "Biennial Reports 1967–1969," 23. The meetings with MSSNY were hailed and noted as a 'historic first." HANYS was asked to approve the first joint statements developed, and subsequently joined the group. Collaboration was also occurring at the national level. Representatives of the AMA and the ANA met for a two day conference in 1964.

73. "52nd Meeting," 163–69; "'64 Legislation," *New York State Nurse* 36 (May 1964): 6; and "NYSNA Board Action," *New York State Nurse* 37 (March 1965): 16.

74. "NYSNA Intersectional Institute," *New York State Nurse* 33 (January 1961): 3.

75. "Biennial Reports 1967–1969," 20; and "What's Ahead in '68: An Overview of NYSNA Action Programs," *New York State Nurse* 40 (May 1968): 3–4.

76. "Biennial Reports 1967–1969," 13; "Toward Quality in Nursing" (Washington D.C.: U.S. Department of Health, Education and Welfare, 1963): 3; and "NYSNA Testifies on Crucial Nursing Shortage," *New York State Nurse* 41 (May 1969): 10.

77. Kalisch and Kalisch, *Advance of American Nursing,* 421–23; and "Biennial Reports 1963–1965," 7.

78. Klappmeier, "Executive Director's Report," 4; and Klappmeier, "Purpose/Practice/Progress," 5

79. References to the Vietnam War were rare. One convention remembered Sharon Lane, the only nurse killed by hostile action in Vietnam, and the *New York State Nurse* announced that NYSNA member Marion A. Tierney had embarked on a 12-month tour of duty as Chief Nurse, U.S. Army in Vietnam, responsible for coordinating all nursing service personnel. ("Lt. Col. Tierney is New Chief Nurse in Vietnam," *New York State Nurse* 38 [September 1966]: 22.) Even news of a bill introduced by Congressman Samuel S. Stratton, at the request of NYSNA, which permitted men to be commissioned as nurses in the regular Army, Navy, and Air Force received only modest coverage in the *New York State Nurse.* ("Congress Passes Stratton Male Nurses Bill," *New York State Nurse* 38 [November 1966]: 19.) No references were found to the civil rights movement or to the assassinations, but the accelerated space program clearly captured the imagination of NYSNA leaders, with references to the program in many speeches and articles.

80. "Proceedings, 54th Meeting of the New York State Nurses Association" (Syracuse, N.Y., 1967, stenotype transcript), A–12–13.

FEATURES

Eleanor C. Lambertsen

1. Eleanor C. Lambertsen, "Who Is the Nurse; Who Are the Others?: An Analysis of the Future of Nursing," *New York State Nurse* 38 (March 1966): 6-9.

Lucille E. Notter

1. Notter, "The Profession's Commitment," 6.

2. "Lucille E. Notter," in *Professionalization of Nursing in New York State: Oral History Interviews with Six Leaders Who Helped to Advance the Mission of NYSNA,* eds. Elizabeth Carter and Jane Fielding (Guilderland, N.Y.: NYSNA, 1988), 89.

3. American Nurses Association Hall of Fame Nomination Form, 1995, NYSNA Archives.

Marion M. Klappmeier

1. "Marion M. Klappmeier Directed NYSNA with Wisdom, Foresight," *New York State Nurse* 41 (March 1969): 11.

2. Marion M. Klappmeier, "Executive Director's Report," *New York State Nurse* 35 (September 1963): 4; and "Miss Klappmeier Submits Resignation," *New York State Nurse* 40 (November 1968): 19.

The Nurses at Westchester Square Hospital

1. "One Request-One Unique Experience-One Momentous Decision," *New York State Nurse* 35 (January 1963): 3-5; "Economic Security Briefs," *New York State Nurse* 34 (September 1962): 6; and Report of Headquarters Staff to the Board of Directors, NYSNA, 7 October 1961, NYSNA Archives. In 1961 non-profit hospitals were exempt from the State Labor Relations Act.

2. "One Request," 5.

3. Klappmeier and Driscoll to Members of the Westchester Square Nurses Unit, Albany, N.Y., 9 November 1962, NYSNA Archives.

4. Report of Headquarters Staff to the Board of Directors, NYSNA, 11 March 1963 and 6 October 1963, NYSNA Archives; "Economic Security Activity Around the Country," *American Journal of Nursing* 65 (January 1965): 140; and "One Request," 5.

EXCERPTS

1. "54th Meeting," A-22.

2. "Education for Nursing Practice: Report of the New York State Nurses Association 1966 Arden House Conference" (Albany, N.Y.: NYSNA, 1966), 5.

3. Peter McLaughlin, "Nurses Feel the Mayor Has Let Them Down," *Daily News,* 9 April 1966.

4. "55th Meeting," 144.

5. "Education for Nursing Practice," 4.

6. "Biennial Reports 1963-1965," 8.

7. "52nd Meeting," 154.

CHAPTER EIGHT

Nursing in 1969

DURING THE 1960S HOSPITALS CONTINUED TO BE THE LARGEST employers of practicing nurses and most new graduates received their initial nursing experience as general duty staff nurses. As part of a team, nurses worked collaboratively with LPNs, nurse's aides, orderlies, and other personnel to coordinate patient care. Nurses planned and implemented care, taking into account cultural and emotional factors as well as physical needs. Teaching of both patients and families was an important aspect of the nursing regimen, as was collaboration with physicians and other health professionals, directing non-professional staff, and utilizing referral systems to plan for care after discharge.

Advancing technology and increasing bureaucracy were making an impact on the traditional role of staff nurses. Increased specialization in medicine and medical advances contributed to growing specialization among nurses and the need to master a host of new skills. Nurses now routinely administered intravenous therapy and blood products, and were delegated more and more responsibility for procedures such as aspiration, inhalation therapy, and irrigation of body cavities. Nurses cared for patients undergoing complex new therapies such as dialysis and participated in revolutionary, exciting developments such as organ transplantation. A variety of costly and sensitive equipment demanded skillful care of both patients and machines. The need to produce statistical reports, incident and accident reports, medication error reports, and incidence of certain diseases and conditions created increased paperwork for nurses. While increased technical skill and participation in ground-breaking new therapies were exhilarating for nurses, the burden of paperwork and other non-nursing functions was demoralizing. In a rapidly changing environment, nurses were a critical component of patient care, yet frequently lacked recognition and respect. Still viewed as subservient to the physician, nurses needed to fight for recognition as valued, independent members of the health-care team.[1]

RIGHT: *Courtesy Alumni Association of Harlem Hospital Center School of Nursing.*

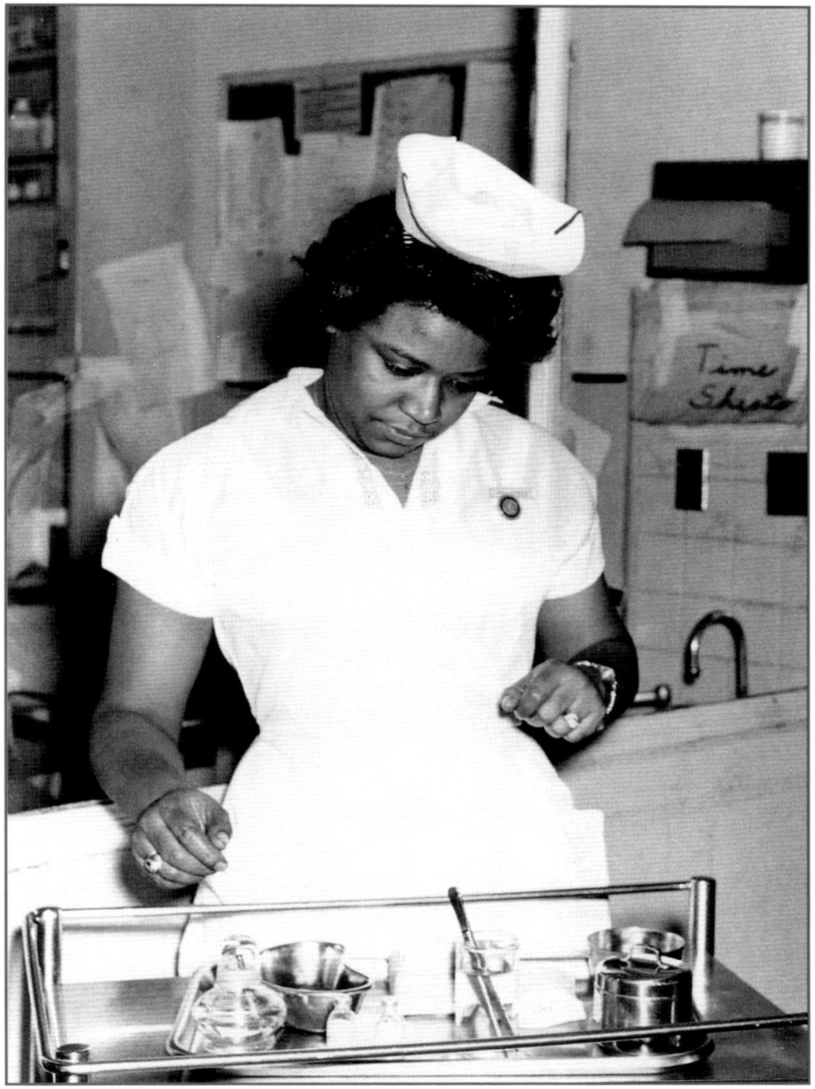

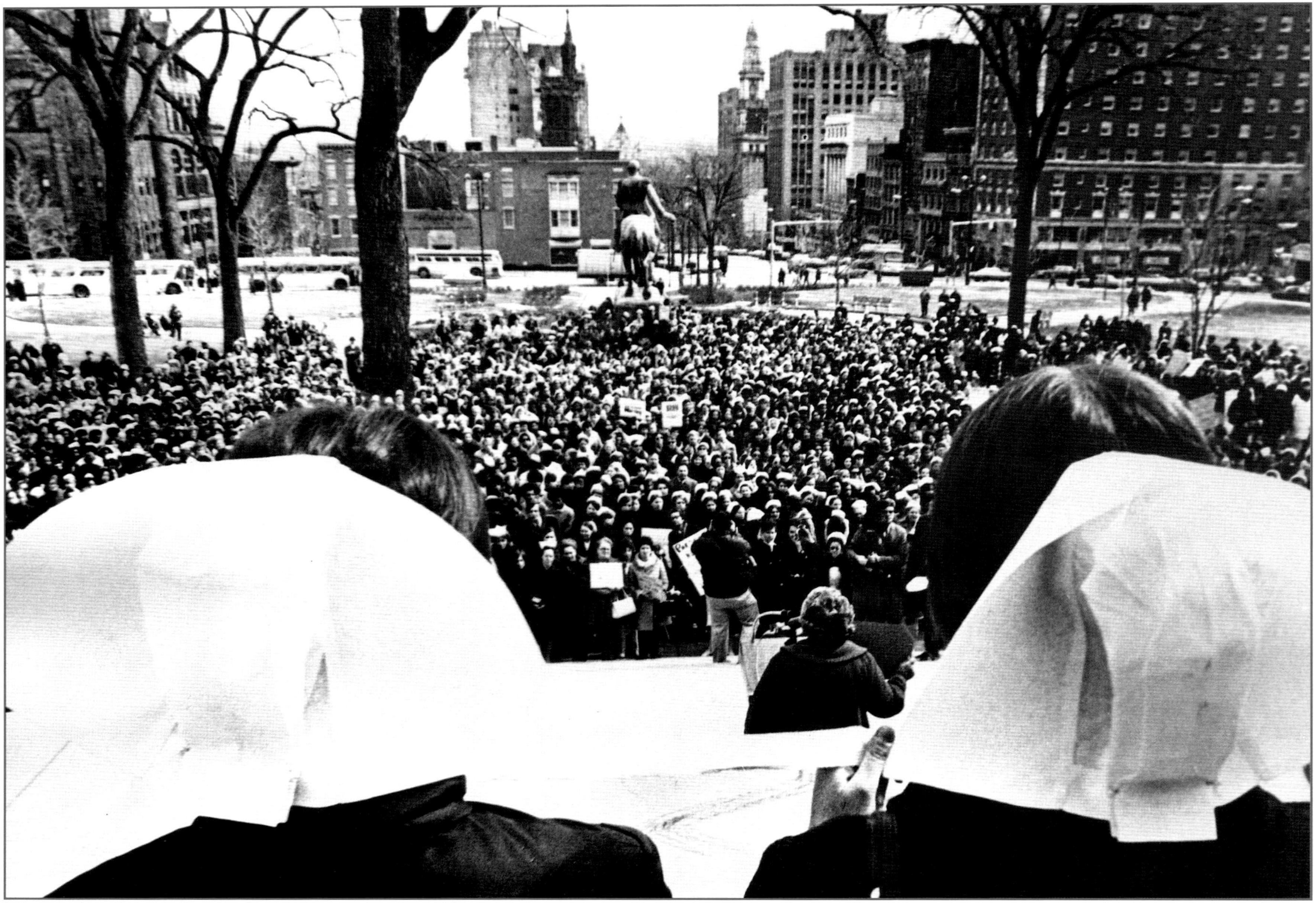

REVOLUTION FOR INDEPENDENCE 1969 ~ 1985

The social turbulence of the 1960s waned, but the effects lingered far into the next decade. In the late 1960s students challenged the "establishment," and the feminist movement urged women to be more assertive and independent. The influence of these movements is evident in remarks made by President Evelyn Peck at NYSNA's 1973 convention. "In the 60's the youth of the country undertook action which to many staid traditionalists was most alarming. They challenged the establishment, they challenged the hypocrisy of lip service to ideals, they questioned the integrity of the leadership. They asked, why. . . No movement can take place in our society and leave one segment untouched unless that segment wishes to die on the vine. The nursing profession . . . has no desire to die on the vine. The New York State Nurses Association has and is still challenging the establishment, each practitioner is questioning his or her right to practice nursing in an independent professional manner . . . The day of standing quiet is over, the nursing practitioner and public in today's society is asking why . . . "[2]

FACING PAGE: NYSNA's *Legislative Bulletin* described the 1971 March on Albany as "a sea of bobbing white nurses caps inundated the State Capitol . . . as thousands of nurses asked that their profession be given proper recognition." *Courtesy the District 14 Collection, Foundation of NYSNA Archives.*

VERONICA M. DRISCOLL
1926 - 1994

Veronica Driscoll was first hired by NYSNA in 1960 as assistant executive director, with responsibility for the Economic Security Program. In this capacity she traveled throughout the state, attending countless meetings, listening to the concerns of nurses, and developing strong beliefs about the profession of nursing and the role of the professional association. In 1967 she left NYSNA to pursue doctoral studies, but returned in 1969 as executive director.

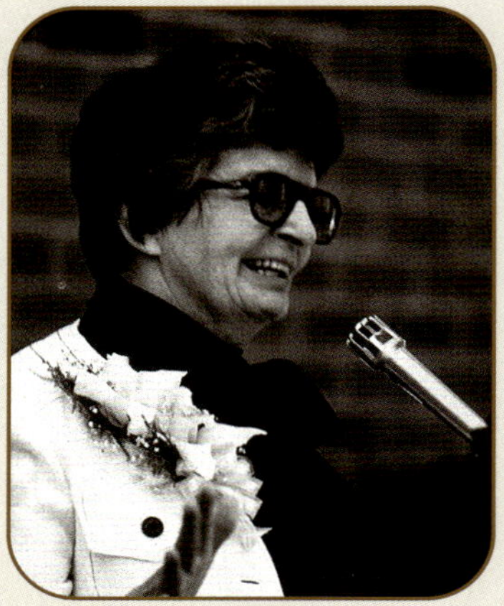

Driscoll coordinated a sweeping reorganization of the association and guided bold initiatives, including a complete reevaluation of the Nurse Practice Act. A believer in the "politics of confrontation," she traveled extensively throughout the state to talk with nurses and promote the work of the association. During her tenure as executive director (1969–1979), a revised Nurse Practice Act was enacted, membership tripled, the role and responsibilities of staff increased, and the association's communication methods were revitalized. Deeply interested in the unique history of NYSNA, Driscoll authored *Legitimizing the Profession of Nursing: The Distinct Mission of the New York State Nurses Association.* Dr. Driscoll became a nationally respected leader, serving as chairman of ANA's Commission on Economic and General Welfare, and receiving ANA's Honorary Recognition Award. She received NYSNA's highest award, Honorary Recognition, in 1979.

Veronica Driscoll was widely sought after as a speaker on nursing issues, and was revered by nurses around the country for her keen intellect, extraordinary vision, courage, and passionate belief in the unique and vital role of nurses.[1]

When Marion Klappmeier resigned in late 1968, the association hired Veronica Driscoll to fill the position of executive director. Driscoll, an energetic, tell-it-like-it-is dynamo, swept into the association with a thorough analysis of the organization and recommendations for change. In rapid succession, she recruited new staff, evaluated the association's financial status, reorganized the staffing structure, created the newsletter *Report,* and initiated an ambitious program of field service. Association staff met with groups throughout the state to address "frank and challenging" questions about the nature of the association. Staff held statewide legislative forums, visited schools of nursing in a "Swing Around the Schools" project, and held a series of informational forums on the Economic Security Program. In 1970 alone the staff's total field service commitment was over thirteen hundred days.[3] Based on information gathered from these grassroots contacts with nurses, Driscoll developed a "broad and aggressive program" involving every program area to create opportunities for greater involvement of individual nurses. ". . . nothing is as essential as a strong relationship between the individual practitioner and the Association itself . . . a profession is severely threatened when deprived of consistent challenge and contribution from the individual practitioner."[4] Driscoll called this effort "venturing," which she defined as a process of self-discovery and reshaping to make NYSNA into "the association we could be."[5]

DECLARATION OF INDEPENDENCE: In the late sixties, NYSNA's Legislative Committee concentrated on a proposed revision of the Nurse Practice Act in anticipation of recommendations by a Joint Legislative Committee to Revise and Simplify the Education Law. Association leaders grew increasingly concerned that the chronic shortage of nurses and a rising public demand for improved health-care services might threaten the traditional system of individual licensure. This concern only increased with the rapid development of the role of physician's assistant and attempts by various groups to define the practice of nursing through legislative proposals. In 1969 the Joint Committee still had not made recommendations, and NYSNA's board appointed a committee to thoroughly study all aspects of the Nurse Practice Act.[6]

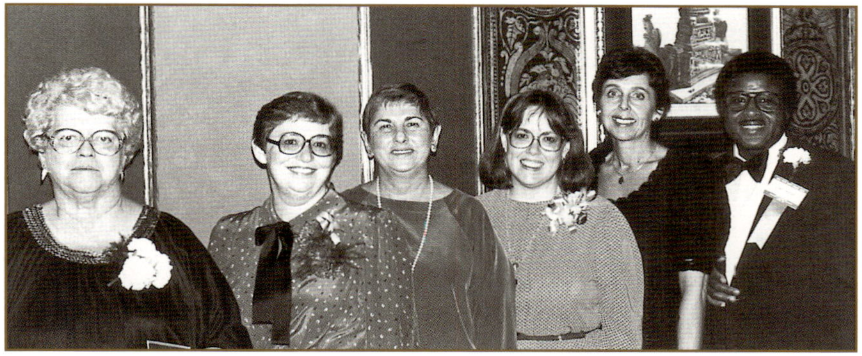

In late 1981 NYSNA's board appointed an ad hoc committee to establish a system of awards to recognize and commend NYSNA members who made extraordinary contributions to the profession. Awards for Nursing Practice, Nursing Service Administration, Nursing Education, Economic and General Welfare, Legislation, and Membership are conferred at an annual awards banquet held in conjunction with the annual convention. The 1983 award winners shown here from left to right are Celia Heffron, Claire Murray, Nina Argondizzo, Diana Mason, Roberta Cohen, and Sidney Morgan.

Convinced that any attempts to revise the current law had to involve a large number of the state's licensed nurses, the committee sent out thousands of questionnaires and held a series of workshops and legislative forums. The committee reported to the board that the current law was "grossly inadequate," and presented recommendations which it believed were historic in nature. The proposed changes were designed to correct inadequacies of the existing act and provide a legal framework within which the profession could adapt to rapid sociological and scientific change. The committee's recommendations included changing titles, adding continuing education requirements as a condition of re-registration, revising stipulations for limited permits, and modifying requirements for appointment to the State Board for Nursing. Most importantly, the committee proposed a new definition of nursing practice which legally recognized nursing as an independent, distinct health discipline. The new definition was, in the committee's opinion, "absolutely essential to the survival of the profession, and thus to the continued existence of nursing care services."[7] The committee viewed the existing definition, last revised in 1938, as archaic. In light of the rapid changes in medical technology, it no longer appropriately recognized the nursing function. The new definition delineated the elements of the nursing process and the independence of the nursing function, and specified the distinctive areas in which the nurse traditionally exercised independent judgment. A critical component of the definition was the inclusion of "diagnosing" as part of the nursing process. This, and the absence of any

LAURA L. SIMMS

Dr. Laura Simms, nurse educator, administrator, and consultant, received her doctorate in nursing education from Teachers College, Columbia University. "An innovator who is not deterred in her efforts by bureaucratic structure," she was one of the first nursing administrators to effectively establish the role of clinical nurse specialist. She served the association in various capacities for many years. As chairperson of the Special Committee to Study the Nurse Practice Act, she guided the development of landmark revisions of the Nurse Practice Act, and spearheaded the drive to secure enactment. From 1975 to 1977, she guided the committee's development of the historic 1985 Proposal. Dr. Simms also served on the Council on Continuing Education, the Governing Council of the Society of Distinguished Practitioners, the Council on Nursing Practice, and on the Foundation's Building Fund Committee.

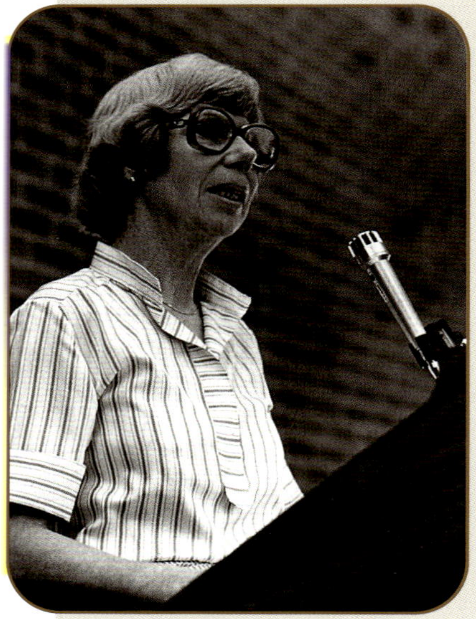

At NYSNA's 1972 convention, Dr. Simms was nominated from the floor for the position of president-elect. In reference to her work on the new definition of nursing, one member noted that ". . . she has demonstrated to us that [the] professional association can be a viable structure for the recognition of nursing's unique functions . . . Through both word and action she has shown us that the nursing profession is a vital social and political force that not only holds answers to improvement of health care in this state, but the collective power to initiate and mandate change . . . But above all, Dr. Simms' fundamental belief is that the primary concern of the profession is practice, whether we be staff nurses, private duty nurses, administrators, educators or supervisors."[1] Simms was elected to the position and served as NYSNA's president from 1973 to 1974. She was the founding president of the Foundation of NYSNA, and served on its board until 1997. She received the association's highest award, Honorary Recognition, in 1978.[2]

reference to physician supervision, were especially significant components of the definition — and highly controversial.[8] At a time when women across the country were striving to overcome traditional dependent and subservient roles, nursing rejected physician domination and defined itself as an autonomous profession.

Members of the Committee to Study the Nurse Practice Act took the proposals to thousands of nurses through forums and meetings, and reported "that the degree of support expressed for the proposals is in essence a mandate . . . and that support of these proposals have been accompanied by an unexpected, but most interesting degree of excitement."[9] Senator Thomas Laverne and Assemblyman Joseph Pisani agreed to introduce legislation incorporating the new definition of nursing and continuing education requirements for re-registration.[10]

The proposed legislation received strong nationwide support. Committee chairperson Dr. Laura Simms addressed nursing groups throughout the country, and letters of support poured into the association, to legislators, and the governor. Eleven state nurses' associations, together with many specialty nursing organizations in New York, officially supported the bill.[11] However, as

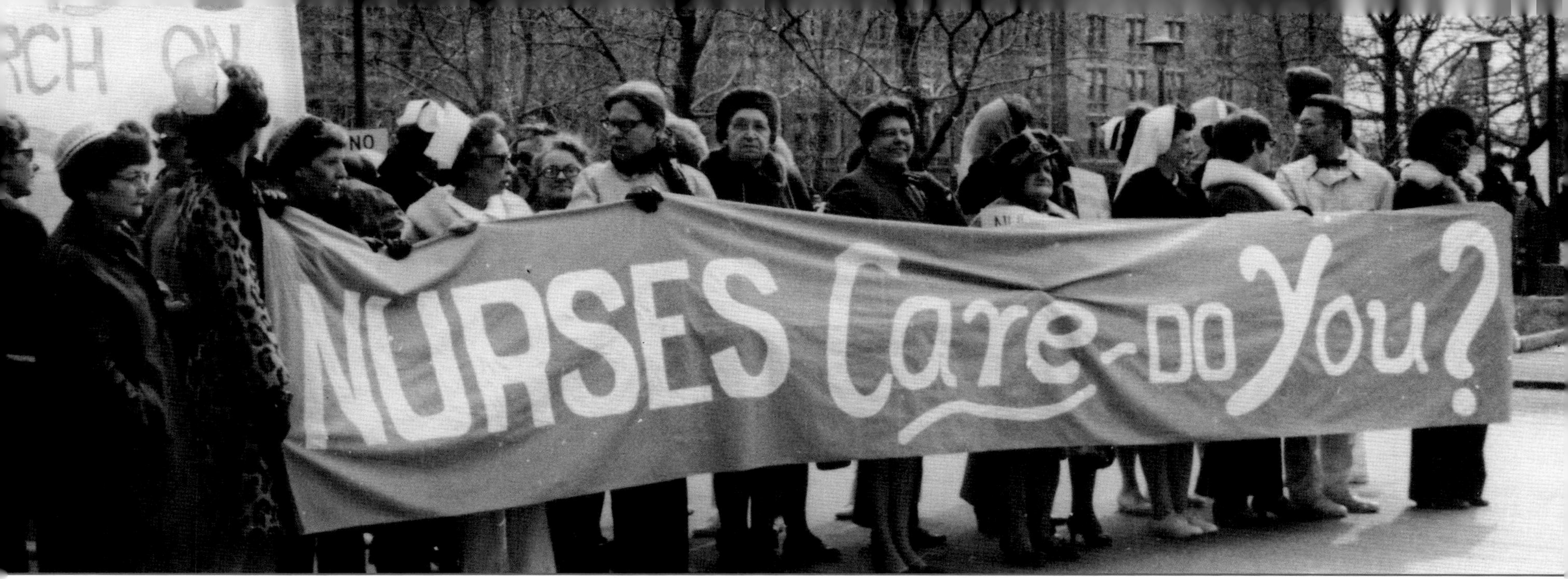

Nurses from around the state joined together in Albany on March 2, 1971.
Thousands of nurses followed these nursing leaders up State Street to the Capitol to demonstrate support for a revised Nurse Practice Act.

the nursing community rallied in support of the proposals, the medical and hospital communities mounted a vigorous opposition campaign. The Medical Society of the State of New York alleged that the bill would permit the unauthorized practice of medicine, and objected to use of the term "diagnose" and the lack of reference to physician supervision.

Repeated attempts by NYSNA to discuss the intent of the proposed new definition with representatives of the medical society were unsatisfactory, and the committee agreed that extraordinary measures were needed to fight the medical society's intense opposition. The continuing education legislation was withdrawn so that all energies and resources could be focused on the new definition. Statewide, nurses united, staging "mini-marches" on hometown legislators, petitioning local newspapers to cover the nurses' point of view, writing to legislators, pounding the pavements for public support, facilitating discussions, and pledging financial contributions.[12] Most dramatically, on March 2, 1971, thousands of nurses, led by Laura Simms, Evelyn Peck, Martha Rogers, and other nurse leaders, marched to the Capitol in Albany in support of the bill. Following the march, nurses sought out legislators to explain the bill's purpose and to request support. "Legislators hastened to become informed regarding the bill within their inner offices, as nurses requested appointments in outer offices. Some legislators, who had been uncommitted regarding the bill prior to the march, indicated definite support for it during conferences with nurses from their home districts."[13]

The medical society remained staunchly opposed. The Assembly Committee on Education urged that the bill be amended, and the association agreed to add the phrase, "and executing medical regimens prescribed by a licensed or other legally authorized physician or dentist."[14] When the bill passed both the Senate and Assembly, members of the medical society and the hospital association flooded the governor's office with messages of opposition. Echoing the fear that the bill would permit nurses to practice medicine, the governor vetoed the legislation.[15] Executive Director Driscoll reported, ". . . the Governor's blow was much too cruel . . . The Medical Society of the State of New York, understandably fearful of losing its time-honored borrowed servant, could hardly be expected to support a definition which would legally authorize the independent practice of nursing—hence, its awesome campaign . . ."[16]

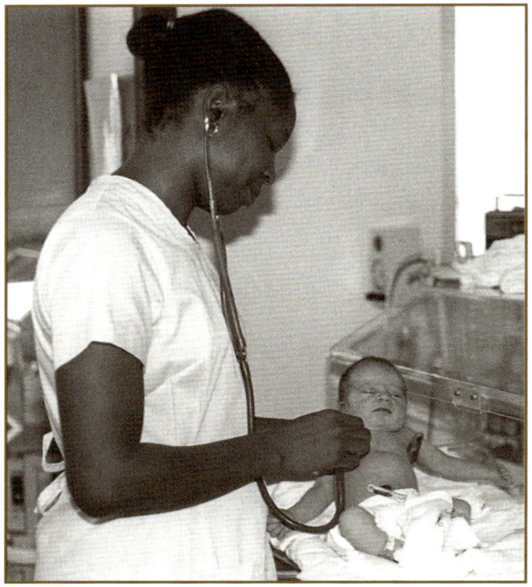

The 1971 veto was both disappointing and alarming. The veto maintained nursing's traditional role, dependent on physician supervision. In addition, recently enacted legislation provided for the practice of the physician's associate under physician supervision within an administrative framework established by the State Health Department. Association leaders viewed these developments as contributing to an alarming trend toward institutional licensure in New York. Institutional licensure called for eliminating individual licensure, and shifting accountability from individual practitioners to a governmental agency. The health-care facility would be regulated by state licensing agencies, after which the administrator would be responsible for appropriate utilization of personnel. Under this proposal, nursing would be placed in the hands of organized medicine, hospital administration, and governmental regulatory agencies.[17] With growing support for institutional licensure, the need for statutory recognition of nursing as an independent profession became even more urgent.

In 1971 President Peck echoed the convention's theme, "Declaration of Independence," by calling for recognition of nursing as an independent, primary, and distinct health discipline.[18] The biennium had been one of the most active in the association's legislative history, and Dr. Simms described it as "nothing short of revolutionary" in the area of nursing licensure. ". . . the nursing community of New York State clearly demonstrated its determination to define nursing practice and to assume responsibility for that practice."[19] Despite the defeat of the proposed definition, leaders hailed the increased recognition of nursing and the demonstration by the nursing community that the profession was an effective political and social force. Simms reported "every cause for optimism . . . the nursing profession is alive, and it is recognized by our politicians . . . the nursing profession has found a mission, and it is a mission to assert its distinctive, purposeful and responsible function . . . nurses have every intention to continue to work with our colleagues in medicine, but we expect to do so as increasingly expert and responsible nursing practitioners and not as servile assistants."[20] Delegates to NYSNA's 1971 convention supported reintroduction of the legislation, unanimously passed a resolution recording extreme distress over the opposition of the hospital association, and declared a statewide "Responsibility Recognition Day."[21]

Hands-on nursing care continued to be the most cherished component of the nursing role.

Responsibility Recognition Day, January 18, 1972, was designated as a day to gather physician support through discussions between indiviual nurses and physicians in the practice setting. Many nurses also chose to eliminate all of their usual independent nursing functions to demonstrate the need for legislation. The project yielded hundreds of letters sent by physicians in support of the bill. Intensive negotiations with representatives of the medical society and the hospital association finally resulted in an amendment supported by all parties. The amendment added, "A nursing regimen shall be consistent with and shall not vary from any existing medical regimen," thus confirming that professional nurses should not undertake the practice of medicine. With the support of the hospital and medical societies, the bill passed and was signed into law. Governor Rockefeller stated, "With the enactment of this measure, the proud, humanitarian profession of nursing receives a new charter in New York State . . . Given the rapid and continuing revolution in medical care in recent decades, what was appropriate in 1938 no longer reflects the capacity of the members of the nursing profession to serve human needs . . . this bill recognizes the expanded and growing role of nursing in modern health-care delivery."[22]

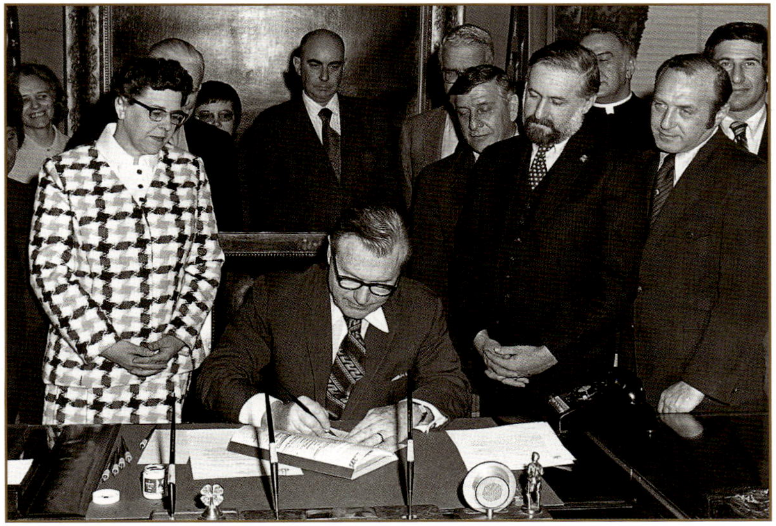

1972 Definition of Nursing

The practice of the profession of nursing as a registered professional nurse is defined as diagnosing and treating human responses to actual or potential health problems through such services as casefinding, health teaching, health counseling, and provision of care supportive to or restorative of life and well-being, and executing medical regimens prescribed by a licensed or otherwise legally authorized physician or dentist. A nursing regimen shall be consistent with and shall not vary any existing medical regimen.

The ground-breaking legislation was widely recognized as establishing statutory authority for the independent practice of nursing for the first time. The association proposed new job descriptions to be included in labor contracts, held conferences to analyze methods and strategies for implementation, and presented regional workshops to assist nurses in analyzing and implementing the scope of nursing practice inherent in the new definition.[23] The new definition of nursing in New York's Nurse Practice Act had widespread impact, becoming a model for many states' legislation. The definition of nursing in ANA's Social Policy Statement of 1983 was also based on New York's definition.

"It's hard to describe, but it was a thrilling time. It was like nothing we had ever lived through."

— *Catherine Leach*[1]

LEFT: NYSNA President Evelyn Peck witnessed Governor Nelson Rockefeller signing landmark legislation in 1972. The legislation defined nursing as a distinct and independent profession. *Photograph by Harry Thayer.*

Legitimized as independent, autonomous practitioners, nurses were optimistic about the future, and about the ability of the professional association to unite with other nursing groups to effect change. This optimism fueled the development of an ambitious association legislative program. Legislation proposed in 1969 as the "RN Project," calling for financial assistance to colleges, universities, and individual nurses seeking additional education, again became a priority. Other legislative initiatives sought third-party reimbursement for nurses and new minimum educational requirements for entry into the profession. The association urged legislation mandating continuing education for re-registration, and sought repeal of the exempt clause in the Nurse Practice Act, which allowed unlicensed mental health aides to administer medication. The association's legislative program was now a formal annual agenda of legislative priorities approved by the voting body, and there were institutes, receptions, lobby days, and other special events to provide opportunities for members and nursing students to meet with legislators. The *Legislative Bulletin* continued to be an important means of communication with members, and a "Leg-Line" was instituted to provide a twenty-four-hour telephone summary of key bills during the legislative session.

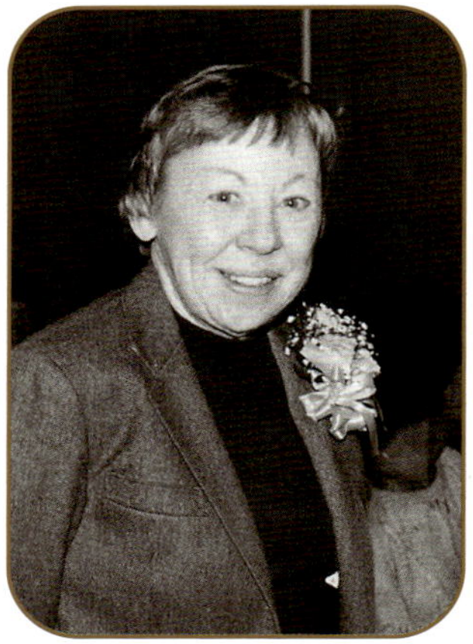

Catherine Leach joined NYSNA staff in 1964. She held the positions of assistant and associate executive director, and in 1969 served as acting executive director. She managed association business and administrative operations, and was the managing editor of association publications. She retired from the position of deputy director for administration in 1985, after twenty-one years of devoted service.

Despite this comprehensive approach to influencing legislation, the association's legislative hopes following the 1972 victory were largely unrealized. The single success in this ambitious legislative agenda was the passage of legislation providing for third-party insurance reimbursement for nursing care services. The legislation, passed in 1985 after a ten-year effort, was viewed by some as too restrictive. Nonetheless, this was landmark legislation that recognized nursing care as a reimbursable component of health care, and encouraged the use of more cost-effective alternatives to hospital and nursing home care. Proposals for financial aid to nursing education were introduced unsuccessfully for thirteen consecutive years, and the exemption to the Nurse Practice Act was never repealed. The continuing education and entry-into-practice proposals were also introduced year in and year out, and generated enormous controversy.[24]

A Storm of Controversy: Mandatory continuing education for nurses was first proposed as part of sweeping changes in the Nurse Practice Act, but was withdrawn in order to focus on passage of the new definition of nursing. At the 1972 convention, President Peck did not waste time gloating over the successful passage of the new definition. Instead, she called for continuing efforts to reform the system of licensure. "Is it not logical that continuing education should be mandatory for maintenance of licensure? It is time to ask ourselves is the purpose of the license to protect our status or is it to protect the public?"[25] Shortly after passage of the new definition in 1972, NYSNA's Board of Directors voted to sponsor legislation to require continuing education approved by the professional association as a condition for re-registration, and to create a permanent body within the association to establish requirements and procedures for approving continuing education programs. A series of forums, characterized by vigorous discussion and significant opposition, were held to present the association's proposals.[26] Mandatory continuing education legislation was introduced in 1975 and was later included in an omnibus mandatory continuing education proposal, but was never enacted.

While mandatory continuing education proposals were defeated, the so-called "voluntary" component of the association's continuing education program flourished. ANA accredited NYSNA as an approval organization and provider of continuing education, and NYSNA received and reviewed thousands of applications for approval of continuing education offerings. In 1981 ANA commended the association for a "model program," with a "high degree of sophistication which constantly improves with time."[27]

NYSNA developed a certification program as another voluntary component of continuing education. Beginning in 1975 psychiatric mental health nurses were certified, and for a brief period gerontological nurses were certified. The Council on Certification engaged in collaborative efforts with ANA and other state nurses' associations, and NYSNA's certification experience significantly influenced the development of ANA's certification program. In 1983 NYSNA's board suspended the program, concurring with the Council on Certification that the certification efforts of ANA and specialty organizations met the certification need and that the continuation of NYSNA's program would not be cost-effective.[28]

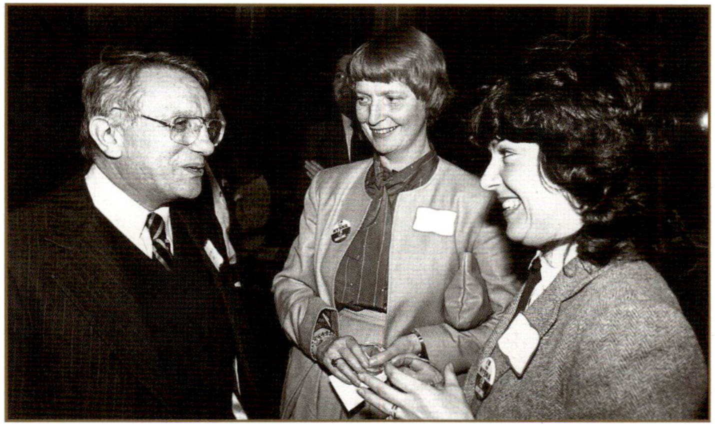

Cecilia Mulvey, NYSNA president from 1983 to 1985, is shown here with legislator Tarky Lombardi at NYSNA's annual Legislative Reception. Dr. Mulvey, center, associate professor at Syracuse University College of Nursing, continued to be active on the district, state, and national levels following her presidency. She received NYSNA's highest award, Honorary Recognition, in 1995.

While work on both the mandatory and voluntary components of continuing education continued, opposition to the association's position on entry-into-practice, developed in the 1960s as "A Blueprint for the Education of Nurses in New York State," was stronger than ever. President Janet Mance described the issue of nursing education as "the single most divisive force within the nursing community today."[29] Nevertheless, the voting body adopted a resolution providing for the development of "a plan for establishing by 1985 the baccalaureate degree in nursing as a requirement for licensure as a registered professional nurse." In 1975 the Special Committee to Study the Nurse Practice Act proposed legislation known as the 1985 Proposal, which called for recognition of two distinct careers in nursing; the baccalaureate prepared "nurse" and the associate degree prepared "practical nurse." The committee recommended "grandfathering" protection of individuals currently licensed or preparing for licensure.[30]

Opposition to the continuing education and entry-into-practice proposals was so strong that groups of nurses — both members and non-members — organized in protest. Both the Concerned Nurses Association and the Empire State Nurses Association vigorously opposed association proposals. Despite numerous informational forums, widespread discussion, and prolonged efforts to build consensus, the profession remained deeply divided. Some believed NYSNA "railroaded" the 1985

Proposal, others believed it "too little too late," while yet another group advised further study.[31] Even the New York State Department of Education maintained that "elevation and standardization of educational requirements for entry into nursing are unnecessary."[32] President Louise Pan remarked, "We all know about the furor that the proposal caused on the outside and inside of the . . . nursing community. We know about the debates, the splinter groups, the high emotions and the low blows . . . Despite all this we all should know and applaud the courage and leadership of the New York State Nurses Association . . . The 1985 Proposal is nursing for the future."[33]

> "The baccalaureate should be the minimum or entry level preparation for nursing . . . we have been putting off this issue for so very long, do let us get on with the business."
>
> — *Jeanne McCrea*[2]

NYSNA was the first state to initiate entry-into-practice legislation, but national interest quickly grew. By 1978 thirty-five other state nurses' associations were actively studying the issue or had adopted resolutions in support of the proposals embodied in the 1985 Proposal, and ANA's House of Delegates had passed a resolution calling for the baccalaureate degree in nursing as minimum preparation for entry into professional practice. Legislation, later known as the "Entry into Practice Bill," was introduced for ten consecutive years, but was never enacted. Nonetheless, NYSNA's organizational units planned for implementation. Councils formulated behavioral outcomes for the two levels of nurses, studied curricula, and planned for the transition of LPNs and RNs seeking additional education. A special task force studied and made recommendations for NYSNA membership requirements if legislation was enacted. Its recommendation to require "nurse" licensure for NYSNA membership, thus preventing future associate degree graduates from membership, was highly controversial.[34]

"EXPANDED" ROLES: In addition to initiating numerous legislative proposals, the association took positions on other legislation affecting the profession. The development of speciality areas such as coronary care units, dialysis units, and intensive care units led to increasing specialization by nurses. This, together with gaps in the health-care system, led to the development of experimental programs in the 1960s which developed roles for "physician extenders," and "expanded" roles for nurses. New programs prepared nurse practitioners to function as primary caregivers in ambulatory settings, and developed roles for clinical nurse specialists in health-care institutions. The association supported the emerging roles and formed organizational units for clinical nurse specialists and primary care nurses, but asserted that these evolving roles were a natural growth of nursing practice, and vehemently objected to the labeling of these roles as "extended" or "expanded."[35] Believing that these roles were already protected by the existing definition of nursing in the Nurse Practice Act, the association opposed legislative proposals seeking to regulate the many emerging health-care roles.

Several proposals were introduced in the 1970 legislature to provide for educational programs and establishment of licensure for the physician's assistant. Noting that admission and curriculum requirements varied widely, NYSNA's board voted to oppose the proposals, and recommended collaborative study with the medical society. Although charged with being reactionary and threatened by the proposed new health-care workers, NYSNA maintained its position that "the present health-care delivery system is chaotic in nature — characterized by inequitable access to services, proliferation of ill-defined occupational titles, and incredible waste of both economic and human resources . . . Introduction of yet another ill-defined worker into such a system can hardly be interpreted as a helpful measure."[36] NYSNA successfully opposed physician's assistant legislation in 1970, but in 1971, legislation was passed establishing the "physician's associate" and "specialist's assistant" roles.[37]

In preparation for the new "expanded" roles, nurses acquired new skills such as performing physical examinations. In 1973 a case concerning the legality of nurses' performing selected parts of physical examinations was brought to the attention of NYSNA and the state departments of education and health.[38] The association maintained that "the practice by nurses of 'expanding' their roles is not new. As health science and technology have advanced, nurses have traditionally incorporated into their practice new tools, techniques and therapeutic measures . . . Those tasks, activities and responsibilities currently being undertaken by registered professional nurses in 'expanding' roles — e.g. physical assessment, history taking, prescription and initiation of therapeutic measures, physician referral, etc. — clearly fall within the scope of nursing practice as defined and authorized" in Education Law.[39]

The Departments of Education and Health were seriously concerned about whether nurse practitioners who were carrying out the "expanded" role were practicing medicine. Numerous legislative proposals supported by the departments were advanced to regulate nurses in these new roles, but the association "regarded the attempt by various groups to revise the Nurse Practice Act to characterize nursing as delegated medical practice as a gross affront to the nursing profession."[40]

By 1982 nurse practitioners in New York had been repeatedly challenged about the legality of their practice, and the controversy over the legal status of their practice had created yet another serious division within the profession. Nurse practitioners organized into a coalition to promote the need for statutory definition and protection of the "nurse practitioner" title, while NYSNA held firmly to its position that nurse practitioners were already protected *as nurses* by the existing Nurse Practice Act.[41] By 1985 the association had succeeded in preventing the enactment of legislation, but enormous amounts of time, energy, and resources had failed to achieve consensus within the nursing community, and the issue was far from resolved.

IMPROVING NURSING PRACTICE: Rapid growth experienced by the Economic Security Program, known as the Economic and General Welfare Program (E&GW) after 1970, continued. In the 1970s nurses at Montefiore, Presbyterian, and Mount Sinai, New York City's largest voluntary hospitals, selected NYSNA as their bargaining representative, as did scores of nurses at smaller institutions. Executive Director Veronica Driscoll commented on the dramatic increase. "We are receiving an unbelievable number of requests daily from groups of nursing practitioners throughout the state for the organization to represent them. Not to just improve their economic status, but to improve the conditions under which they practice as professionals."[42] In one year alone, twenty-one new councils were certified. By 1983, over twenty-nine thousand nurses in 154 employment settings were covered by NYSNA agreements.[43]

Indeed, after gaining dramatic economic concessions in the 1960s, nurses shifted their focus to nursing practice issues and their status as nursing practitioners. To mark this shift in the program's development the term "local units" was changed to "Councils of Nursing Practitioners." Proposed contract provisions began to stress innovations in defining nursing practice and guaranteeing a real voice for nurses in the practice setting. Mount Sinai outpatient nurse Audrey McAllister pointed out that nurses were more concerned with their status as practitioners than with economic issues, but hospital officials opposed nurses' proposals to define nursing practice, claiming these proposals were "infringing on management rights."[44]

In fact, the primary association-wide objective for 1971 was to support and assist nurses in implementing the nursing role. The association was gravely concerned that "a serious erosion of the 'nursing' role has occurred . . . Expected to function as quasi-administrators and 'jacks of all trades,' nurses have been forced to abandon their direct patient care role. It is well-documented that over 60% of the nursing practitioner's time is spent in non-nursing care functions. This scandalous and persistent inappropriate utilization has perpetuated the popular myth of a nursing shortage . . ."[45] Gradually, negotiated contracts began to include nursing practice provisions, such as decreasing non-nursing functions, and the establishment of committees on nursing practice to develop practice standards and make recommendations on staffing patterns.

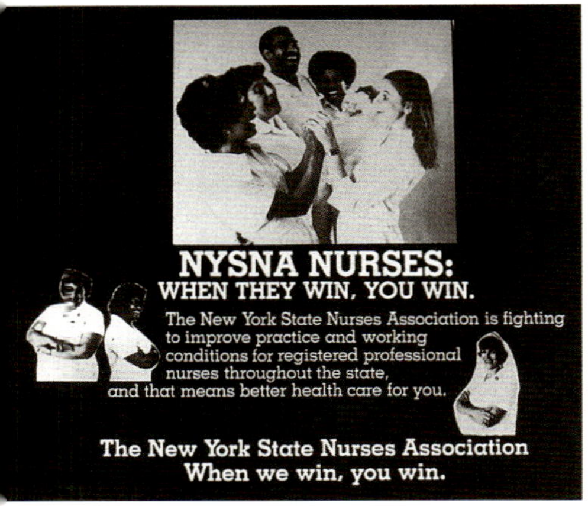

NYSNA publicity campaigns emphasized the value of nursing care to the public.

Determined to assist nurses in practicing within the new definition of nursing practice, program director Eileen M. McCaul declared, ". . . many of the City institutions do not recognize the registered professional nurse's lawful obligation for implementation of nursing diagnosis and treatment and do not, in any way, permit the nursing practitioner to carry out this obligation . . . the registered professional nurses employed by the City of New York wish to emphasize that the period of the great nursing compromise is over. These practitioners are prepared to take every necessary step to improve the quality of nursing care services in City institutions — and will not settle a contract on terms that do not assure them that dramatic, indeed radical progress will be made in permitting nurses to carry our their obligations to patients." On behalf of the nurses, NYSNA submitted specific contract items, including revised position descriptions reflecting the new legal definition of nursing.[46]

"If anyone sitting in here tonight thinks that we would leave, abandon our patients in critical areas, you're mistaken, because we do not propose to strike and to see that consumers and patients are left uncared for."

— *Haywood Gill*[3]

CHALLENGING THE NO-STRIKE POLICY: Conditions in New York's municipal hospitals, now administered through the Health and Hospitals Corporation (HHC), continued to receive attention. In 1970 NYSNA joined with the Committee of Interns and Residents and District Council 37 of the State, County, and Municipal Employees unions in an attempt to raise the level of care in the hospitals. Through "long and historic efforts," this coalition developed a "set of sweeping proposals designed to improve utilization of health manpower in the Department of Hospitals of the City of New York," and protested budget cuts. "We consider that our hospitals are, in fact, being subjected to a budgetary bombing leading to their imminent destruction."[47]

When the steady economic growth of the postwar years slowed in the early 1970s, the situation in the HHC hospitals worsened. The recession hit New York City harder than most areas, and as bankruptcy threatened the city, a freeze was imposed on city wages and thousands of municipal employees were laid off. Frustration among nurses escalated. At NYSNA's 1976 convention, Miriam Gonzalez, on behalf of the Council of Nursing

Practitioners of the Health and Hospitals Corporation, introduced a resolution to remove the no-strike clause from NYSNA policies. Proponents of the resolution spoke graphically of situations which prompted the resolution and contended that rescinding the policy would increase nursing's "clout" in collective bargaining efforts. "We happily gave up our six percent cost of living increases because of the crisis. We're only concerned with giving quality patient care and every nurse practitioner in this room feels the very same way. We need some help."[48] The proposal was highly controversial. To many nurses, the thought of nurses on strike was unacceptable, and opponents argued that withholding nursing services "is in direct and total conflict with the legal and ethical responsibilities of professional nursing practitioners," and urged nurses to focus their efforts on "influencing those responsible for the current mismanaged and politicized health-care field."[49] After an extensive and highly charged debate, the resolution was defeated.

Following the convention, the Board of Directors considered at length the concerns expressed by the voting body, particularly the "overwhelming feeling of despair and frustration projected by nurses as they related their attempts to protect patient interests amid a trend of lowered health standards, personnel cutbacks and financial stringencies."[50] The board authorized a task force to examine impediments to the delivery of quality nursing care and analyze the implications of the no-strike policy. The task force appointed by the board included bargaining unit members and representatives from every major organizational unit to insure broad examination of the issues. The task force recommended "major long-term changes in nursing education, the professional socialization of nursing practitioners and the organization and delivery of nursing care services." In addition, recognizing that "in certain instances, the existence of the No-Strike Policy may inhibit rather than facilitate necessary modification of nursing employment and practice conditions and, thereby, jeopardize rather than protect the welfare of patients," the task force recommended the no-strike policy be rescinded, and developed policies and procedures to protect patients during "voluntary withholding of nursing services."[51] The 1977 voting body accepted the recommendation, and affirmed the professional right of nurses to strike unless prohibited by law.

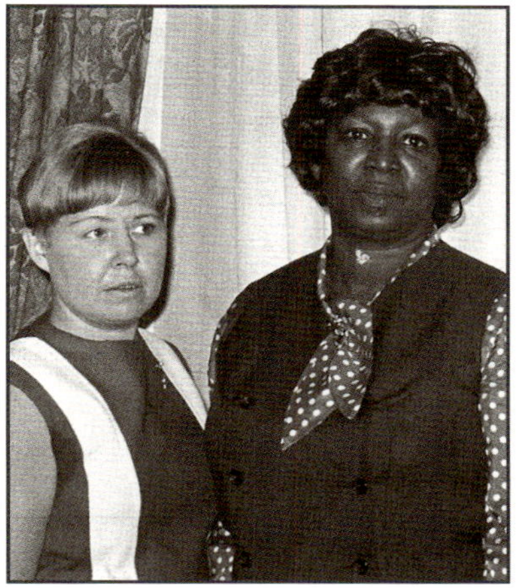

Eileen McCaul on the left and Clara Zeller on the right are shown here in 1970 following negotiations with the City of New York. McCaul was NYSNA's director of the Economic Security Program from 1969 to 1979. Zeller was chairperson of the Department of Hospital's unit council.

The first strikes in NYSNA's history commenced on February 1, 1980, when negotiations over staffing, mandatory overtime, non-nursing functions, and other issues dragged on at Kingsbrook Medical Center, Maimonides Medical Center, and Presbyterian Hospital. Nurses believed that "strike action was the only means of demonstrating to hospital management that critical economic and practice issues had to be resolved."[52] By February 5 new contracts had been accepted, and nurses at all three facilities returned to work. "The major point throughout this situation has been quality patient care . . . The new agreements reflect both patients' and nurses' legitimate rights. Through these agreements the delivery of that essential social service — professional nursing care — will be enhanced."[53]

Meanwhile, frustration was again mounting at New York's municipal hospitals, where nurses were experiencing critical staff shortages, a dangerous and unsanitary working environment, lack of supplies, rat and roach infestations, outdated equipment, and a host of other unacceptable conditions.[54] Nurses held rallies and informational picketing. Finally, on October 10, 1980, nurses, frustrated and angered by a lack of progress in negotiations, staged wildcat strikes and job actions at many of the hospitals. Because the Taylor Law prohibited nurses employed in the public sector from striking, the action was unlawful, and although sympathetic to the nurses' plight, association staff was bound by voting body action which prohibited the sanctioning of illegal strikes. Executive Director Cathryne Welch discussed the association response to the job actions. "There was no denial by this Association of the conditions operant now in the Health and Hospitals Corporation—and operant for literally months and years — which led to a frustration level beyond description. There was no denial that bargaining had been difficult and that the City's position was untenable. Nor was there abandonment of those nurses by this association at any moment."[55] Nurses later expressed understanding of NYSNA's actions when Maggie Jacobs, chairman of the Executive Council of NYSNA's Council of Nursing Practitioners in HHC, introduced a resolution reaffirming commitment to and support of the association and its goals.

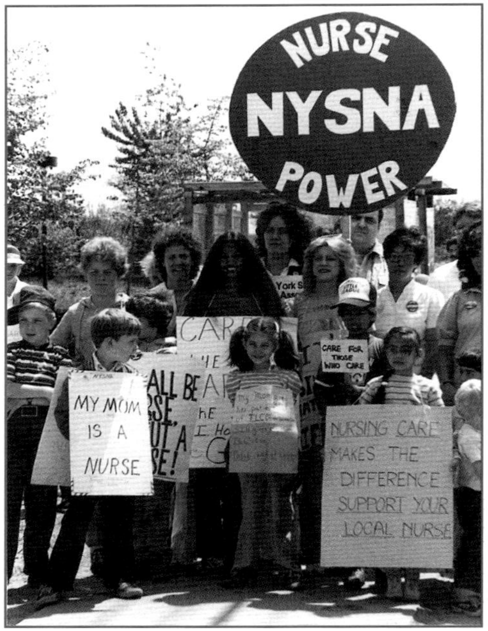

Staten Island nurses and their families rallied during a 1983 strike.

Raids by Competing Unions: During the economic recession of the 1970s, many labor unions faced declining membership and turned their attention to nurses. The American Federation of Teachers (AFT), AFL-CIO, launched a million dollar national effort to organize nurses, and District 1199 of the National Health and Human Service Employees Union stepped up its efforts to do the same. The association was challenged thirty-four times in 1979 "by other labor organizations attempting to increase their membership ranks and their financial status by making a whole host of promises to nurses we represent."[56] The AFT began a well financed campaign to decertify NYSNA at HHC and cause decertification elections in the majority of NYSNA units throughout metropolitan New York City and Long Island. Raiding activity was subsequently launched in virtually every region of the state by a wide variety of unions. Newly appointed Executive Director Cathryne Welch refuted the charges by competing labor organizations that NYSNA was weak, ineffective, elitist, and management dominated. "NYSNA sets the pattern and model for appropriate terms and conditions of practice and employment of registered professional nurses and health-care agencies throughout this state whether it is the elected bargaining representative or not. NYSNA is highly representative of the nursing population in this state . . . the overwhelming majority of its members are in staff nurse and other non-managerial, non-educational positions."[57]

The raiding threats necessitated extraordinary vigilance, but NYSNA prevailed in the majority of representational elections. Of particular importance was the overwhelming defeat in 1980 of the teachers' union and 1199 in a decertification election to determine representation of the HHC nurses, the largest public sector state nurses' association bargaining unit in the country. In 1981 President Beletz hailed the victory at HHC, "as a reinforcement of our major beliefs, that only nursing will control nursing; that only nurses can speak for and represent nurses and nursing."[58]

"We have been harassed. We have been wined, we have been dined, we've been given the opportunity to have shrimps, and sandwiches and other things . . ."

— *Margaret Hobson*[4]

Representing more nurses than any other U.S. labor organization, NYSNA maintained its position as the "strongest and most effective representative of nurses," but by the end of 1984 NYSNA's Economic and General Welfare Program, now under the direction of Kathleen Hoover, was stretched to its limit.[59] The economy continued to lag and employment among nurses vacillated. The poor economy and increased recruitment of foreign nurses led to unemployment among nurses for the first time since before World War II. However, the number of graduating nurses was in decline as both hospital diploma programs and college and university programs closed, and by 1980 the "nursing shortage" was again in the news. Institutions hired nurse recruiters and engaged in massive advertising campaigns to bolster their ranks. Hospitals were forced to confront new realities when consumers demanded improved services and questioned the alarming increase in expenditures for hospital care, and protested the growing differences in care given to the rich and the poor.[60]

Public officials attempted to control health-care costs through regulation of hospital-care costs and the unchecked hospital construction of the postwar period. In 1983 New York passed legislation creating a new system of hospital reimbursement which used a prospective, case-based method of payment for hospital care rather than payment based on actual patient-care costs. NYSNA worked to incorporate nursing care in the reimbursement formula by convening panels of expert nurses who worked in cooperation with consultants and staff from the Department of Health to determine the level of nursing care that the typical patient in each of over seven hundred diagnostic related groups was likely to need. These determinations of "Nursing Intensity Weights" promoted recognition of the value of nursing care in the reimbursement framework. In 1993 New York remained the only state that factored the level of nursing care into the reimbursement formula.[61]

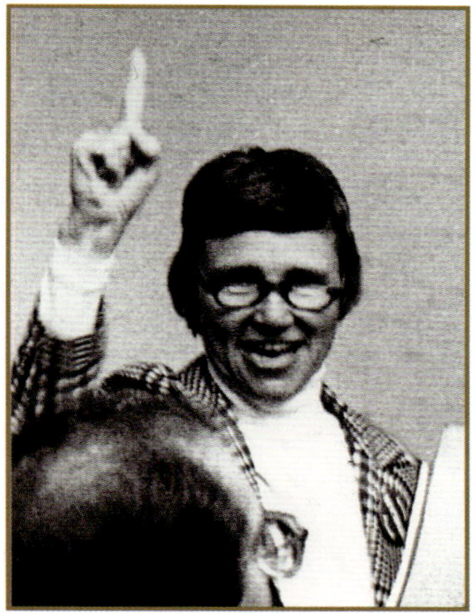

Cathryne A. Welch was a charismatic and devoted executive director. The force of Dr. Welch's leadership far outlasted her five year tenure. Following her resignation from NYSNA, she became the executive director of the Foundation of NYSNA. She received NYSNA's Honorary Recognition Award in 1986 and ANA's Distinguished Membership Award in 1996.

Changes in the hospital reimbursement methodology created an atmosphere of austerity and uncertainty. Threats of hospital closings and news of mergers demoralized nurses and seriously complicated the representation of nurses. As if that weren't enough, the National Labor Relations Act was amended to extend coverage to employees of voluntary hospitals, which led to an increase in unit clarification petitions. The petitions claimed certain supervisory titles should be excluded from contracts, while NYSNA contended that these titles should remain since nursing supervisors were not comparable to industrial supervisors. Concerns were also raised about the legality of participation of directors of nursing in the activities of the association, and the voting body passed resolutions affirming support for the E&GW program and for a "united professional

Foundation of the New York State Nurses Association

The Foundation of the New York State Nurses Association, established as a charitable corporation in 1975, continues to carry out its mission to strengthen the nursing profession's services and increase public knowledge of the nursing profession. The Foundation works to improve health care and public understanding of nursing through its Center for Public Education, strives to improve nursing practice through nursing research via its Center for Nursing Research, and preserves and promotes the history of the profession through its Center for History. The Foundation's Center for History serves as the repository for all of the association's archival records, and NYSNA has worked cooperatively with the Foundation on numerous other public education, research, and historical projects through grants and shared services. In 1988 NYSNA's Council on Nursing Research and the Foundation collaboratively published *Professionalization of Nursing in New York State: Oral History Interviews with Six Leaders Who Helped to Advance the Mission of NYSNA.* The Veronica M. Driscoll Center for Nursing continues to showcase the ongoing contributions of nursing by housing the Foundation's archive center, library, conference facilities, and offices.

association."[62] District 14 member Mary Biris commented, "As members of the council of nursing practitioners, we understand the continuing concern of the directors of nursing services in relation to their roles in the professional organizations of nursing. We are assured that with the wisdom and guidance of the Boards of Directors of this association, those concerns will be explored and that a satisfactory solution will be reached whereby all nurses will be able to live and participate in our multi-purpose organization."[63] These dilemmas continued to be of concern to the association into the next decade.

STRUCTURAL REFORM: In 1969 declining membership, the formation of an increasing number of special interest groups, and low visibility of NYSNA led the board to

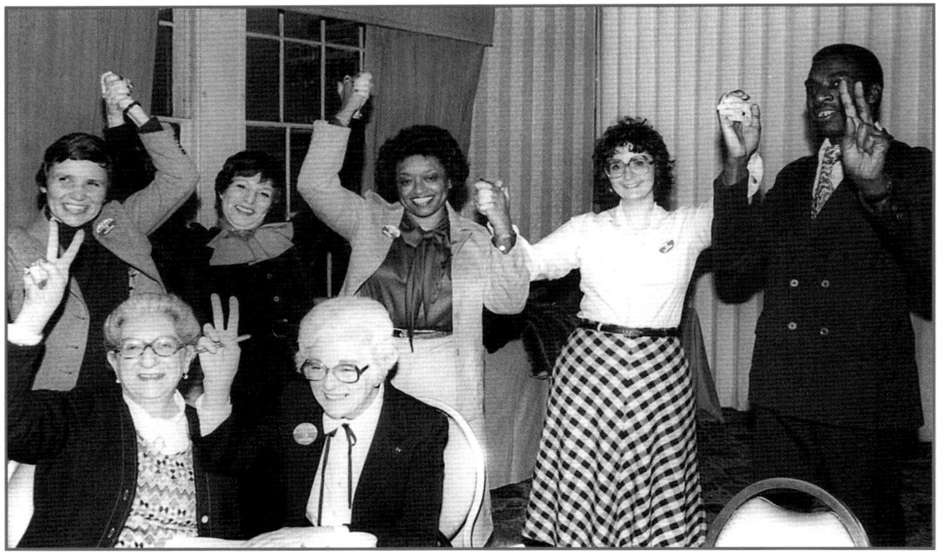

ABOVE: In 1980 ANA President Barbara Nichols met with three hundred members of NYSNA bargaining units to discuss the efforts of trade unions seeking representation of the HHC nurses. Shown standing from left to right are Cathryne Welch, Elaine Beletz, Barbara Nichols, Kathleen Nokes, and Charles Hargett. Seated are Ruth Harper and Sister Mary Meehan. *Photograph by Diane J. Mancino.*

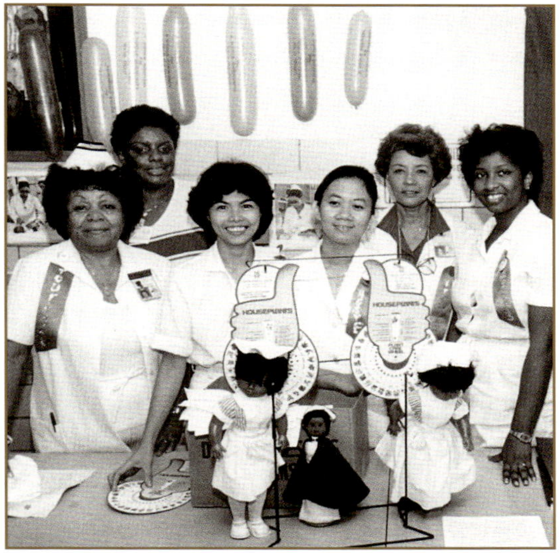

Hospitals sponsored displays such as this one to recruit nurses during the nursing shortage in the 1980s. Nurse recruiters were also sent abroad to bring foreign nurses to New York hospitals. *Courtesy Alumni Association of Harlem Hospital Center School of Nursing.*

appoint a committee to study the association's purpose, structure, and functions. The committee spent hours of exploration, deliberation, and soul searching, as it confronted the recurring issues of misinformation, misconceptions, distance required to attend meetings, lack of communication, and the need for nurses to get involved, especially at the local level. Bylaws' amendments presented to delegates at the 1971 convention included many of the committee's recommendations. Committee chairman Edward Wray urged the delegates to act on the recommendations. "The future of organizations and institutions which remain unresponsive to the rapidly changing needs of their membership and society is predictable. They will crumble and die. Let us not approach our future with suicidal inefficiency and delay. Now is the time for innovation and bold changes!"[64]

The bylaws proposals were indeed bold, and included elimination of sections as the primary organizational units, the creation of councils and nursing practice conference groups, and establishment of the position of president-elect. New organizational units were established, most notably a Lay Council, a Council on Nursing Research, and a Committee on Ethical Practice. Perhaps most significantly, biennial conventions were changed to annual meetings, and the traditional representative House of Delegates was replaced with an "open convention" which provided for a voting body made up of all accredited members in attendance.[65] Another recommendation which was to have a significant impact on both NYSNA and the future structure of ANA, called for experimentation with the long standing tri-level membership structure.

When Veronica Driscoll became executive director, she was seriously concerned about declining membership. Nurses were confused by the membership structure which provided combined district, NYSNA, and ANA membership, and there was increasing concern that members would be lost as a result of a growing philosophical split over association positions. If that wasn't enough, ANA, in the midst of its own financial crisis, increased its dues 100 percent.[66]

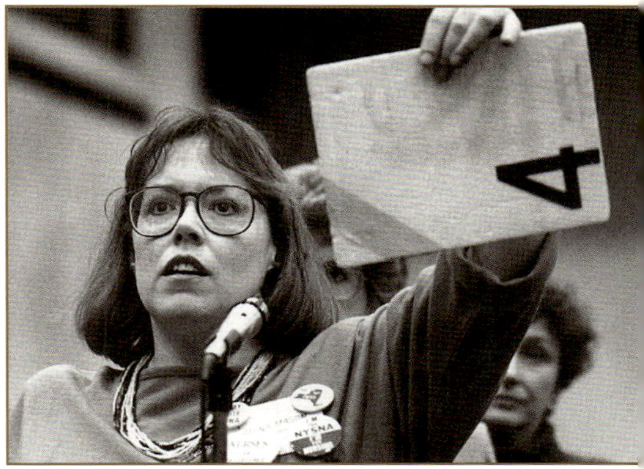

Convention goers like Diana Mason, shown here, debated numerous controversial proposals at ANA and NYSNA meetings.

In 1970 the board approved an experimental program to offer direct NYSNA membership, and a pilot project to offer direct, district-only membership. The board viewed the projects as necessary, extreme measures to revitalize membership. Despite charges by ANA that the experiments were in conflict with ANA bylaws, NYSNA's board reaffirmed its belief in the legality and necessity of the projects. Ongoing discussions with ANA resulted in a three-year joint project which gathered information on the experimental direct-member programs. Data demonstrated that through the direct membership option more nurses became involved and that membership in one level of the organization promoted membership in other levels.[67] In fact, the association's membership nearly doubled between 1974 and 1984, due to direct membership options and to mandatory membership provisions negotiated in collective bargaining agreements.

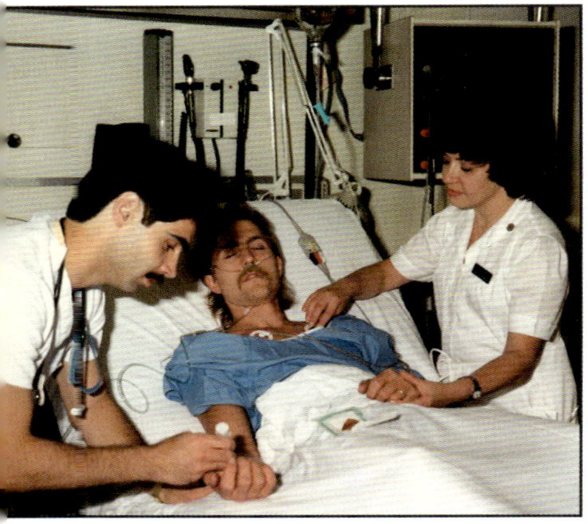

ABOVE: In 1984 NYSNA's Image Campaign brought nursing to the attention of the public. Photographs such as this one were visual reminders of the complex and vital roles nurses played.

Despite the demonstrated success of direct membership, there continued to be conflict between ANA and NYSNA over bylaws issues. Other state associations agreed that their financial difficulties stemmed from ANA's membership structure, and in 1978 representatives of the Eastern Seaboard Regional Executive Conference, a group of association presidents from ten northeastern states, recommended that ANA become a federation of state nurses' associations rather than a membership corporation of individuals.[68]

ANA responded with a proposal to dramatically revise its structure, but the proposal was not for a federation model, but for a conglomerate model. The "new" ANA was proposed as a federation of labor organizations representing health-care workers, with a second national organization proposed as a conglomerate of credentialing, research, political, and other groups. President-elect Susan Fraley stated, "In all candor, the 'conglomerate' structure appears to guarantee complete and total organizational disaster," and NYSNA's voting body adopted a resolution opposing the proposal.[69] At ANA's 1982 convention, delegations from New York and Washington led a movement which resulted in defeat of the conglomerate proposal and adoption of a modified federation.[70] Thus, ANA's unit of membership became the constituent state nurses' association rather than the individual nurse.

GROWTH AND PLANNING: The new-found pride and hopefulness of nurses following the successful 1972 legislative campaign was short-lived. Efforts to maintain the unity of nursing groups through increased communication and the formation of a State Alliance of Nursing Organizations were not powerful enough to counteract the controversial issues of continuing education, entry-into-practice, and "expanded" roles. The growing divisiveness, along with union raiding activities, attempts by the State Board for Nursing to create standards of practice, and various legislative initiatives, threatened the work of the association.

Despite these challenges, there was tremendous growth and activity. Membership more than doubled, association staff grew from fifteen in 1969 to eighty in 1983, and the association and Foundation of NYSNA built a new headquarters. The association was exceedingly active as it responded to the needs of a growing membership and a rapidly changing heath-care system. Staff and organizational units sponsored educational events and responded to daily requests for guidelines, clarification, and advice on nursing practice issues. Staff and members collaborated to formulate position statements, develop a peer review system to assist nurses in evaluating nursing care, and design a nationally recognized quality assurance model. The association expanded collaboration with health-care facilities on health-care standards, and finally developed procedures for handling alleged violations of the Code of Ethics. New organizational units were formed, and a task force was established to develop a peer assistance program for chemically dependent nurses.[71]

A Measure of Professional Pride

By 1970 association office space was grossly inadequate, and a Committee to Study Needs for Headquarters Office recommended the construction of a facility to meet both current and future needs. A "Center for Nursing" was proposed as "a center for library, research, conference and association office facilities. A center for recording of the profession's past and for the developing of the profession's future."[1] The Foundation of the New York State Nurses Association, whose establishment was proposed by NYSNA, raised funds through special events and individual contributions, and the proposed building was constructed on a wooded site in Guilderland, New York. Dedicated in 1977, the Center for Nursing represented for many "new life and renewed vigor, new approaches to old problems, and new hope for the future."[2] In 1979 the center was renamed the Veronica M. Driscoll Center for Nursing in tribute to Driscoll's leadership. The association's new headquarters was much more than a building, it was a symbol of the strength and vitality of nursing, and a tribute to a living legend. Cathryne Welch described the center as a "living testimony to the dignity and perpetuity of the nursing profession and to the faith of nurses themselves in themselves, their practice and their organization."[3]

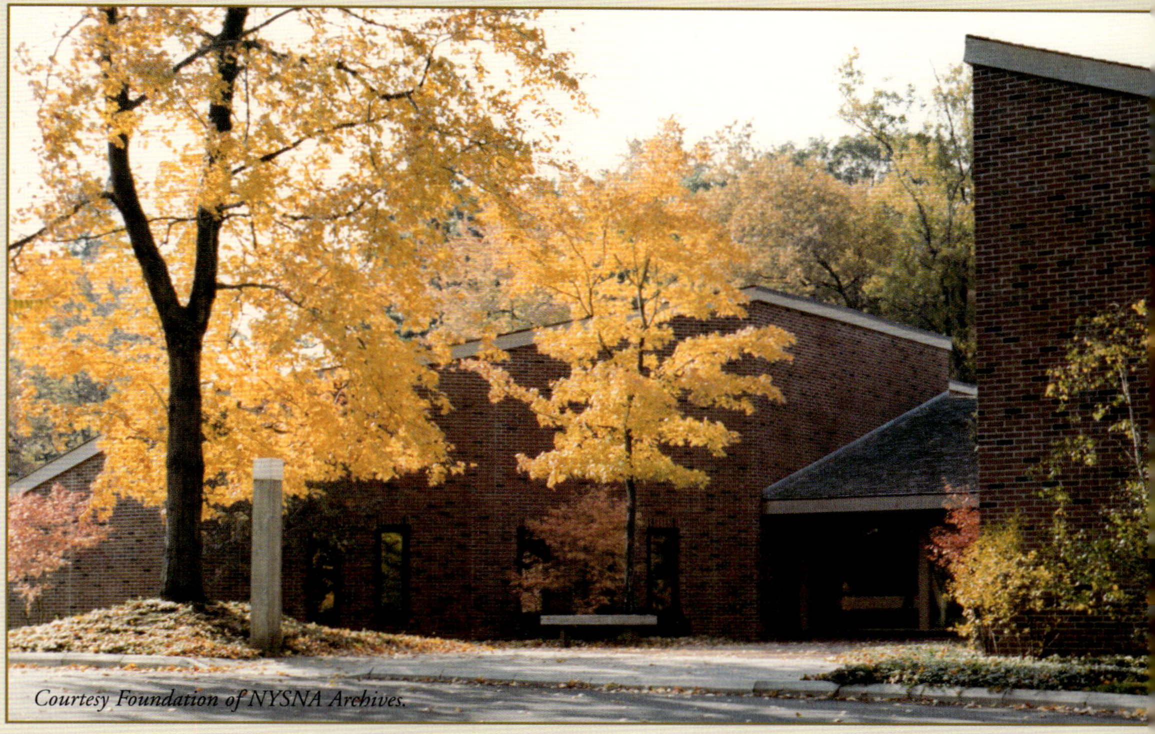

Courtesy Foundation of NYSNA Archives.

The work of the association became more focused on systematic analysis, evaluation, and planning when Cathryne Welch was hired as the director of Planning and Research in 1969. The Council on Nursing Research was formed, and research priorities were developed. In 1972 NYSNA became the first state nurses' association to hire a full-time librarian, and the library began lending materials, participating in regional interlibrary loan systems, and preparing bibliographies. Later, under the direction of Warren Hawkes, director of the Library, and Julie Pavri, archivist, NYSNA developed the first comprehensive archives and records management program housed in a state nurses' association. This program enabled nurses, students, and the public to have access to the extensive historical records and holdings of the association. In 1978 the Council on Research began the continuing practice of compiling information on nursing research through its Clearinghouse on Nursing Research in New York State, published in the *Journal of the New York State Nurses Association.*[72]

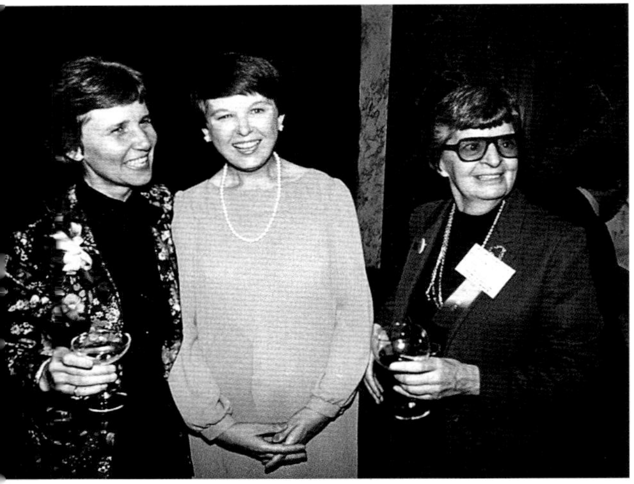

LEFT: New Executive Director Martha Lane Orr is shown here at center with her predecessors Cathryne Welch at left and Veronica Driscoll at right.

With the resignation of Executive Director Cathryne Welch in 1984, another stage in the life of the association came to an end. During the distinguished tenure of Executive Directors Driscoll and Welch, the association experienced exhilarating successes and bitter defeats. President Susan Fraley admitted to "battle fatigue" in 1982, after struggling to ward off numerous threats. ". . . we cannot continue to argue item for item among ourselves and still expect to advance nursing . . . we have grasped the frightening reality that as we continue to divide ourselves internally a tragic vacuum in professional leadership occurs." In 1983 Fraley proposed an organizational self-assessment to "reorient the association's preoccupation with defense to a more effective unifying programmatic effort." The needs and resources assessment provided a framework for strategic planning to prepare the organization to resolve "unfinished business," and face new challenges in the years ahead.[73]

CHAPTER NOTES

TEXT

1. Laura L. Simms, "The Role of the Staff Nurse in Nursing Service," *New York State Nurse* 38 (January 1966): 2–4.

2. "New York State Nurses Association 1973 58th Convention" (Rochester, N.Y., 1973, stenotype transcript), A 18–22.

3. "Swing Around the Schools" Report to the Board of Directors, NYSNA, 24 June 1971, NYSNA Archives; Economic Security Program Informational Forums' Report to Board of Directors, NYSNA, 24 June 1971, NYSNA Archives; and "New York State Nurses Association 1971 Convention" (Buffalo, N.Y., 1971, stenotype transcript), A 10.

4. "Program of Action," *Report* 1 (January 1970): 1.

5. "Venturing," *Report* 1 (January 1970): 1.

6. "By Jove—Perhaps We've Got It!" *Report* 2 (January 1971): 1; and Legislative Program Report to Board of Directors, NYSNA, 11 June 1970 and 17 December 1970, NYSNA Archives. A recodification of the Education Law, based on the work of the joint legislative committee, was finally introduced in 1970. This omnibus professions bill was vetoed by the Governor, and introduced again in 1971.

7. "1971 Convention," D 57–58. Questionnaires were distributed to all directors of nursing service, all directors of schools of nursing, nurses in two hospitals and one public health agency in each district, and faculty and senior students in nursing education programs in every district. Responses (based on a 49 percent return) indicated there was not a "groundswell of dissatisfaction with the Act," nor was there familiarity or understanding of the content of the law. The committee viewed these findings alarming "in light of the advances in science and technology and increasing demands for redefinitions of roles of all health workers." There was also considerable diversity of opinion about the purpose and adequacy of the law. However, there was strong support for improving the educational preparation and functioning of all personnel providing nursing care. The committee concluded there was a sufficient degree of commitment to facilitate changes in the Nurse Practice Act. (Questionnaire on The Nurse Practice Act: A Summary Report of Findings, 2 February 1970, NYSNA Archives.)

8. Driscoll, *Legitimizing the Profession,* 59, 64.

9. "1971 Convention," D 58.

10. "1971 Convention," D 59. Other committee proposals were included in the omnibus professions bill.

11. Special Committee to Study the Nurse Practice Act Report to the Board of Directors, NYSNA, 18 March 1971, NYSNA Archives; and "1971 Convention," D 61.

12. *NYSNA Legislative Bulletin* (2 April 1971): 1. One nurse anonymously donated $2,500 to the cause.

13. Legislative Program Report, NYSNA, 18 March 1971, NYSNA Archives.

14. Driscoll, *Legitimizing the Profession,* 61–62.

15. "1971 Convention," D 61.

16. Veronica M. Driscoll, "The Practice of Nursing Remains Illegitimate — But Who Cares?!" *Report* 2 (July–August 1971): 1.

17. "The First Step Toward Institutional Licensure," *Report* 2 (July–August 1971): 3. At its December 1971 meeting, the Board of Directors accepted the Committee on Legislation's recommendation that NYSNA oppose the concept of institutional licensure and urged ANA to adopt and publish a position on this issue. (Board of Directors Minutes, NYSNA, 16 December 1971, NYSNA Archives.)

18. "1971 Convention," A 7–8. NYSNA proposals which had been included in the omnibus professions bill were enacted.

19. Ibid., D 54–55.

20. Ibid., D 61–62; and "Additional Biennial Reports to the House of Delegates 1969–1971" (Albany, N.Y., 1971, mimeographed), 4. "Nursing practitioner" (not to be confused with "nurse practitioner," a term not yet widely used) was a term frequently used during this period as a synonym for registered nurse.

21. Driscoll, *Legitimizing the Profession,* 63.

22. "New York State Nurses Association 1972 Annual Reports" (Albany, N.Y., 1972, mimeographed).

23. Kalisch and Kalisch, *Advance of American Nursing,* 452; and "New York State Nurses Association 1974 Annual Reports," (Albany, N.Y., 1974, mimeographed), 17–19. Less than two years after passage of the new definition, the rationale for the First National Conference on Classification of Nursing diagnoses stated, "The nursing diagnosis has been recognized professionally and legally as a major component of nursing practice, as in the definition of nursing included in the New York State Nursing Practice Act." ("Annual Reports of the New York State Nurses Association 1972–1973" [Albany, N.Y., 1973, mimeographed], 29.)

24. Board of Directors Minutes, NYSNA, 8 December 1969, NYSNA Archives; "58th Convention," D 12; "Annual Reports Supplement to the 1979–1980 Book of Reports" (Guilderland, N.Y., 1980, mimeographed), 1; and Veronica M. Driscoll, "The Continuing Saga of Nursing's Failed Professionalization: The New York Story, 1973–1985," in *Critical Issues in American Nursing in the Twentieth Century: Perspectives and Case Studies,* ed. Darwin H. Stapleton and Cathryne A. Welch (Guilderland, N.Y.: Foundation of NYSNA, 1994), 119–20.

25. "New York State Nurses Association 1972 Convention" (Kiamesha Lake, N.Y., 1972, stenotype transcript), B 17.

26. Board of Directors Minutes, NYSNA, 15 June 1972, NYSNA Archives; and "Annual Reports 1972–1973," 14.

27. "Annual Reports 1980–1981 New York State Nurses Association" (Guilderland, N.Y., 1981, mimeographed), 15.

28. "The New York State Nurses Association Annual Reports 1974–1975" (Albany, N.Y., 1975, mimeographed), 13–15.; "Annual Reports Supplement 1982–1983" (Guilderland, N.Y., 1983, mimeographed), 17–19; and Board of Directors Minutes, NYSNA, 19–20 September 1985, NYSNA Archives.

29. *Entry into Professional Practice: The Arden House Conference* (Albany, N.Y.: NYSNA, 1975), 5.

30. "Annual Reports 1974–1975," 43–47.

The proposal included a revised definition of nursing, fully supported by the medical society, which eliminated all references to medical and dental regimens. ("New York State Nurses Association Convention" [Syracuse, N.Y., 1975, stenotype transcript], B 15.) The proposed titles were later changed to "registered associate nurse" and "registered professional nurse."

31. "Convention, 1975," A 15 and B 17–20.

32. "The New York State Nurses Association Annual Reports 1977–1978," (Albany, N.Y., 1978, mimeographed), B 2.

33. "61st Annual Convention, New York State Nurses Association" (New York, N.Y., 1976, stenotype transcript), B 28.

34. "American Nurses' Association Board Announces Support of NYSNA 1985 Legislation; Nationwide Survey Shows 72% of States Now Involved in Entry into Practice Issue," *Report* 9 (March–April 1978): 1, 5; and "House of Delegates Passes Entry into Practice Resolutions; National Officers and Directors Elected," *Report* 9 (July–August 1978): 1. The House also directed that by 1980 ANA clearly identify two categories of nursing practice, and approved a grandfathering proposal. In January 1986 North Dakota was the first state to implement the recommended standardization through State Board for Nursing regulations.

35. "1972 Convention," D 12–13.

36. "Will the Real Physician's Assistant Please Stand Up?" *Report* 1 (September 1970): 3; Cathryne A. Welch, Statement of the New York State Nurses Association to Board of Regents Legislative Conference, Albany, N.Y., 10 September 1970, NYSNA Archives; Board of Directors Minutes, NYSNA, 19 March 1970, NYSNA Archives; and "P.A.'s Perhaps . . . But First Things First," *Report* 2 (April 1971): 4.

37. "Additional Biennial Reports 1969–1971 (Albany, N.Y., 1971, mimeographed).

38. "The 'Expanded Role of the Nurse' Becomes the Focus of Interest of Several External Groups," *Report* 6 (April–May 1975): 1. The Department of Education ordered nurse employees of the New York Telephone Company to cease and desist performing certain parts of physical examinations. NYSNA protested the action, but in the middle of the debate New York Telephone acceded to the Department's order. (Driscoll, "The Continuing Saga," 121–22.)

39. Position re: Resolution of the "Nurse-Practitioner Question," 4 March 1975, NYSNA Archives, 1–2.

40. Driscoll, "The Continuing Saga," 121.

41. Board of Directors Minutes, NYSNA, 21–22 April 1983, NYSNA Archives.

42. "1972 Convention," B 26.

43. "1974 Annual Reports," 33–36; and "Annual Reports, the New York State Nurses Association 1982–1983" (Guilderland, N.Y., 1983, mimeographed), 50. The reported increase was for the September 1973 to September 1974 time period.

44. "Nurses Guaranteed Right to Govern Nurse Practice," *American Journal of Nursing* 71 (January 1971): 11.

45. "Let the Record Show," *Report* 2 (January 1971): 5; and "1971 NYSNA Program of Action," *Report* 2 (January 1971): 4.

46. "The Great Nursing Compromise is Over!" *Report* 3 (June 1972): 4, 6.

47. NYSNA, District Council 37, and Committee of Interns & Residents to Health and Hospitals Corporation and the Office of Labor Relations, 4 June 1970, NYSNA Archives; "Coalition for Care," *Report* 1 (June 1970): 1, 3; and "New York City Hospitals in Crisis Over Budget," *American Journal of Nursing* 69 (May 1969): 913. The Committee of Interns & Residents initiated the joint deliberations, and continued to support the nurses' concerns in November 1970, when a group of two thousand indicated they would plan to list deaths "attributable to the shortage of nurses." (*American Journal of Nursing* 70 [November 1970]: 2276.)

48. "61st Convention," C 3–36–37.

49. "New York State Nurses Association Annual Reports 1976–1977" (Guilderland, N.Y., 1977, mimeographed), B 7. The final report of the task force summarized the discussion at the 1976 convention.

50. Ibid.

51. Ibid., B 16–20. The task force included representatives from organizational units on nursing practice, nursing service administration, ethics, and nursing education.

52. "Major Improvements in Practice Conditions Won as RNs Ratify New Contracts; 3 Strikes End," *Report* 11 (January–February 1980): 1, 3.

53. Ibid., 3.

54. "HHC/City Nurses Express Frustration; Await Panel Report," *Report* 11 (November–December 1980): 3.

55. Ibid.

56. "The Opportunity is Ours–If We Want It!" *Report* 10 (May 1979): 1; and "Annual Reports Supplement to the 1978–1979 Book of Reports" (Guilderland, N.Y., 1979, mimeographed), 3–5. Both AFT and 1199 were rapidly losing members in New York State, and NYSNA saw these new campaigns as a move to improve their financial status through increased membership.

57. "65th Convention, New York State Nurses Association" (Grossingers, N.Y., 1980, stenotype transcript), A 42–43; and "Annual Reports 1982–1983," 50–51.

58. "66th Convention, New York State Nurses Association" (Rochester, N.Y., 1981, stenotype transcript), A 34.

59. "Annual Reports Supplement 1979–1980," 7–8.

60. Advisory Council Report to Board of Directors, NYSNA, 8 June 1971, NYSNA Archives; "Some Thoughts to Ponder About 'The Nursing Shortage'" *Report* 11 (May–June 1980): 3; and Opdycke, *No One Turned Away,* 162 Between 1960 and 1980, national expenditures for health care rose from $27 billion to $248 billion, or from 5.3 percent of the gross national product to 9.4 percent. The number of nursing programs in New York dropped from 139 in 1969, to 98 in 1980.

61. "What You Need to Know About Hospital Reimbursement," *Report* 24 (May 1993): 8; "NYSNA Panel Sets Nursing Care Levels for DRG Reimbursement System," *Report* 24 (March 1993): 3; Update on Activities Related to the Nine Action Proposals and Implementation Strategies, Report to the Board of Directors, NYSNA, 26–27 July 1989, NYSNA Archives; and Report of the Executive Director, 29 October 1994, 3. The New York Prospective Hospital Reimbursement Methodology system was known as NYPHRM.

62. "New York State Nurses Association 59th Annual Convention," (Lake Placid, N.Y., 1974, stenotype transcript), B 33.

63. "Convention, 1975," D 6.

64. "Biennial Reports of the New York State Nurses Association 1969–1971" (Albany, N.Y., 1971, mimeographed), 15–18.

65. "1971 Convention," B 55–D 53; and "Proposed Amendments to New York State Nurses Association Bylaws," *Journal of the New York State Nurses Association* 2 (Summer 1971): 53–66. The "open convention" was a hotly debated issue, which was defeated on the first vote, and passed at the end of the meeting when it was re-introduced. Some committees were disbanded, including the Committee on Service Funds and the Anne L. Hansen Loan Fund. Remaining funds were distributed to Nurses House and the association's library.

66. Driscoll to Robert H. Jones, 29 July 1970, NYSNA Archives. In July 1970 only 18 percent of the state's actively practicing registered nurses were NYSNA members.

67. Patricia H. Collins to Veronica M. Driscoll, Buffalo, N.Y., 17 September 1970, NYSNA Archives; Board of Directors Minutes, NYSNA, 24 September 1970, NYSNA Archives; "A Revitalization Attempt," *Report* 2 (May–June 1971): 1.; Board of Directors Minutes, NYSNA, 18 February 1971, NYSNA Archives; "1974 Annual Reports," 46–51; "Annual Reports 1976–1977," C 1–2; and "ANA and NYSNA Interpretation of Bylaws Differ," *Report* 9 (March–April 1978): 3.

68. Board of Directors Minutes, NYSNA, 19–20 September 1977, NYSNA Archives.

69. "Conglomerate Model for ANA Draws Voting Body Opposition & Resolution," *Report* 12 (November–December 1981): 3–4.

70. "NYSNA Members Elected to Office During ANA Convention in Washington," *Report* 13 (July–August–September 1982): 3.

71. "1974 Annual Reports," 18–19; "Annual Reports 1975–1976," 30–31; and "Annual Reports 1982–1983," 26.

72. "The NYSNA Library — A Benefit of Membership," *Report* 7 (January–February 1976): 7. In 1970, the *New York State Nurse* was replaced as the association's official publication by the *Journal of the New York State Nurses Association* and the newsletter *Report.* ("The New York State Nurses Association Annual Reports 1977–1978" [Guilderland, N.Y., 1978, mimeographed]; and "New York State Nurses Association 1983 Voting Body Business Sessions" [Albany, N.Y., 1983, stenotype transcript], A 18–20.)

73. Susan J. Fraley, "President's Address," *Journal of the New York State Nurses Association* 13 (December 1982): 7.

FEATURES

Veronica M. Driscoll

1. Board of Directors Minutes, NYSNA, 6 October 1969, NYSNA Archives; "Confrontations," *Report* 1 (December 1969): 2; and "Veronica M. Driscoll," in *Professionalization of Nursing in New York State: Oral History Interviews with Six Leaders Who Helped to Advance the Mission of NYSNA,* ed. Elizabeth Carter and Jane Fielding (Guilderland, N.Y.: NYSNA, 1988), 115-26.

Laura L. Simms

1. "1972 Convention," B 38-42.

2. "Harper and Simms Receive Honorary Recognition," *Report* 9 (November 1978): 11; and Curriculum Vitae, NYSNA Archives.

A Measure of Professional Pride

1. "A Measure of Professional Pride . . . Support the Center for Nursing," *Journal of the New York State Nurses Association* 8 (December 1977): 43.

2. "A Measure of Professional Pride: Center for Nursing Officially Dedicated," *Report* 8 (June–August 1977): 8–9.

3. "67th Annual Convention, New York State Nurses Association" (Albany, N.Y., 1982, stenotype transcript), A 39; "NYSNA to Build Own Office by 1972," *Report* 1 (June 1970): 1; and "A Center for Nursing: A Measure of Professional Pride," *Report* 5 (December 1974): 4–5.

EXCERPTS

1. "Catherine Leach, Deputy Director, Retiring After 21 Years With NYSNA," *Report* 16 (March-April 1985): 3.

2. "59th Annual Convention," C 38.

3. "61st Annual Convention," C 4-15.

4. "New York State Nurses Association" (Syracuse, N.Y., 1979, stenotype transcript), B 35.

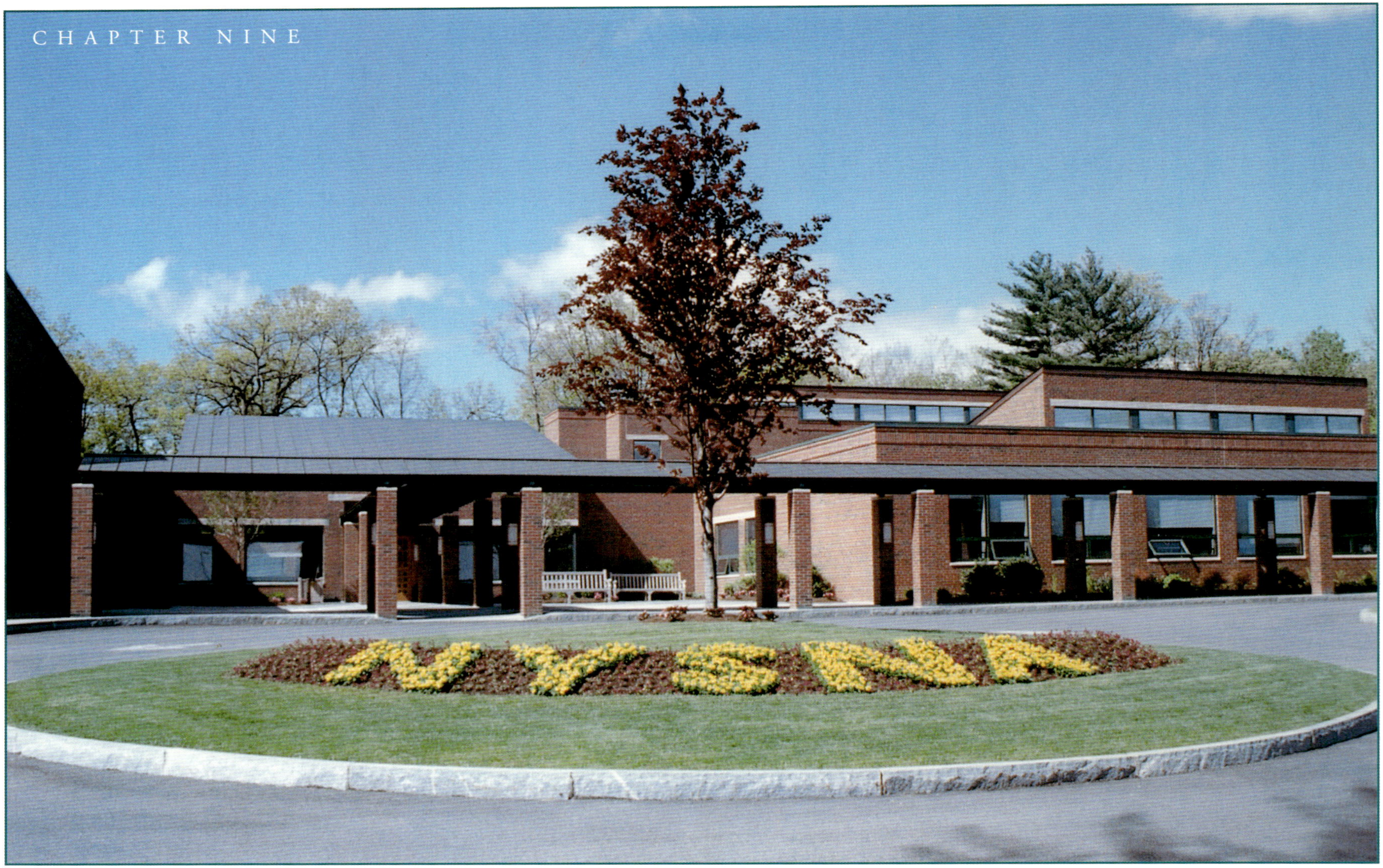

CHAPTER NINE

In 1995 NYSNA built new expanded headquarters in Latham, New York.
Photograph by Mark Genovese.

STRIVING FOR REFORM 1984 ~ 2000

Attendees at the 1984 convention recognized the resignation of Cathryne Welch, and welcomed Martha Lane Orr as the association's new executive director. The voting body addressed the long-standing, unresolved issues of entry-into-practice legislation, exempt clause repeal, financial support for nursing education, affirmation of primary care nurses, and the utilization of unlicensed personnel. Members also addressed emerging concerns: the needs of chemically dependent nurses, nursing entrepreneurship, and foreign nurses. Many of these issues remained on the association's agenda throughout the 1990s, and together with the Action Plan based on the Nursing Needs and Resources Assessment, constituted a challenging agenda.[1] The escalating nursing shortage, ANA membership proposals, and a National Labor Relations Board (NLRB) decision placed even more demands on the association's resources.

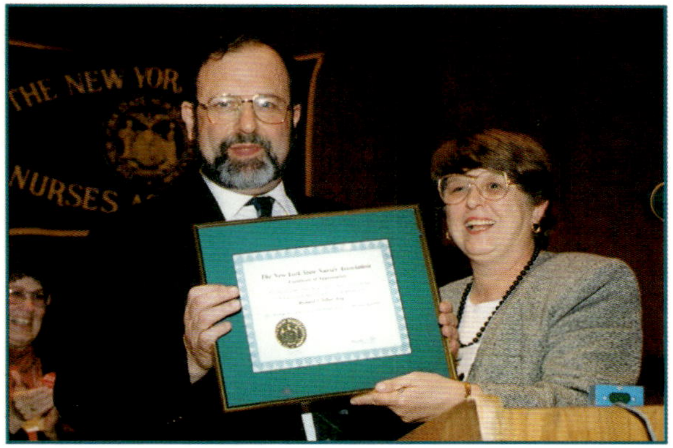

ABOVE: Richard Silber, NYSNA's legal counsel for many years, received a certificate of appreciation in 1994 from Martha Orr for distinguished service to the association.

THE NORTH SHORE DECISION: Executive Director Orr's first significant challenge was an NLRB decision regarding NYSNA's representation of nurses at North Shore University Hospital. Registered nurses at North Shore overwhelmingly elected NYSNA in 1977, but the hospital quickly filed a motion to revoke NYSNA's certification, charging supervisory and management domination. After years of hearings and legal maneuvering, the NLRB released a decision in 1985 that revoked the certification. The ruling accepted earlier opinions that statutory supervisors were actively involved in the governance of NYSNA, and that the collective bargaining process was not sufficiently insulated from governance of the association. NYSNA maintained that the NLRB misinterpreted the structure and function of NYSNA as a multipurpose professional association. Nonetheless, NYSNA's long-time legal counsel Richard Silber, of the Harder, Silber and Bergan legal firm, recommended a series of steps to remove any *appearance* of insufficient insulation of the collective bargaining program. The board instituted a variety of administrative policies, recommended the elimination of the Council on Economic and General Welfare, and established a task force to plan for a delegate assembly of nurses in NYSNA collective bargaining units.[2] Orr was optimistic that the association would withstand the threat of the NLRB decision. "I am confident that we will preserve and protect the multi-purpose nature of this Association and the membership right of all nurses. We will persist in our efforts. We will maintain our efforts to demonstrate that the nurses whom we represent are autonomous; they are independent, and this Association will prevail."[3]

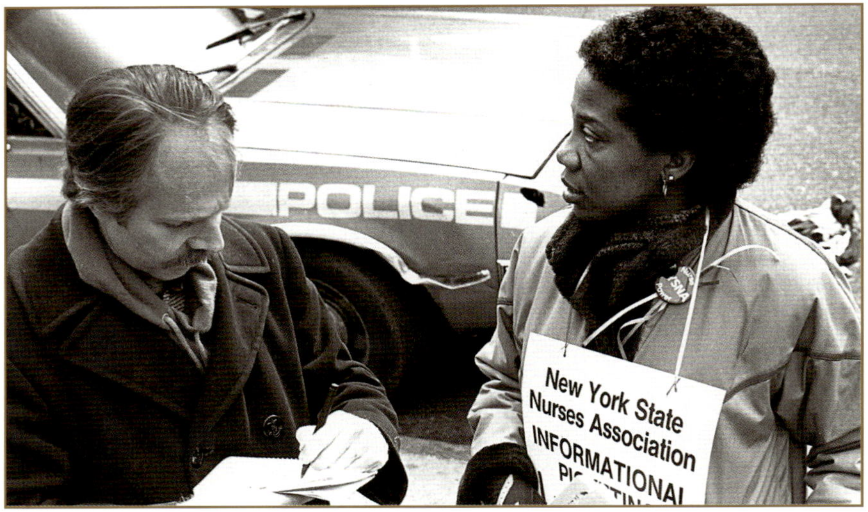

Maggie Jacobs, long-time chair of the bargaining unit at Kings County Hospital and former NYSNA secretary, protested conditions. *Photo by Ricky Flores.*

The newly elected Delegate Assembly held its first meeting in 1988, and elected Marva Wade as its first chairperson. Over the years the Delegate Assembly developed into an important resource for bargaining unit nurses. Through meetings four times a year, the assembly provided a forum for making recommendations on collective bargaining issues to staff, and instituted an annual Delegate Assembly Award. The Delegate Assembly was instrumental in establishing a Protected Action Fund which provided financial support for individuals or bargaining units on strike or in difficult negotiations. Funds were also used for media advertisements to combat layoffs and downsizing. In 1993 Delegate Assembly chair Audrey Ludmer noted that the Delegate Assembly provided nurses represented by NYSNA with the "power and resources to affect policy and develop statewide strategies."[4]

CONFLICT WITH THE AMERICAN NURSES ASSOCIATION: NYSNA was the largest of the fifty-three constituent members of ANA, and took its national leadership responsibilities very seriously. In 1986 ANA's House of Delegates anticipated passage of entry-into-practice legislation creating two statutory categories of nursing personnel (the "professional" baccalaureate prepared nurse, and the "associate" prepared nurse), and requested analysis of membership eligibility of these two levels of nurses. NYSNA had already studied this issue in relation to its own membership, and maintained that such consideration was premature until the issue of entry-into-practice was actually resolved. NYSNA's earlier task force recommended that NYSNA membership be restricted to professional nurses, and NYSNA's board supported an all professional model for future ANA membership.[5] Despite the unanimous opposition of the New York delegation, ANA's 1987 House of Delegates adopted bylaws which required state associations to offer membership to non-professional nurses. NYSNA President Ellen Burns commented, "The vote in the House of Delegates does violence to our tradition. We were organized as a society of professional nurses. If we diversify, we will dilute our resources, fragment our purpose, and diminish our impact."[6]

> "The times demand that we stay unified and use our energies collectively to solve the serious problems facing the profession and the health-care system."
>
> — *Diana Mason*[1]

Believing the bylaws fundamentally altered the nature, composition, and mission of ANA, NYSNA's board took an unprecedented step, and courageously approved a resolution to withdraw as a constituent member of the ANA. Forums held to discuss the proposal revealed little opposition to maintaining an all professional membership association, but serious disagreement over the proposed withdrawal. The 1987 voting body overwhelmingly voted to postpone consideration of withdrawal.[7]

In 1988 NYSNA's voting body again postponed action pending the report of ANA's Commission on Organizational Assessment and Renewal (COAR). Former NYSNA President Cecilia Mulvey, a member of the commission, congratulated the association "for bringing forward the membership issue, which forced a creative rethinking of ANA."[8] The COAR report made sweeping recommendations on ANA's structure, functions, and organizational relationships. In acting on the report, ANA's 1989 House of Delegates reinstated RN licensure as a requirement for membership, although membership remained an option for "future second-level practitioners," thus permitting states that enacted two levels of nursing practice to admit non-professional nurses as members.[9] Although some NYSNA members were dissatisfied with ANA's resolution of the issue, NYSNA maintained its historic ties to the national organization.

ADVANCED NURSING PRACTICE: The growth of opportunities in specialty nursing practice and "expanded" practice continued, and nurses forged new modes of independent practice in response to advancing medical technology and an increasingly complex health-care system. NYSNA supported these efforts on several fronts. In 1984 NYSNA formed a task force to explore mechanisms of establishing a business operation, models of entrepreneurial endeavors, funding sources, trends, and impediments to moving nurses out of the traditional employee role. NYSNA even considered forming a "nursing corporation" to establish practice centers to make quality nursing care directly accessible to the public. While the plan was never realized, the association actively supported nurses in innovative practice. NYSNA held regional workshops, published *Nursing Entrepreneurship in New York State,* and formed the Functional Unit of Nurse Entrepreneurs.[10]

Nurses providing primary care services were hampered by an inability to prescribe, and the 1985 voting body adopted a resolution on the need for prescriptive privileges for nurses. Meanwhile, an advanced nursing practice bill, endorsed by the Coalition of Nurse Practitioners, was introduced into

MARTHA L. ORR

Martha Orr was hired as NYSNA's executive director in 1984. Orr had extensive experience as a practicing clinical nurse specialist, and was widely regarded for her expertise in dialysis and transplant nursing. She also was experienced in organizational work, administration, and teaching. In her first address to NYSNA's voting body, Orr expressed her pleasure at the opportunity to "bear witness to the vitality, the commitment, and the enthusiasm of an organization that can justifiably claim to be the brightest and the best of the state nurses associations . . . I have discovered the dimensions of excellence are rewritten every day by those who passionately believe that this organization can, does, and is expected to provide the leadership needed to realize nursing's goals."[1]

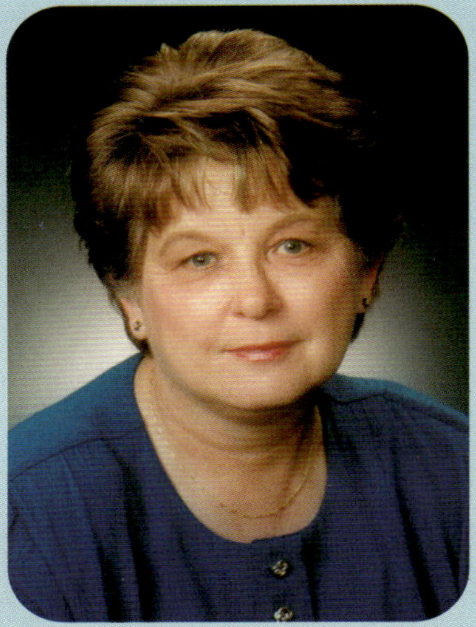

Orr has served longer than any previous NYSNA executive director. She has faced many challenges, including personnel shortages, health-care restructuring, and competing labor unions. Through empathetic listening she has heard the concerns of New York's nurses. Through her eloquent addresses, she has reconciled diverse interests and inspired both members and staff to work together for nursing, for nurses, and for the public. During her tenure, membership reached an all-time high of over 35,500, and staff grew to over 125. NYSNA formed a political action committee, a program for chemically dependent nurses, and a delegate assembly of nurses represented for collective bargaining. Orr facilitated a strategic planning process, and carefully monitored implementation of association goals, including the construction of a new headquarters building. Through challenges and triumphs, Orr has celebrated and contributed to the sustained history of accomplishment that characterizes the New York State Nurses Association.[2]

the legislature. NYSNA's Functional Unit of Primary Care Practitioners was eager for the association to develop legislation designed to resolve problems faced by primary care nurses. The board, however, believed the bill restricted the practice of nurses and placed advanced practice nurses under physician control. NYSNA vigorously opposed the legislation, but in 1988 New York's Nurse Practitioner Bill was signed into law. The law established a certification system, and authorized nurse practitioners to diagnose illness and physical conditions, perform therapeutic and corrective measures, and write prescriptions in collaboration with a physician and in accordance with written practice agreements and protocols.[11]

Despite its opposition to the bill, once it was enacted, NYSNA worked tirelessly with state agencies to clarify regulations and remove obstacles to certification. NYSNA provided information on the new law in *Report*, and sponsored courses to help nurses meet certification requirements. NYSNA also fought for full prescriptive privileges when the federal Drug Enforcement Agency refused to issue numbers to New York nurse practitioners, thus blocking their ability to prescribe controlled substances. NYSNA initiated an intense letter writing campaign which resulted in an opinion by New York's attorney general supporting full prescriptive privileges for nurse practitioners.[12]

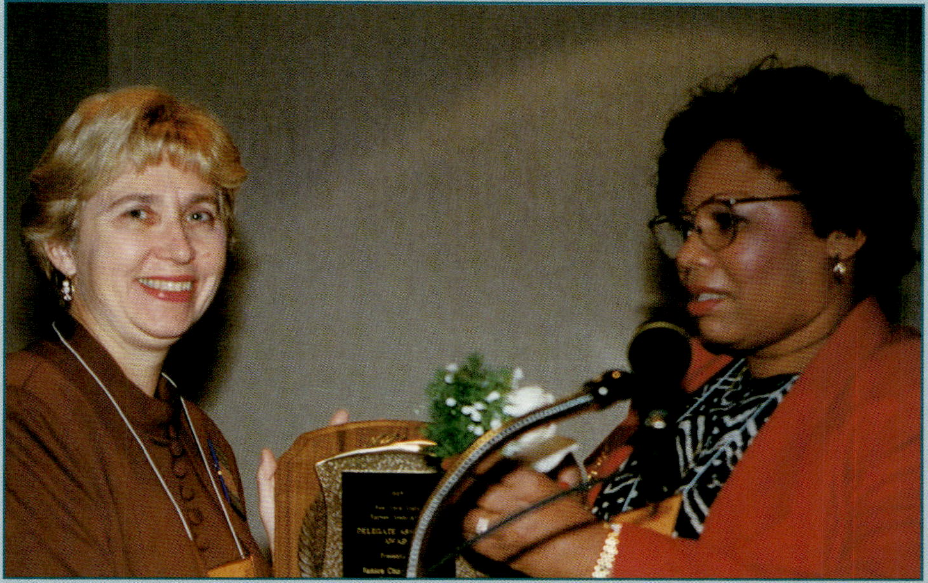

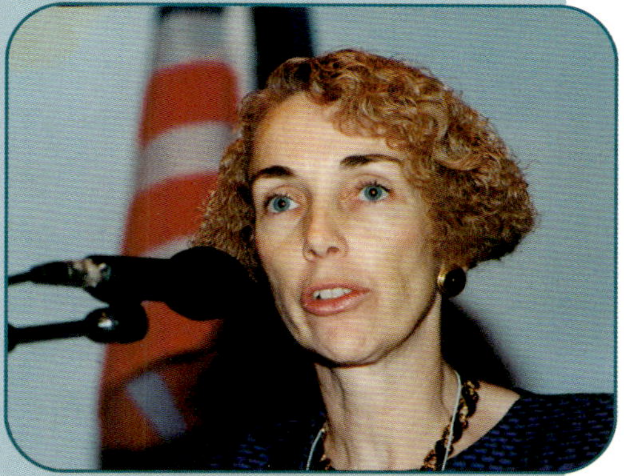

RIGHT: Mary Eileen Callan, a family nurse practitioner from Rochester, served as NYSNA president from 1993 to 1995. An active participant in NYSNA's political action committee, Callan ran for the New York State senate in 1996. *Photograph by Steve Fink.*

LEFT: Janice Viola received the Delegate Assembly Award in 1995 from Verlia Brown, right.

NYSNA also continued to work for legislation to guarantee reimbursement. The 1985 third-party reimbursement law permitted direct reimbursement for non-institutional services of nurses, but only for groups that requested a policy rider. NYSNA supported legislation which would provide mandatory coverage (i.e. not require the rider) and managed care legislation which included reimbursement for nurses. In 1998 NYSNA was cited by ANA for its key role in the passage of federal legislation providing for direct Medicare reimbursement for services rendered by advanced practice nurses.[13]

Proposals for health-care reform in the early 1990s focused new attention on primary care nurses and made provisions for the growing role of advanced practice nurses. Enrollments in nurse practitioner programs soared, and NYSNA published information for members and facilitated career transition.[14]

NURSING'S PERENNIAL PROBLEM: By 1986 the nursing shortage was again reaching crisis proportions. President Ellen Burns commented on this perennial problem. "We have suffered through shortages all of my professional life . . . Today we are dealing not only with a shortage of numbers, we are dealing with a shortage of the right kind of prepared nurses to care for a different kind of patient population than we have ever had before . . . An increased demand for nurses, particularly those with special skills, now coexists with declining enrollments and graduations."[15] Lucrative careers in business, law, medicine, engineering, and other professions that did not require night and weekend work or rotating shifts drained the nursing profession of many prospective students, and nursing had to look to non-traditional groups to bolster its ranks.[16]

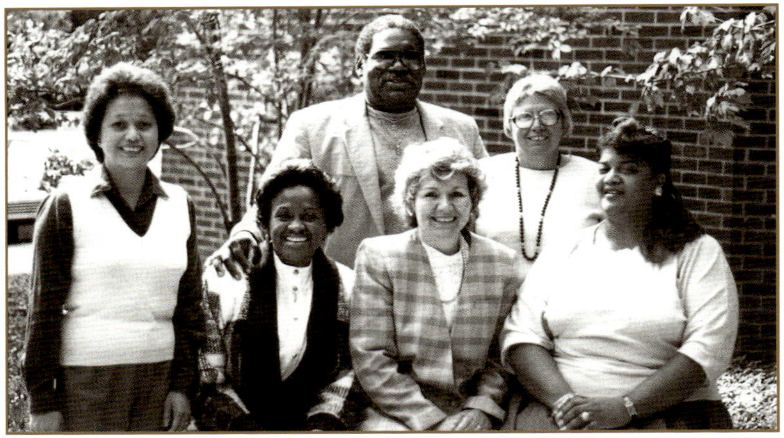

ABOVE: The Council on Human Rights monitored a variety of issues, including minority recruitment and retention in nursing and cultural diversity. Shown here is the 1987 council with NYSNA staff, Elizabeth Carter. From left to right are Lolita Compas, Dorothy Ramsey, Claude Willis, Kathleen Colling, Elizabeth Carter, and Barbara May.

The 1986 voting body adopted resolutions to increase nursing school enrollment and plan for the recruitment and retention of minorities and men into nursing. Recruitment activities were launched through regional planning groups and district nurses' associations, and included presentations to guidance counselors, students, and second-career adults. The association strongly supported the development and retention of an ethnically diverse nursing workforce. When nursing scholarship legislation repeatedly failed, NYSNA facilitated the development of the Lombardi Scholarships in Nursing, funded by the Medical Society of the State of New York, to provide financial support for non-traditional students. Nursing school enrollments of minority students increased as did enrollments of other non-traditional students such as men, single parents, second-career students, and English as-a-second-language students. After a five-year decline in enrollments, the trend began to reverse in 1988. By 1992 many schools of nursing had waiting lists, and nearly half the associate and bachelor's degree programs reported the number of older students was at least equal to that of recent high school graduates.[17]

To complement the intensive recruitment campaign, the association launched a massive lobbying effort to promote nursing's solutions to the nursing shortage: higher salaries, better benefits, career ladders, relief from non-nursing duties, and a more collaborative health-care environment.

"... We have buttons all over the place that say, Nursing Shortage is Dangerous to your Health. I would add to that ... [the] nursing shortage is a virulent organism that is threatening the viability of the nursing profession ... "

— *Lolita Compas*[2]

"More and more patients need total care, and it is impossible to do everything we have to do."

— *Cynthia Bottoms-Suarez*[3]

The award winning "Band-Aid Campaign," designed by director of the Legislative Program, E. Joyce Gould, was announced at a press conference in February 1989. Nurses were urged to send a "band-aid gram" — a band-aid attached to a letter — to legislators and the governor. Band-aid grams proclaiming the message, "The nursing shortage hurts! A band-aid is not enough," swamped most legislators' offices. NYSNA leaders met with Governor Cuomo to share concerns, feature articles describing the contributions of nurses to health care appeared in nearly every major state newspaper, and NYSNA's communications department coordinated members' participation in local radio and television coverage. Several legislators accepted invitations from members in their respective districts to "Keep Pace with a Nurse" to learn first hand about nursing by spending time with a nurse in the practice setting.[18]

THREATS TO LICENSURE: Proposals designed to alleviate the nursing shortage proliferated. The practice of "downsubstitution," whereby practical nurses and unlicensed personnel were assigned tasks formerly carried out by registered nurses, increased and new categories of unlicensed personnel emerged. Government officials revived proposals for institutional licensure and the waiver of licensure requirements. NYSNA vigorously maintained that blaming standards and licensure for personnel shortages was a smoke screen. The real issues included inadequate salaries, poor working conditions, lack of upward career mobility, and the rising need for personnel.[19]

"If we are replaced by technicians, there is no way patients will get the care they need."

— *Monica King*[4]

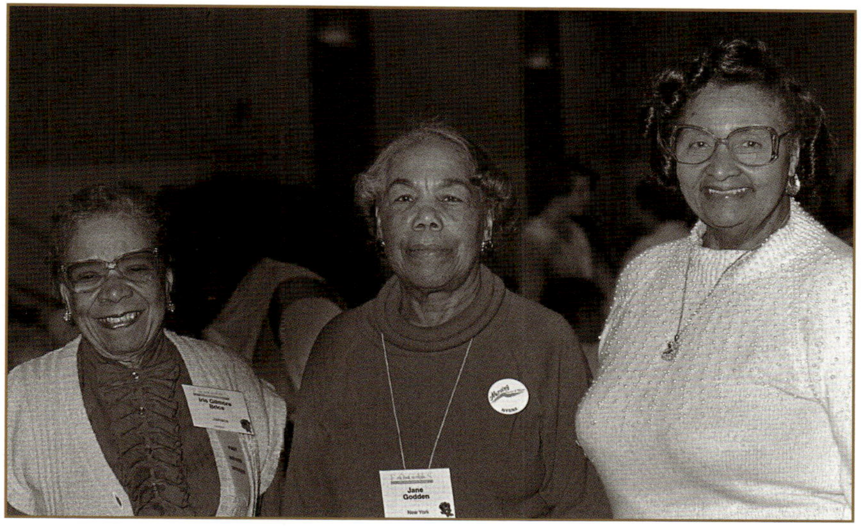

ABOVE: Many retired nurses such as Iris Brice, Jane Godden, and Etta Miller, shown here from left to right, faithfully attend NYSNA conventions. *Photograph by Marilyn Anderson.*

The American Medical Association's (AMA) response to the nursing shortage focused on the creation of a new category of unlicensed health-care worker, the Registered Care Technologist (RCT). The AMA proposed three levels of RCTs, trained in programs of two to eighteen months' duration to provide bedside care and carry out physician orders. NYSNA's voting body passed a resolution on the inappropriateness of nurses training and supervising RCTs, and established a network of nurses to address RCT program development. The RCT proposal elicited a striking display of unity as the nation's nurses vigorously opposed the proposal, and the RCT program was never implemented.[20]

In 1988 the New York State Health Department's Labor-Health Industry Task Force on Health Personnel proposed a host of recommendations to address the health-care crisis. NYSNA supported many of the recommendations, but vigorously objected to proposed demonstration projects that fostered institutional licensure and a reassessment of scope of practice requirements and other regulations seen as barriers to the utilization of health professionals. President Juanita Hunter commented, “If implemented, these recommendations would destroy the distinctions between the registered professional nurse and other health-care workers. Institutions would be allowed to assign tasks to non-professionals which registered professional nurses normally would be expected to perform. In addition, a review of scope of practice requirements could eventually invalidate our Nurse Practice Act.”[21]

NYSNA’s 1990 voting body took issue with the task force’s emphasis on efficiency and cost-containment, its lack of concern for quality care, and its support of increased use of less qualified personnel. Resolutions opposing the report called for the association to resist Department of Health efforts to usurp the role of the State Education Department in the regulation of nursing, strongly oppose institutional licensure, and continue to protect the Nurse Practice Act. NYSNA organized labor groups, pharmacists, physicians, and other health-care professionals to oppose waiver of licensure, and when a bill allowing waiver of professional licensure in certain demonstration projects was introduced in 1991, members were urged to step up opposition. Thanks to intense lobbying, letter writing, and coalition building, the provision was removed.[22]

FOREIGN NURSES: During the nursing shortage hospitals recruited thousands of foreign nurses. These nurses, working on temporary visas, comprised as much as 30 percent of the nursing staff of some New York hospitals. Many were poorly informed about their rights as workers and the implications of their visa status. Although the association believed the importation of foreign nurses was an inadequate solution to the nursing

BELOW: Verlia Brown, head nurse at Kings County Medical Center in Brooklyn, was elected to ANA’s Board of Directors in 1994. She was the first New York staff nurse and the first member of an NYSNA bargaining unit to hold such a high ANA office. Brown is shown here, third from right, with, from left to right, Elizabeth Mahoney, Linda O’Brien, Jean Heady, Cecilia Mulvey, Sharon Bidwell-Cerone, and Patricia Holloman.

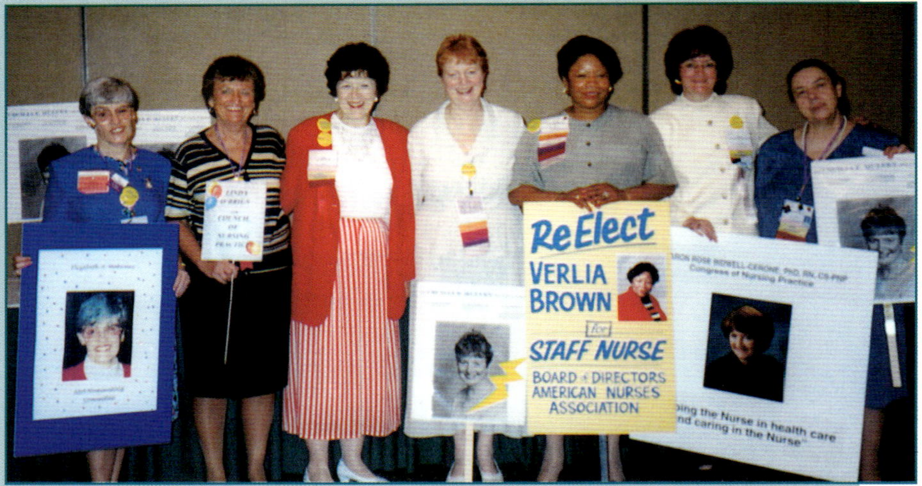

RIGHT: First Lady Hillary Rodham Clinton addressed NYSNA’s 1999 convention. Clinton is shown here with, from left to right, NYSNA parliamentarian Eugene Bierbaum, State Assembly Speaker Sheldon Silver, and NYSNA President Barbara Joyce.

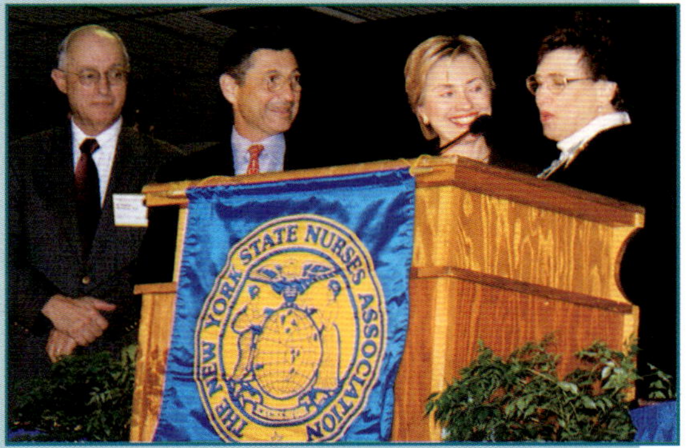

shortage, it provided information and support to these nurses. NYSNA worked to extend visas, lobbied for the Nurse Immigration Relief Act, held workshops on cultural diversity, developed relationships with organizations of nurses from other countries, and convened a Task Force on Foreign Nurse Issues to plan concerted action. A publication, *Foreign Nurses: What You Need to Know About the U.S.*, compiled information and resources for newly arrived foreign nurses.[23]

A CHANGING WORK ENVIRONMENT: The nursing shortage, escalating cost containment measures, increased levels of patient acuity, and the emergence of new health threats changed the work environment. Nurses faced understaffed units and unreasonable patient assignments that threatened their ability to maintain standards of care. Virulent new organisms such as drug-resistant tuberculosis threatened nurses' own health as well as that of their patients. NYSNA worked to protect nurses from a variety of hazards, and to alleviate the shortage through improved salaries and working conditions.[24]

In response to increasing frustration over demanding workloads, the voting body passed resolutions on the rights of nurses to refuse unreasonable patient assignments. The association developed Protest of Assignment forms to register nurses' concerns over unsafe assignments, document unsafe conditions, and emphasize to the employer the shared risk.[25]

Two important strategies of the association to alleviate the nursing shortage were to raise salaries and improve benefits through collective bargaining. In 1988 significant gains were made when NYSNA and New York City's Health and Hospitals Corporation (HHC) reached agreement

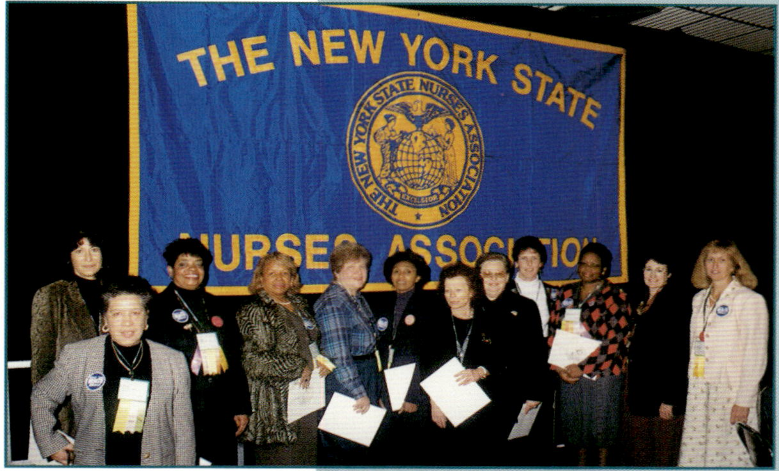

In 1998 NYSNA established a Leadership Institute to recognize members who have demonstrated sustained leadership in the association. Shown here are twelve of the 1999 inductees. From left to right are Amy Wysoker, Miriam Gonzalez, Marva Wade, Camille Petty, Ruth Korn, Cecilia Pennyfeather, Susan J. Fraley, Claire Murray, Denise McKee, Helen Dunwell Inniss, Ann Marie Cartwright, and Joanne Billott. Not pictured are Nettie Birnbach, Diane Giordano, Barbara May, and Madeline A. Naegle.

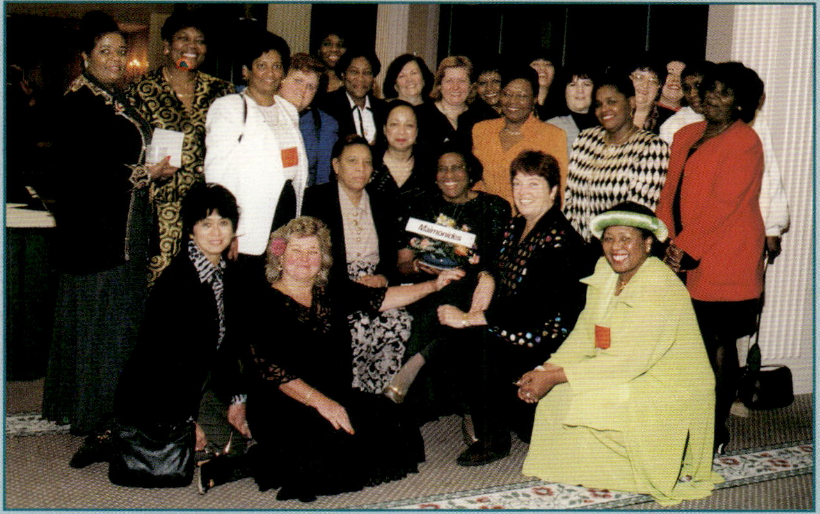

Nurses from Maimonides Medical Center gathered for a group photograph at NYSNA's 1998 convention.

on a new contract which put HHC nurses' salaries on a par with the private sector. This "parity" was critical to improving the recruitment and retention of nurses in the HHC system.[26]

"The development of two levels of nursing practice and clear avenues of education and evaluation to achieve them is long overdue . . . The nurses of New York State must unify in their ownership of this issue."

— *Madeline Naegle*[5]

Raising the salaries of experienced nurses was especially important to retain highly skilled veteran nurses. At the peak of the nursing shortage in 1989, NYSNA negotiated landmark salary increases. Contracts negotiated at Mt. Sinai, St. Luke's-Roosevelt, and Presbyterian Hospitals in New York City set new standards for the salaries of experienced nurses and brought national attention to NYSNA's collective bargaining program. At Presbyterian the salary of veteran nurses with over seventeen years of experience rose to more than $50,000. Marianne Kerner of the negotiating team stated, "The nurses here feel their worth has finally been realized. The more experienced nurses think it has been a long time coming, but that the hospital has finally acknowledged something."[27]

The 1989 contracts also directly addressed nurses' concerns over staffing and unsafe assignments. The Presbyterian contract eliminated mandatory overtime and limited floating, the practice of arbitrary, temporary reassignment to unfamiliar patient care areas. St. Luke's-Roosevelt Medical Center nurses went out on strike over inadequate staffing, and won a contract that included a joint staffing committee. The committee was composed of six representatives from management and six representatives from the Council of Nursing Practitioners. The committee's role was to review and evaluate the need for increased nurse staffing, and make recommendations to nursing administration. The contract was the first in the nation in which management guaranteed the establishment of staffing ratios and initiation of other measures if the shortage continued.[28]

NYSNA set the pace for increased salaries, improved benefits and pensions, and improved practice conditions. By 1990 nurses represented by NYSNA at every level and every title received pay equal to or higher than other New York nurses. At Mt. Sinai Medical Center, the base staff nurse salary negotiated for 1995 reached $50,100, more than double what it was in 1984. Salaries for experienced nurses rose from $27,277 in 1985 to as high as $75,100.[29] The association also made significant gains in New York's rural north country. By 1991 NYSNA represented nurses at eleven of the fifteen north country hospitals. Collective bargaining raised salaries for these historically severely economically disadvantaged nurses as much as $7,700 higher than nurses employed by hospitals in Syracuse and Albany, where few nurses were represented.[30]

"In this environment of cost containment, RNs are being asked to compromise patient care."

— *Sr. Mary Finnick*[6]

The emergence of the HIV epidemic and AIDS in the early 1980s, an increase in hepatitis cases, and the re-emergence of particularly virulent strains of tuberculosis placed nurses at considerable risk. The association held workshops to provide up-to-date information, printed articles in *Report,* issued nursing practice alerts, and promoted the availability and use of prevention safety equipment such as needleless devices and vaccines.[31]

"We knew that nurses' role in staffing decisions was an issue whose time had come, and we wanted to be agents of change. I'm proud of the staffing language we won. In fact, I'm proud and happy to be a nurse."

— *Mary Gilbert*[7]

As the HIV epidemic intensified, conflict arose over how to prevent HIV infection without violating rights of health-care workers or patients. NYSNA opposed proposals for mandatory testing of health-care workers, but did support voluntary, anonymous testing. The association urged all nurses to scrupulously follow universal precautions when caring for patients, and kept nurses up-to-date on infection control guidelines through workshops and publications. NYSNA joined the Coalition for Safe Health Care to protest recommendations that health-care workers testing positive for HIV stop performing "exposure prone" procedures.[32]

In addition to infectious diseases, nurses were exposed to hazardous medical devices, indoor air pollutants, radiation, and patient violence.[33] Stress and burnout from changing shifts, ethical conflicts, and other demands also affected the health of many nurses. In 1986 and again in 1991, NYSNA received grants from the New York State Department of Labor totaling $162,000 to alert nurses to environmental dangers and teach them to protect themselves. The award winning program, designed and implemented by Barbara Garrett, director of the Nursing Education Program, included workshops, brochures, and other projects to focus nurses' attention on occupational safety and health. Another grant was received in 1998 to educate nurses on another emerging occupational hazard, latex allergy.[34]

HEALTH CARE FOR ALL: By 1990 the nursing shortage had eased. Nonetheless, New York's health-care system was in crisis. Emergency rooms were overcrowded, costs were skyrocketing, and there were serious shortages of many services such as nursing home beds and home care. Over two million New Yorkers had no health insurance, and millions more were inadequately insured. NYSNA joined with the Hospital Association of New York State and other health organizations to protest Medicaid cuts, and joined coalitions of health-related organizations, consumers, and health-care workers to promote adequate hospital reimbursement and a more efficient and compassionate system of health care.[35]

"If our professional Association doesn't focus on issues important to RNs, we will lose our credibility."

— *Glenda Marshall*[8]

NYSNA's 1989 voting body overwhelmingly adopted a resolution introduced by Montefiore Hospital CNP chair Judy Sheridan-Gonzalez, calling for the establishment of a national health system. NYSNA joined coalitions such as the New York State Health Care Campaign to support accessible, high quality care for all New Yorkers, and participated in drafting legislation. Nurses attended rallies and flooded the Capitol with postcards and petitions in support of the New York Health bill. Although the bill was not enacted, the campaign, "Stop the Bleeding — with Health Care for All," raised public awareness of the health-care crisis.[36]

Indeed, concern over health care swept the country during the 1992 Presidential campaign. President Bill Clinton, newly elected, formed a task force under the leadership of First Lady Hillary Rodham Clinton to prepare proposals for health-care reform. The nursing community was gratified that

BELOW: Judy Sheridan-Gonzalez, chairperson of the Council of Nursing Practitioners at Montefiore Hospital since 1986, spoke at NYSNA's 1994 convention. *Photograph by Steve Fink.*

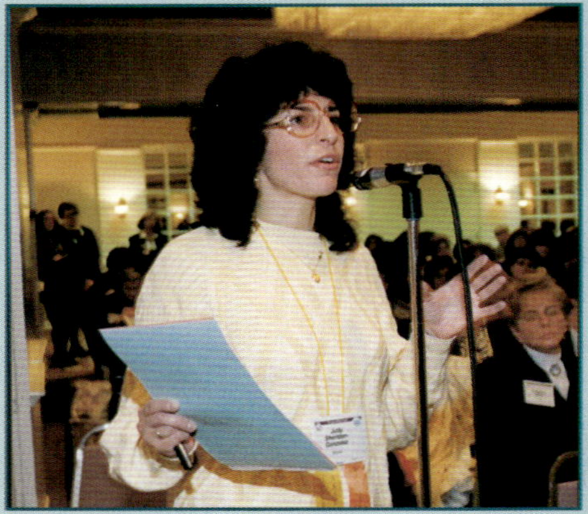

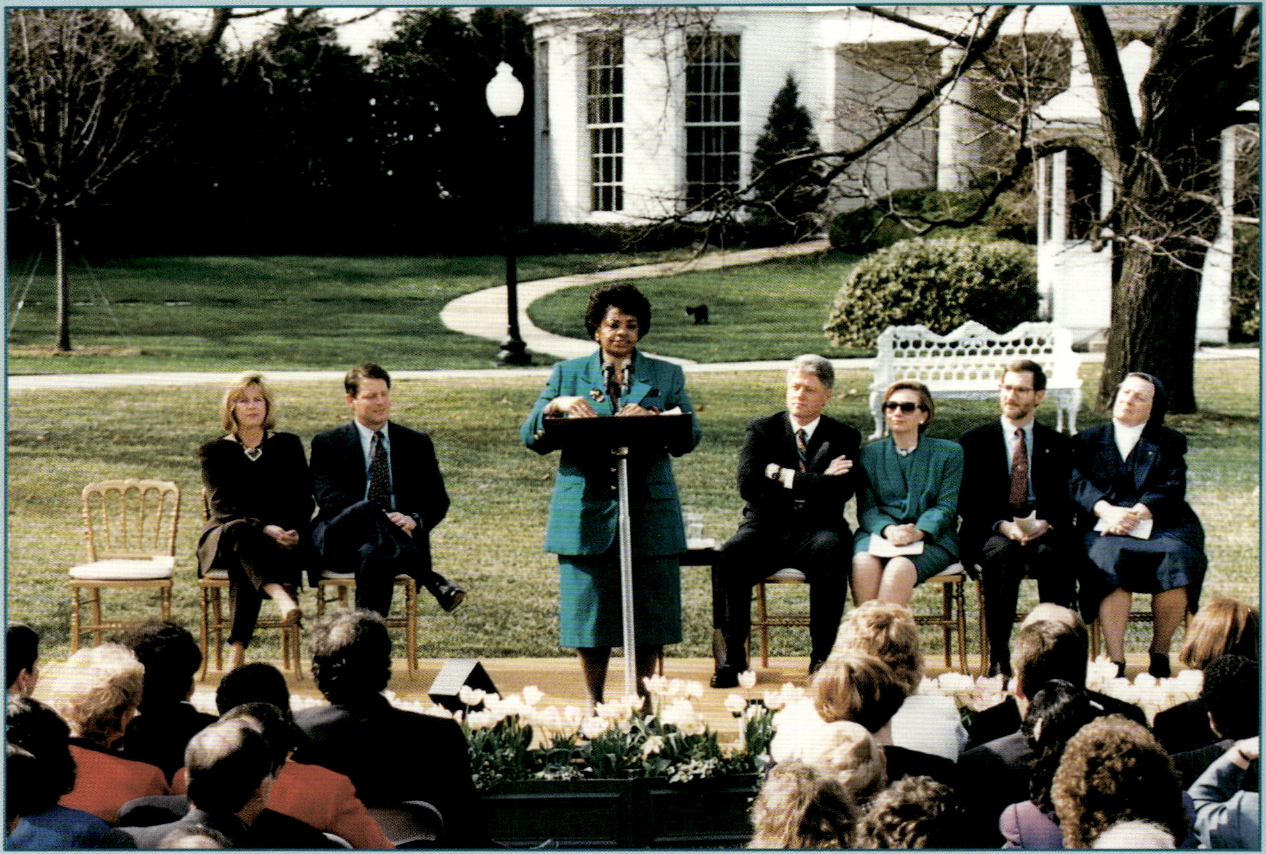

RIGHT: Marva Wade, shown here speaking at a White House Summit on Health Care Reform in the White House Rose Garden, was the first bargaining unit nurse to be elected NYSNA president.

nurses, including NYSNA members Mary Mundinger and Judith Leavitt, were chosen to participate on a review panel to comment on the proposals. The Clinton plan proposed a fundamentally restructured health-care system to increase access, assure high quality care, and control costs. The plan emphasized long-standing nursing priorities, including primary and preventive care, guaranteed health care for everyone, and recognition of nurses as legitimate providers of primary care.[37]

It was an exhilarating time for nursing. Nurses had unprecedented access to national policy makers, and enjoyed significant public credibility and visibility. In 1993 NYSNA President Nettie Birnbach was among a group of nurses from around the nation at a White House meeting with Hillary Rodham Clinton, and in 1994 President Mary Eileen Callan and President-elect Marva Wade met with President and Mrs. Clinton and other health-care providers at a White House Summit on Health Care Reform. Wade, an operating room nurse at Mt. Sinai Medical Center, was one of

RIGHT: Nurses at Presbyterian Hospital held a one-day strike in 1996 to protest the replacement of RNs by unlicensed personnel.

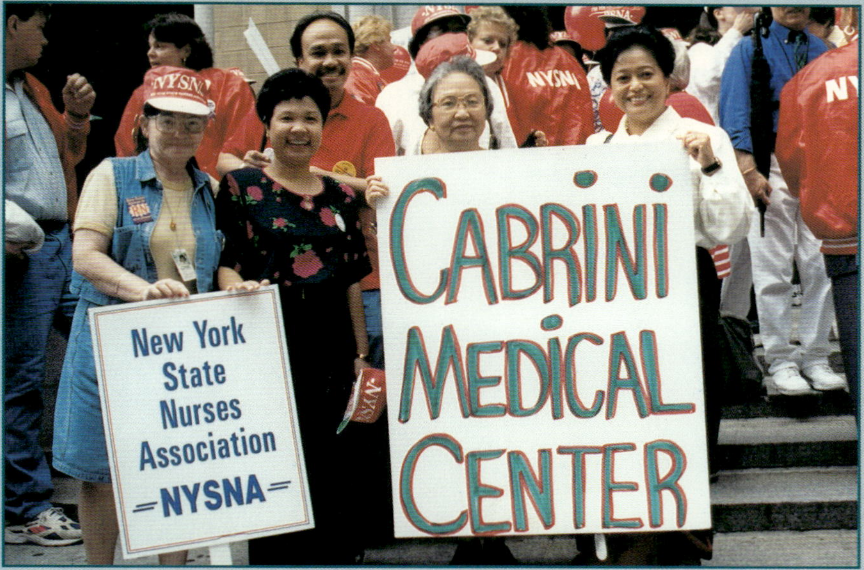

ABOVE: Nurses at Cabrini Medical Center and other nearby hospitals supported colleagues at Presbyterian Hospital in 1996. Nurses at Presbyterian protested replacement of RNs by unlicensed workers.

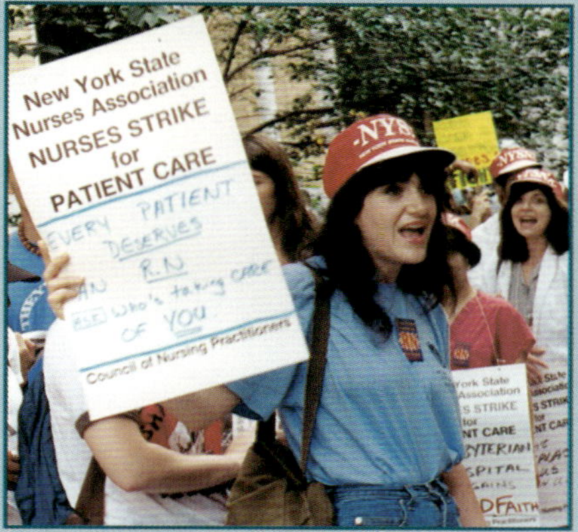

BELOW: Over fifteen hundred NYSNA members, including these nurses from Bellevue, joined nurses from around the country in a 1995 Washington, D.C., rally to protest the growing substitution of unlicensed health-care workers for registered nurses. NYSNA chartered nineteen buses to bring members to the rally.

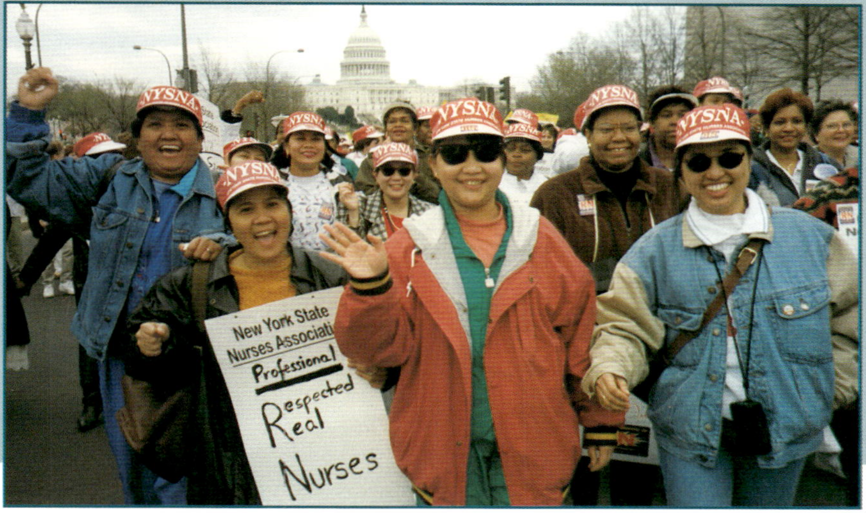

only three speakers to address the group. "Based on my years of experience as a nurse, I know how the current health-care system fails people, each and every day. But I am afraid that policymakers are only focusing on how we finance care and will not address the important question of how to improve the way we deliver care. The priorities are wrong in today's health-care system— and everyone suffers because of it . . . We enthusiastically support the President's plan and we will continue to work to make health care a right that cannot be denied or taken away."[38]

Federal legislative proposals for health-care reform proliferated, and NYSNA featured detailed information on the various plans in *Report* and in special lobbying packets. But as support built within nursing, opposition grew within many powerful groups. The medical establishment, big business, the insurance industry, and pharmaceutical companies supported some provisions but fiercely opposed others. The biggest and most expensive lobbying campaign in history, together with political infighting, the complexity of choices, and growing fears among the public, took a heavy toll on the reform movement. No comprehensive reform plan was enacted, but for the first time in history, the profession of nursing played a forceful role in the national debate. NYSNA vowed to continue its efforts to enact a single-payer plan providing comprehensive health-care coverage for all of New York's citizens.[39]

A TURBULENT HEALTH-CARE SYSTEM: A poor economy and looming reform catapulted the health-care system into turmoil, and increasingly hospitals faced restructuring and downsizing. The Department of Health urged hospitals to reduce acute-care beds and offer other services such as long-term care, psychiatric care, and substance abuse services. Cost containment measures and the increasing replacement of registered nurses with unlicensed personnel created uncertainty over the future and threatened to seriously undermine the quality of patient care. Many New York hospitals slashed services and jobs to reduce massive deficits, and financially pressed hospitals tried to eliminate hard-won benefits from contracts and weaken staffing requirements. NYSNA was successful in reducing layoffs and replacements by skillful and determined collective bargaining, and by targeting other forces that had an impact on nurses' jobs, such as the state budget, insurance industry policies, and public opinion.[40] NYSNA fought on several legislative fronts to support a state budget that provided needed services, a reformed system that provided access to preventive care, a managed care environment that promoted patient information and provider accountability, and an equitable system of professional regulation.[41]

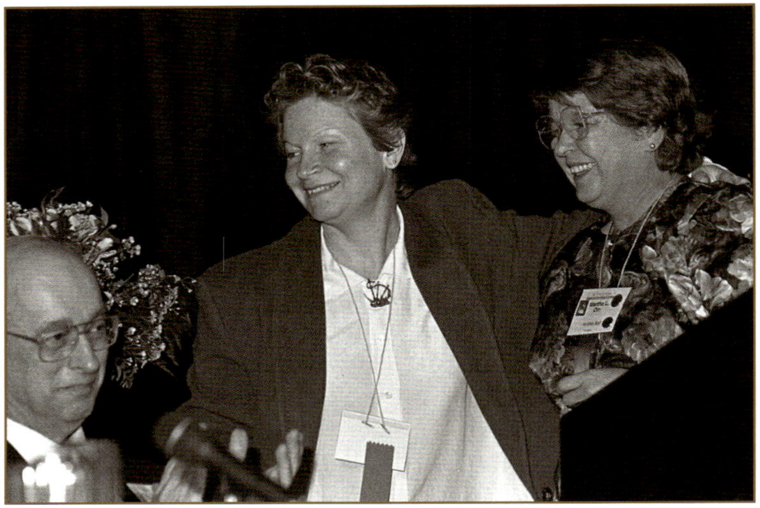

Associate to the Executive Director Wendy M. Burbank, center, is one of many non-nurse staff members at NYSNA. Throughout the association's history, these staff members have contributed to the work of the association with dedication and commitment. Burbank is shown here with Eugene Bierbaum and Martha Orr. *Photograph by Marilyn Anderson.*

In 1994 New York City's Health and Hospitals Corporation announced plans to cut services and thousands of jobs in an effort to reduce its massive deficit. NYSNA joined with other municipal unions to protest these cuts that would devastate patient care. Three thousand layoffs were avoided, but less than two years later, HHC again announced staff cuts. NYSNA efforts saved many jobs, but five hundred RNs were laid off and hundreds of others were displaced to new assignments. NYSNA participated in a coalition, Campaign to Save Our Hospitals, to insure the continuation of care for the poor, and organized a massive citywide rally at HHC's twenty facilities. Half-page ads were taken in local newspapers, warning "What is a city hospital without RNs? It's a morgue."[42] Martha Orr emphasized the patient care focus of the protests. "If we are not at the bedside, if we are not there to deliver the care, our patients will suffer . . . is it also about our jobs? You bet it is. But it is mostly about caring for people and wanting to be there for them. And my hat's off to all of these nurses who have been out in the street trying to fight back and to enlist public support."[43]

Other New York hospitals pushed to reduce nursing staff and increase unlicensed personnel. Mt. Sinai Medical Center wanted the right to replace 40 percent of its RN staff with unlicensed workers. The bargaining unit organized demonstrations, a "work-to-rule" action, and ran advertisements highlighting the danger of RN replacement in *The New York Times.* As a result, the hospital received hundreds of phone calls, and the contract was successfully settled without the replacement demand. Presbyterian Hospital also demanded language allowing the hospital to replace RNs with unlicensed personnel. Management committed millions of dollars to hire a "union-busting" law firm and "strike-busting" replacement nurses, but after a one-day strike, advertising in *The New York Times,* and sustained bargaining, agreement was reached. The new contract allowed replacement of fewer RN positions than were likely to become vacant, and *only* if NYSNA or a neutral panel certified replacements as cost-effective and safe for patients.[44]

Despite these successes, the use of unlicensed workers skyrocketed. NYSNA issued position statements on the role of the nurse regarding unlicensed personnel and developed guidelines for the qualifications, training, and performance of nurse's aides. Under the direction of Karen Ballard, director of the Nursing Practice Program, staff reviewed dozens of training program curricula and job descriptions. NYSNA alerted the State Board for Nursing and often the media when job descriptions violated registered nurses' scope of practice, and frequently won changes that protected both nurses and patients. Staff and members presented testimony on the danger to patients of the inappropriate use of unlicensed personnel, offered workshops for registered nurses on delegation and supervision, and provided information through articles in *Report.*[45]

NYSNA worked to help members adjust to this rapidly changing health-care system, and urged nurses to stay informed about emerging trends and prepare to explore new areas of practice. The Legislative Program lobbied to include retraining funds for nurses in hospital reimbursement legislation, and the Economic and General Welfare Program worked to provide training and guaranteed job security in negotiated contracts. Job opportunities for nurses in acute-care facilities decreased, and experts predicted increasing employment opportunities for nurses in home care. NYSNA collaborated with Pace University and Molloy College to develop continuing education programs to prepare nurses to work in the home environment. Nurses working outside the traditional acute-care setting turned to NYSNA for collective bargaining representation. Across the state, nurses in hospice programs, specialty settings, home care, and ambulatory care clinics organized for representation.[46]

In 1996 unemployment among nurses continued to rise. NYSNA provided six months' complimentary membership to laid-off nurses, and NYSNA's board authorized the establishment of a career center to assist members in identifying job opportunities and acquiring new skills to facilitate career transitions. Career center staff provided individual counseling, prepared a workbook, *Tomorrow's Solution for Today's Nurse: The Nursing Career Development Process,* held career planning workshops, formed networking groups, and listed jobs and career planning information on the newly developed NYSNA internet web site at www.nysna.org.[47]

Despite widespread restructuring during the 1993–1997 period, fewer than eight hundred of NYSNA's more than thirty-one thousand bargaining unit members were laid off. This outstanding record of protecting jobs was due to determined negotiating, lobbying, and nurses walking the picket lines to stand up for patients and the profession of nursing. The health-care crisis, however, persisted. Martha Orr addressed the 1997 convention. "In the past year, the crisis has deepened, and our anxiety as nurses can now be better characterized as alarm. Nurses are hurting, patients are suffering, the public seems apathetic, government seems uninterested and unwilling to take action, and there is no end in sight."[48]

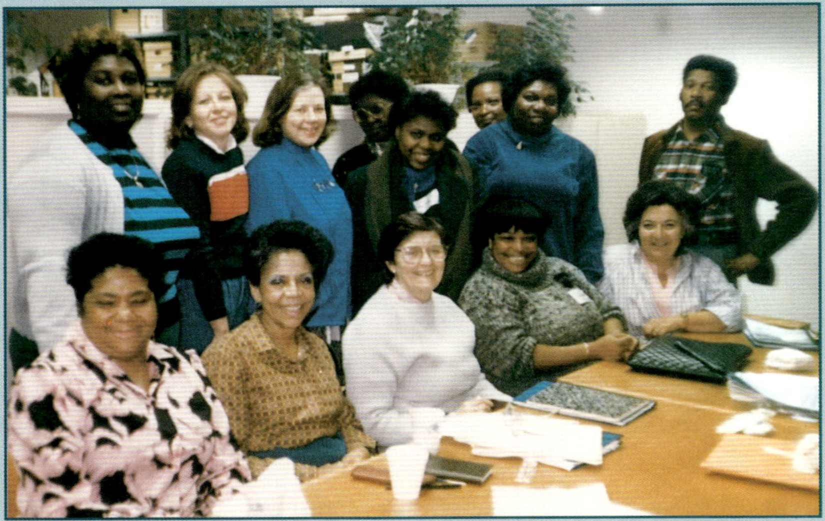

Bargaining unit negotiating teams, such as this 1988 HHC team, devote their time and energy working for improved working conditions.

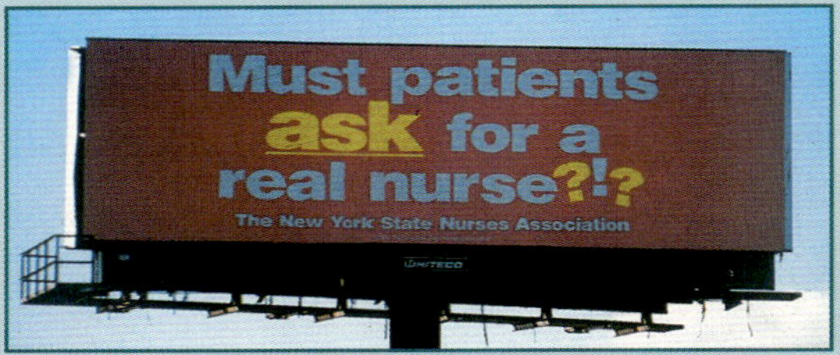

This billboard in downtown Albany drew attention to NYSNA's media campaign.

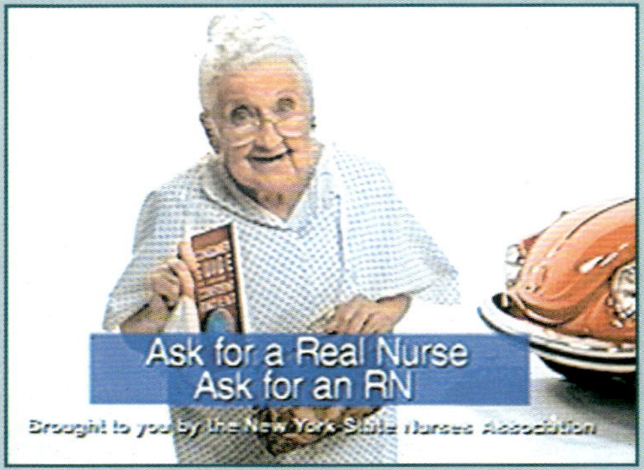

The "Ask for a Real Nurse, Ask for an RN" campaign brought the unique role of registered nurses into the public eye.

Ask for a Real Nurse: NYSNA's most visible response to the health-care crisis was its massive public relations and advertising campaign, guided by Director of Communications Anne Schott. In 1994 the voting body was alarmed over the effects of restructuring and overwhelmingly authorized an aggressive media campaign that explained in detail why registered nurses were both cost-effective and necessary to quality patient care. In a special edition of *Report,* sent to every RN in New York, nurses were urged to tell patients they were registered nurses and proudly display buttons and bumper stickers proclaiming the message, "Every Patient Deserves a Registered Nurse." Radio and television commercials, and subway and bus posters featuring the message, "Ask for a Real Nurse, Ask for an RN," targeted the metropolitan New York area. In the campaign's first year, thousands of consumers called a toll-free number for tips on evaluating nursing care in hospitals. As a result of the campaign, patients called hospitals with staffing questions and asked caregivers, "Are you an RN?"[49]

The campaign was so successful, it was expanded to other areas of the state, and included billboards and ads in magazines and newspapers. Thousands more consumers requested hospital evaluation kits and other information. During the three-year campaign, over $2.5 million was spent on the "Ask for a Real Nurse, Ask for an RN" campaign, the largest such campaign by any nursing organization. The award-winning project heightened public awareness of the value of registered nurses, and brought pressure on health-care facilities to provide registered nurses for patient care. Most importantly, NYSNA members felt they were actively doing something to improve the quality of care for their patients, and to protect their own careers during this turbulent time.[50]

Forging New Coalitions: Health-care restructuring continued at a rapid pace across the state. Some hospitals closed, others were bought out, and there were mergers, consolidations, and affiliations. Health-care systems and networks were formed, and NYSNA negotiating teams faced a more powerful administrative base at the bargaining table. It was necessary to develop new strategies to protect nurses in the workplace.[51]

In 1998 NYSNA and 1199 (the National Health and Human Services Union/SEIU) agreed to share a federal training grant to support the retraining of RNs, to develop a common approach to restructuring, and to cooperate in other arenas to protect patient care and health-care workers. Economic and General Welfare program director Carolyn McCullough explained, "Today's tough economic health-care climate — in which the livelihoods of all hospital workers are under threat — has made it necessary for former rivals to cooperate."[52]

NYSNA was instrumental in establishing another coalition which led to a national restructuring of nursing's labor activities. In 1997 NYSNA collaborated with eight other state nurses' associations with large collective bargaining programs to form the State Nurses Association Labor Coalition. The coalition recognized the need for a united response to trade unions that were launching massive drives to organize and represent nurses. According to McCullough, "If that trend had been allowed to continue, trade unions could ultimately have claimed more RN members than the ANA and the right to speak for registered nurses."[53] The coalition worked with ANA to strengthen economic and general welfare programs and establish and implement a national labor agenda. Coalition members supplied staff and resources to each other in organizing drives, decertification campaigns, and negotiations, advocated for substantial increases in ANA resources, and commissioned a study of the possible effects of affiliation with an international union or with the AFL-CIO.[54]

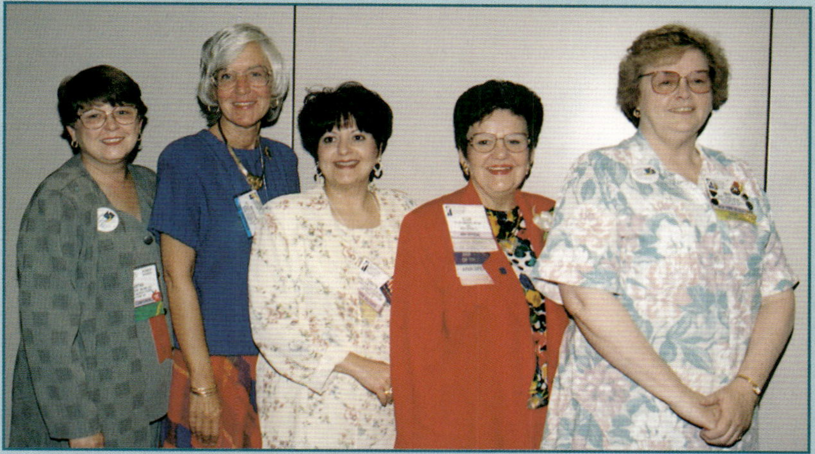

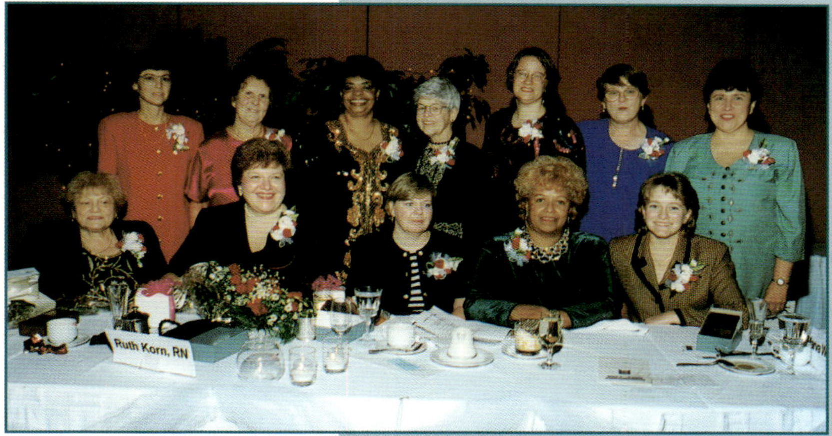

ABOVE: Past and present leaders of NYSNA's E&GW Program gathered at the fiftieth anniversary celebration of ANA's Economic and General Welfare Program. From left to right are Executive Director Martha Orr, Kathleen Hoover, Carolyn McCullough, Ellen Sanders, and Mary Finnin.

ABOVE LEFT: Each year members are honored for outstanding nursing leadership. In 1996 award winners were, seated from left to right, Teresa Domanic, Ruth Korn, Marianne Herner, Camille Petty, Marca Capuano, and standing Nancy Iafrati, Margaret Hobson, President Marva Wade, Jane Fielding, Anna Mary Hudock, Executive Director Martha Orr, and President-elect Barbara Joyce. *Photograph by Michael Sisti.*

The work of the State Nurses Association Labor Coalition led to a proposal to create a new labor entity to offer nurses across the country an opportunity to be represented for collective bargaining by their professional association. NYSNA President Barbara Joyce, Executive Director Orr, and Delegate Assembly chair Edward Goldberg were among the NYSNA delegation deeply involved in building national consensus in support of the proposal. The 1999 ANA House of Delegates overwhelmingly voted to alter ANA's structure by creating United American Nurses, a new labor division within ANA.[55]

POLITICAL INFLUENCE AND SOPHISTICATION: Entry-into-practice legislation was the central element in the association's Action Plan, based on the needs and resources assessment of the early 1980s, and was the focus of the association's 1985 legislative agenda. Dr. Elizabeth Carter, appointed special associate for the Entry Into Practice Project, led the association's efforts to build consensus on this divisive issue. Despite these efforts, and after years of discussion, New York's nurses remained divided, and no entry-into-practice legislation was enacted. There was, however, a steady decline in hospital-based nursing programs and by 1989 a majority of nurses were educated in institutions of higher learning. Standardizing nursing education and promoting the baccalaureate degree as the minimum entry requirement for RNs remained association goals throughout the 1990s.[56]

"Now we'll be part of PAC and I think that can only give us more power, more clout, and I don't think it degrades us in any way, I think it makes us a more powerful people."

— *Margaret Leonard*[9]

By the late 1980s NYSNA's annual legislative agenda had moved from its entry-into-practice focus to a broad program which included monitoring all legislative and regulatory initiatives affecting the health-care system. The association became increasingly skillful at utilizing legislative, regulatory, and political strategies to address a wide range of issues. NYSNA co-sponsored a major conference on the role of nurses in shaping public policy on health care, held political skills workshops, and developed networks to increase NYSNA's legislative influence by matching an association member with each congressman and state legislator.[57]

The formation of a political action committee further contributed to NYSNA's political sophistication and influence. New York State Nurses for Political Action (NYS-NPA), formed in 1976, received financial and in-kind contributions from NYSNA. NYS-NPA requested formal affiliation with NYSNA, and recommended that a formal relationship between the two groups correspond to the relationship between ANA and ANA-PAC. The 1992 voting body passionately debated a board recommendation that NYSNA form a political action committee, and ultimately adopted bylaws creating NYSNA-PAC.[58]

NYSNA-PAC's first Board of Trustees, under the leadership of chairperson Connie Vance, developed a process and criteria for endorsing candidates. The committee quickly demonstrated effective use of grassroots activism, visibility, and dollars to influence the election process to benefit both consumers and the profession of nursing. By the end of the 1994 campaign, both major political parties recognized NYSNA as a valuable ally.[59]

NYSNA's increasing political influence was matched by increasing success in securing appointed positions in state policy-making groups for its members, and by 1993 was a significant force in New York's health-care policy development. Representatives attended hundreds of official meetings, and provided testimony on issues ranging from HIV/AIDS and domestic violence to health-care reform. On the federal level, association members actively participated in the development of health-care reform proposals, and worked with New York Congressman Hinchey on the federal Patient Protection Act.[60] President Nettie Birnbach commented, "The visibility of nursing at the policy setting table is greater than ever before and unparalleled opportunities lie before us."[61]

IMPAIRED PRACTICE: In the 1980s NYSNA formed a Task Force on Alcohol and Substance Abuse in the Profession of Nursing to address the needs of nurses whose practice was impaired by drug or alcohol abuse. As chairperson of the task force from 1982 to 1986, Madeline Naegle, NYSNA president from 1989 to 1991, was instrumental in the development of this innovative program. The task force developed guidelines for hospital-based employee assistance programs, prepared informative literature, and provided consultation to institutions and individuals. NYSNA published a *Peer Assistance Manual* to assist all nurses in helping colleagues, and developed programs to protect patients and assist nurses in preserving their licenses, overcoming addiction, and returning to practice.[62]

In 1992 the board approved expansion of the program to include regional outreach efforts, new educational materials, consultant services, and support services to nurses. The expanded Statewide Peer Assistance for Nurses (SPAN) Program hired full-time professional staff and a part-time regional consultant in District 14 to select and train nurse advocates to work with impaired nurses, and services were expanded to include nurses suffering from mental illness or exposed to HIV.[63] The advocate program was eventually extended into all five New York City boroughs as well as Nassau and Suffolk Counties. In 1998 funds for the program were included in the New York State budget. The funding was vetoed by the governor, but following intense lobbying from nurses, $150,000 was designated for the program through special funds.[64] In 1999 similar funding was included in the budget and signed by the governor.

STRENGTH AND STABILITY: The 1985 to 1999 period was a turbulent time. Despite the oftentimes overwhelming threats to nursing and to the association, NYSNA grew into a remarkably strong, stable, and complex organization. In 1991 a restructuring of NYSNA dues provided for regional rates based on negotiated salaries of represented nurses, and provided reduced dues for members in several categories.[65] The new structure was designed to be more equitable for the membership, while assuring a sound financial base for association activities. A concerted effort to increase non-dues income, such as grants, further contributed to NYSNA's financial health.

Programs were developed in the 1990s to increase member involvement. A leadership development program instituted in 1991 provided a series of planned experiences to develop organizational skills and encourage more active participation in the association's leadership. Many leadership fellows, such as Marion Spector and Ann Converso, went on to serve on the Board of Directors, and to assume a variety of positions of leadership at the state, district, and national levels. A two-year fellowship program for nurses interested in research was developed in 1996 to prepare members for involvement in association research activities.[66]

NYSNA's newsletter and journal became more sophisticated, and numerous high-quality brochures, pamphlets, and booklets were published. The *Journal of the New York State Nurses Association* was transformed into a peer-reviewed journal of scholarly articles published twice each year, and *Report* developed into a full-color newsletter providing information on association activities and in-depth analysis of current nursing issues. Published ten times each year, *Report* received numerous awards for excellence from the *American Journal of Nursing* Company.[67]

NYSNA worked on countless fronts to meet the information needs of nurses. When legislation mandated training in child abuse and infection control for re-registration, NYSNA developed workshops and video-taped

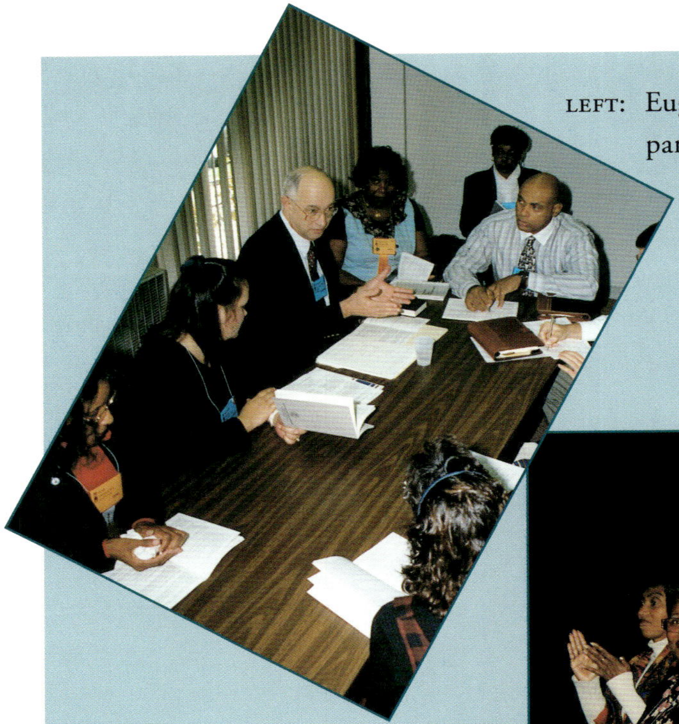

LEFT: Eugene Bierbaum, long-time NYSNA parliamentarian, attended conventions and conducted workshops for members.

RIGHT: Erie County Medical Center nurses picketed against layoffs in 1993.

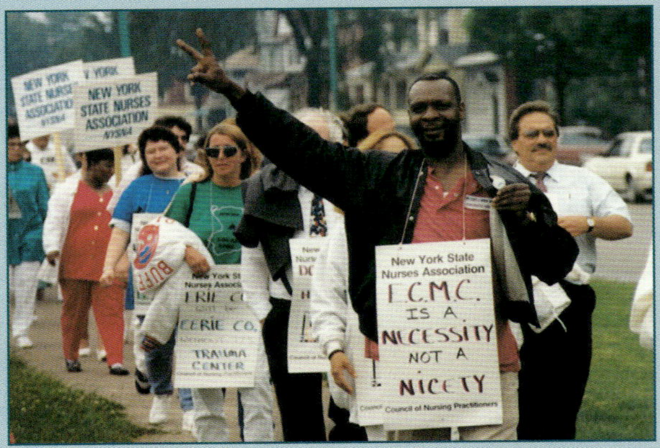

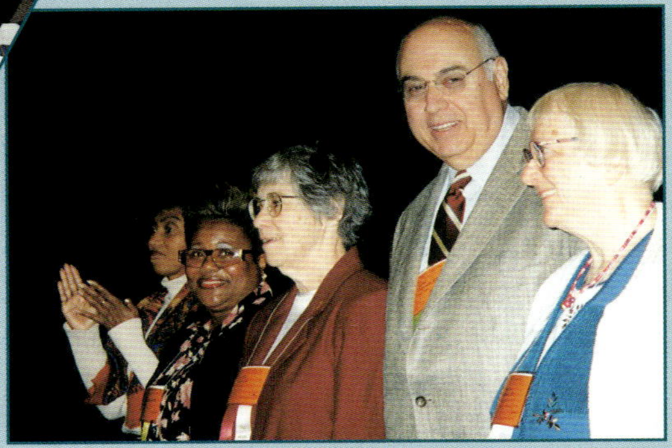

LEFT: In 1999 Robert Piemonte, shown here with Joan Cumberbatch, Sister Mary Finnick on the left, and Nancy Sweeney on the right, was elected to serve as NYSNA president, effective in 2001. Piemonte is the first man elected to serve as NYSNA president. Previously, Paul Hageman served as NYSNA president from 1978 to 1979, fulfilling an unexpired term.

programs to assist nurses in meeting these mandatory continuing education requirements. Staff in the Nursing Practice and Services Program responded to thousands of requests for information on nursing practice issues, and developed position statements and nursing practice alerts on scope of practice and ethical issues.[68] The association's library provided information to staff, members, and the public.

In its tenth decade, as in each decade in the association's history, NYSNA worked for the passage of numerous legislative proposals and opposed others, endured periods of declining membership and enjoyed times of rapid growth, fought to improve the salaries and working conditions of nurses, and held onto its goal of providing the highest quality nursing care to the citizens of New York. Throughout the years, members demonstrated both a respect for the association's past and a vision of its future. At NYSNA's 1999 convention, President Barbara Joyce urged fellow members to continue a long tradition of preparing the profession for the future. "Who is nursing to be in the new era upon us? Who are we *really* to be in the next millennium? . . . As we stand together on the threshold of the new millennium, may we continue to 'seek a newer world'—the one which nursing envisions for health care in the 21st century."[69]

NYSNA has achieved many profound successes throughout its history, yet as the year 2000 unfolds, many of the same challenges persist. The association was founded to secure legislation which would regulate the

By 1992 the association's membership had reached an all-time high. The 1992 Strategic Plan called for adequate physical facilities to meet the association's growing membership and staff, but space at the Center for Nursing would not accommodate so much as one additional employee. With great reluctance, the Board of Directors accepted the architects' judgement that the building could not be expanded, and considered proposals for building or leasing additional space.[1] The proposal evoked mixed reactions from members — pride that the association had grown and and developed, and reluctance to abandon the beautiful Center for Nursing. The association donated to the Foundation of NYSNA the land on which the Center for Nursing was built.

After reviewing numerous options, the association purchased a site in Latham and worked with the architectural firm of Mallin Mendel Associates to develop plans for a new building. Having designed the Center for Nursing, architect Benjamin Mendel was uniquely qualified to collaborate with NYSNA on the new headquarters.

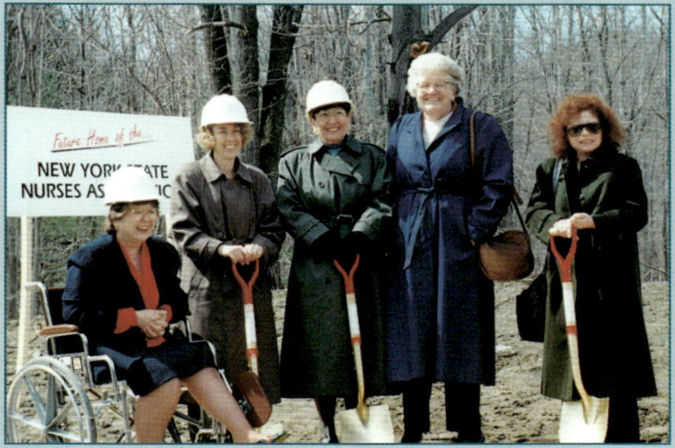

ABOVE LEFT: Executive Director Martha Orr on the left was joined by, from left to right, President Mary Eileen Callan, and former NYSNA Presidents Nettie Birnbach, Ellen Burns, and Susan Fraley at groundbreaking ceremonies for NYSNA's new headquarters.

ABOVE RIGHT: The new headquarters provided extensive conference and meeting facilities, with state-of-the-art audio and video capabilities.

Association staff moved into the new facilities in June 1995, and the building was formally dedicated on September 15. In delivering the keynote speech, former President Madeline Naegle said, "our new building makes a clear statement about the permanence and ongoing activity of the association."[2] The new facility was a 41,000-square-foot brick structure, designed around a series of courtyards, that provided both office space for NYSNA staff and extensive facilities for association meetings and conferences.[3]

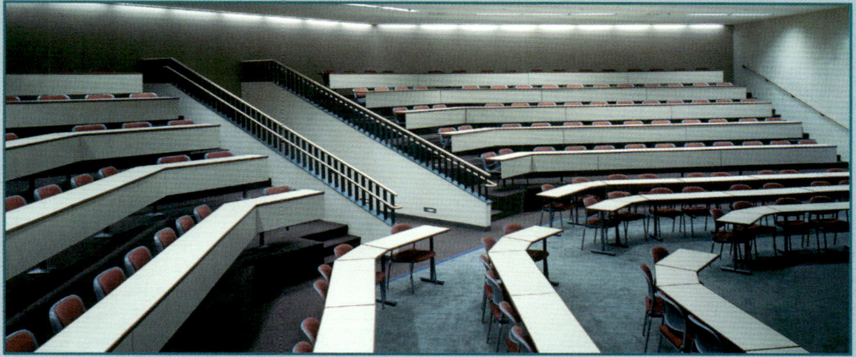

Martha Orr reported on the completion of the new building at the 1995 Convention: "This marks the completion of many years of dreaming, planning, and hard work by too many to name. The building is a testimony to the courage and leadership of our boards of directors and finance committees over the past five years. It is a statement of trust in our future. It is an expression of pride in the profession of nursing. It is an acknowledgment, with gratitude, for the contributions of professional nurses to the health care of people. The design of the building reflects all of these values. It embraces our history in its continuity of spirit with our former headquarters, the Center for Nursing. Its openness, light, richness of color, spaciousness and comfort are the embodiment of our profession's caring tradition and the diversity of our practitioners."[4] ■

profession and protect the public from untrained nurses. As the association prepares to enter its one hundredth year, an emerging nursing shortage is once again raising the specter of the increased use of unlicensed personnel. The failure of health-care reform opened the door for a market-driven system of health care, and the resulting financial pressures on the health-care system have again brought about intolerable working conditions for registered nurses. Once again staffing conditions are a top priority. New challenges will certainly emerge as the century unfolds. These challenges will demand the same courage, perseverance, and innovative solutions that have brought the association through its first one hundred years. ■

CHAPTER NOTES

TEXT

1. "Voting Body Passes 11 Resolutions," *Report* 15 (November–December 1984): 9–11; "NYSNA Voting Body Approves 1985 Legislative Program," *Report* 15 (November–December 1984): 2; and "Nursing Needs & Resources Action Plan Approved As Guideline For Future," *Report* 15 (November–December 1984): 1. The Action Plan was a nine-point plan that focused the attention and work of the association.

2. "NYSNA Responds to North Shore Ruling," *Report* 16 (May–June 1985): 2, 6; Board of Directors Minutes, 6–7 June 1985, NYSNA Archives; "Active, Fast-paced NYSNA Convention Draws Over 800"; and "Voting Body Approves Bylaws Amendments & Legislative Program," *Report* 16 (November–December 1985): 1, 4. The 1985 voting body endorsed the task force in a resolution, and voted to eliminate the Council on Economic and General Welfare. ("Resolutions Passed By Voting Body," *Report* 16 [November–December 1985]: 10.)

3. "The New York State Nurses Association 70th Convention" (Albany, N.Y., 1985, stenotype transcript), A 36. NYSNA's legitimacy as a labor organization was also challenged by Highland Hospital, but in 1988, after an eleven-year legal battle, the NLRB and the Federal Court ruled that NYSNA was in fact an appropriate and legitimate labor organization, and operated in a manner that avoided conflicts of interest. ("NYSNA Wins Major Legal Victory," *Report* 19 [November–December 1988]: 1.)

4. "Message from the Chair," *Statewide* 10 (May 1993): 3; and *Forty Years of Collective Bargaining*, 23–24.

5. Board of Directors Minutes, NYSNA, 7–8 January 1987, NYSNA Archives; and "NYSNA Board of Directors Deliberates Future Membership of the Association," *Report* 18 (March–April 1987): 2. Many were confused, and failed to understand that the term "associate nurse" did *not* refer to current associate degree graduates, but to the proposed technical nurses of the future who would be associate degree prepared and not licensed as registered nurses. *Report* clarified: "NYSNA welcomes as members all RNs regardless of their educational preparation, and will continue to do so. Anyone who is currently an RN will remain an RN and a valued member of NYSNA despite any changes in educational requirements for licensure. That is — and always has been — NYSNA's position." ("Who May Belong to NYSNA and the ANA?" *Report* 19 [January–February 1988]: 3.)

6. "Should Our Association Be for RNs Only?" *Report* 18 (July–August 1987): 1. The "associate" nurse was also often referred to as the "technical" or "non-professional" nurse.

7. Board of Directors Minutes, NYSNA, 10–11 July 1987, NYSNA Archives; "Membership Divided on Issue," *Report* 18 (September–October 1987): 1; and "Voting Body Reaffirms Professional Association," *Report* 18 (November–December 1987): 1.

8. "ANA Proposes Major Organizational Restructuring," *Report* 20 (May 1989): 1.

9. "Voting Body Postpones Action on Withdrawal from ANA," *Report* 19 (November–December 1988): 1; and "ANA House of Delegates Adopts COAR Report and Approves Dues Increase," *Report* 20 (August 1989): 1. NYSNA opposed many of the report's recommendations, but was unsuccessful in affecting change.

10. Board of Directors Minutes, NYSNA, 4–5 January 1985 and 6–7 June 1985, NYSNA Archives; and "Entrepreneurship Booklet Available," *Report* 17 (May–June 1986): 1.

11. "Resolutions Passed," 10; and Board of Directors Minutes, NYSNA, 5–6 June 1986, and 26–27 July 1989, NYSNA Archives.

12. "New Law Will Alter Requirements for State's Nurse Practitioners," *Report* 20 (March 1989): 1; "NYSNA Achieves Gains for Nurse Practitioners," *Report* 21 (March 1990): 3; and "Persistence on DEA Numbers Pays Off," *Report* 23 (July 1992): 3. NYSNA's Functional Unit of Primary Care Practitioners was changed to the Functional Unit of Nurse Practitioners to conform with the statutorily protected title of "nurse practitioner." (Board of Directors Minutes, 14–15 June 1989, NYSNA Archives.)

13. "Third-Party Reimbursement Bill Introduced in Congress," *Report* 29 (May 1997): 6; *New York State Nurses Association Annual Report 1996–1997* (Latham, N.Y.: NYSNA, 1997), 4; and "NYSNA Honored for Role in National Medicare Victory," *Report* 29 (January 1998): 1.

14. "Nurses Prepare for Changes in Health Care," *Report* 25 (March 1994): 1, 13.

15. *Conference on Recruitment and Retention in Nursing, Arden House May 13–14, 1987* (Guilderland, N.Y.: New York State Nurses Association, 1987), 1.

16. Linda H. Aiken and Connie Flynt Mullinix, "Special Report. The Nurse Shortage: Myth or Reality?" *New England Journal of Medicine* 317 (September 1987): 641–46; and John K. Iglehart, "Health Policy Report: Problems Facing the Nursing Profession," *New England Journal of Medicine* 317 (September 1987): 646–51. While starting salaries for nurses had been raised to a level comparable to those of other college graduates, salaries for experienced nurses were only about $7,000 more than the average starting salary.

17. "Voting Body Passes Eight Resolutions, Affirms Initiative to Recruit Students into Careers in Professional Nursing," *Report* 17 (November–December 1986): 8; Update on Activities Related to the Nine Action Proposals and Implementation Strategies, Report to the Board of Directors, NYSNA, 26–27 July 1989, NYSNA Archives; "Winners of First Lombardi Scholarships in Nursing Are All Young Mothers," *Report* 21 (August 1990): 11; "Survey Reveals Enrollment in RN Programs is Up Statewide," *Report* 20 (December 1989): 3; and "Nontraditional Students Filling the Nursing Programs," *Report* 23 (March 1992): 4.

18. "NYSNA Launches Campaign to Eliminate Nursing Shortage," *Report* 20 (March 1989): 1; "Campaign to Eliminate Nursing Shortage Begins with Albany *BAND-AID* Protest," *Report* 20 (April 1989): 1; and "The New York State Nurses Association 74th Annual Convention" (Albany, N.Y., 1989, stenotype transcript), 12–13. The campaign won the 1990 American Society of Association Executives' Award of Excellence for Government Relations. ("Band-Aid Campaign Wins National Award," *Report* 22 [January–February 1991]: 9.) The Keep Pace with a Nurse program continued long after the nursing shortage eased as a valuable mechanism for enhancing legislators' understanding of nursing.

19. "Cuomo Backs Waiver of Licensure," *Report* 22 (March 1991): 1, 7.

20. "Nurses Unite to Oppose AMA Plan for Registered Care Technologist," *Report* 19 (July–August 1988): 1; "Resolutions Adopted by 1988 Voting Body," *Report* 19 (November–December 1988): 8; and "Nurses Win Struggle Over RCTs," *Report* 21 (August 1990): 1.

21. "From the President . . ." *Report* 19 (January–February 1988): 2; and "Task Force Offers Scholarships — and Insults," *Report* 19 (January–February 1988): 1. NYSNA supported task force recommendations for higher salaries, particularly for experienced nurses, a portable pension system and improved benefits, increased funding for nursing education, active statewide recruitment programs, and prescriptive privileges for qualified nurses. ("NYSNA Works to Shape Solutions to Nursing Shortage," *Report* 19 [May–June 1988]: 1.)

22. "Resolutions Passed by the 1990 Voting Body," *Report* 21 (December 1990): 14; "Bill that Allows Waiver of RN Licensure Introduced in Assembly," *Report* 22 (May 1991): 7; and "Waiver of Licensure: NYSNA Wins Early Battles — But the War is Not Over," *Report* 22 (July 1991): 1.

23. "NYSNA Task Force Working for Foreign Nurses," *Report* 21 (August 1990): 1; *40 Years of Collective Bargaining*, 24–25; and "Welcome to the Multicultural Workforce," *Report* 24 (December 1993): 1.

24. "New York State Nurses Association 71st Convention" (Lake Placid, N.Y., 1986, stenotype transcript), B 23–24.

25. "Voting Body Passes Eight Resolutions Affirms Initiative to Recruit Students into Careers in Professional Nursing," *Report* 17 (November–December 1986): 8; and *40 Years of Collective Bargaining*, 22.

26. "City Nurses Win Breakthrough Contract," *Report* 19 (July–August 1988): 1.

27. "Presbyterian Hospital Nurses Win Landmark Contract," *Report* 20 (June 1989): 1; "Landmark Contract at Presbyterian Hospital

Brings Veteran Nurses Over $50,000," *Statewide* 6 (Spring 1989): 1; and "74th Annual Convention," 14.

28. *40 Years of Collective Bargaining,* 24; and "St. Luke's–Roosevelt Nurses Win Strike for Improved Staffing Levels — and *Better* Patient Care," *Report* 20 (July 1989): 1.

29. "When it Comes to Great RN Contracts NYSNA Sets the Pace," *Report* 21 (January–February 1990): 1; and "RN Salaries HIt New Highs," *Report* 24 (May 1993): 1.

30. "NYSNA Adds to North Country Dominance as Elizabethtown RNs Win Representation," *Report* 22 (August 1991): 1; and "1990 Voting Body Business Sessions" (Lake Placid, N.Y., 1990, stenotype transcript), B 14.

31. "Resolutions Passed by the 1990 Voting Body," *Report* 21 (December 1990): 15; and "1990 Voting Body," B 15.

32. Should All Health Care Workers Be Tested for HIV/AIDS?" *Report* 22 (September 1991): 1, 6; and "NSYNA Joins Coalition to Oppose Mandatory HIV Testing and Disclosure," *Report* 22 (October–November 1991): 1.

33. In 1991 the incidence of occupational injuries in nursing and personal care facilities alone was 15.5 per one hundred full-time workers — higher than the rates in mining and heavy construction. ("Protect Yourself from Workplace Hazards," *Report* 23 [August 1992]: 1.)

34. "Association Wins Major Grant to Support Occupational Safety and Health Program," *Report* 17 (November–December 1986): 1; "Occupational Hazards Workshops Scheduled for May and June," *Report* 18 (January–February 1987): 1; "New York State Nurses Association [76th Convention]" (Long Island, N.Y., 1991, transcript), 8; and *New York State Nurses Association Annual Report 1998–1999* (Latham, N.Y.: NYSNA, 1999), 6.

35. "Nurses Rally in Albany to Demand Health Care for All!" *Report* 21 (June 1990): 1; and "Nurses Rally in Albany on Health Awareness Day," *Report* 21 (May 1990): 1.

36. "Voting Body Affirms National Health System," *Report* 20 (December 1989): 1; "Landmark New York Health Bill Passes State Assembly: Strong RN Lobbying Pays Off," *Report* 23 (July 1992): 1; and "NYSNA Supports NYHEALTH: Affordable Health Care For All!" *Report* 22 (July 1991): 6.

37. "Two NYSNA Members Appointed to Clinton's Health Review Panel," *Report* 24 (May 1993): 3; and "Clinton Health Plan is a Get Well Card for Americans," *Report* 24 (October–November 1993): 1.

38. "Callan and Wade Attend White House Summit on Health Care Reform," *Report* 25 (April 1994): 8; and "Clinton Plan a Get Well Card," 1.

39. "New York State Nurses Association, 27 October 1994" (Niagara Falls, N.Y., 1994, transcript), 17; "Nurses Demand *Real* Health Care Reform," *Report* 25 (June 1994): 4; and "Whatever Happened to Health Care Reform?" *Report* 25 (October–November 1994): 7.

40. "Is Reform a Threat to the Staff Nurse?" *Report* 25 (April 1994): 1; *Annual Report 1996–1997,* 6; and "Negotiating in a Stormy Sea," *Report* 26 (August 1995): 7.

41. Report of the Executive Director to the Voting Body, 31 October 1997, NYSNA Archives.

42. "Nurses' Rally Helps Halt 3,000 Layoffs," *Report* 25 (December 1994): 16; *1995–1996 Annual Report* (Latham, N.Y.: NYSNA, 1996), [8]; and "Will New York City Abandon Care for the Poor?" *Report* 27 (May 1996): 1.

43. "The New York State Nurses Association 81st Annual Convention" (Buffalo, N.Y., 1996, transcript), 121.

44. *1995–1996 Annual Report,* [7]; and "Columbia-Presbyterian Drops Plan to Replace RNs," *Report* 27 (October–November 1996): 1.

45. Board of Directors Minutes, NYSNA, 9–10 January 1986, NYSNA Archives; "NYSNA Blows Whistle on Improper Use of Technicians," *Report* 27 (April 1996): 1; "Legislators Hear Reports of Illegal, Unlicensed Practice," *Report* 28 (March 1997): 1; and "Delegation & Supervision," *Report* 28 (May 1997): 1.

46. "Putting Jobs to Bed," *Report* 25 (January–February 1994): 7; "Opening the Door to Home Care," *Report* 26 (July 1995): 1; "81st Annual Convention," 116; and *1995–1996 Annual Report,* [8].

47. "81st Annual Convention," 115–16; Report of the Executive Director, 1997; "Facing a Career Crisis? Now There's Help!" *Report* 28 (May 1997): 4. NYSNA's web site was developed in 1997, and provided meeting and workshop schedules, news releases, summaries of articles, position statements, and nursing practice alerts. (*Annual Report 1996–1997,* 9.)

48. Report of the Executive Director, 1997.

49. "Concern Over Health Care Restructuring Dominates Convention," *Report* 25 (December 1994): 4; "Concern for Patients Spurs Nurses to Action," *Report* 26 (January–February 1995): 1; "Why NYSNA is Leading a Campaign to Promote the RN," *Report* 26 (January–February 1995): 14–15; "Ask for a Real Nurse, Ask for an RN," *Report* 26 (March 1995): 4; "No Experience Necessary," *Report* 26 (March 1995): 16; and Report of the Executive Director, 20 October 1995, NYSNA Archives. This was the first time an NYSNA publication was sent to every registered nurse in the state. The special, expanded issue of *Report* was co-sponsored by the State Education Department, and included several pages devoted to education department news. Recommended questions for consumers included, "Will I be cared for by a registered nurse? Will an RN give me my medications and do my treatments? How many other patients will be assigned to the RN who is caring for me? What other workers will be involved in my care?" ("Consumers Respond to NYSNA Advertising Campaign," *Report* 26 [April–May 1995]: 5.)

50. "'Ask for an RN' Campaign Goes Statewide," *Report* 27 (February 1996): 4; "NYSNA Tells Consumers . . . Get Your Free Hospital Evaluation Kit," *Report* 28 (February 1997): 1; *Annual Report 1996–1997,* [8]; and "New Media Campaign Ready to Roll," *Report* 29 (January 1998): 1.

51. "A New World of Health Care—Part II," *Report* 28 (February 1997): 8–9.

52. "NYSNA, 1199/SEIU Enter New Era of Cooperation," *Report* 29 (April 1998): 1.

53. "ANA House of Delegates Votes to Create National Nurses Union," *Report* 30 (July–August 1999): 1.

54. "Who Will Speak for Professional Nursing?" *Report* 29 (October–November 1998): 11.

55. "ANA to Create National Nurses Union," 1.

56. Board Minutes, January 1985 and June 1985; "Dr. Elizabeth Carter to Coordinate NYSNA Entry into Practice Project," *Report* 16 (November–December 1985): 1; Update on Action Proposals; New York State Nurses Association Strategic Plan 1992–1997, Latham, N.Y., 1992, NYSNA Archives; and "NYSNA Sets Course to New Millennium," *Report* 28 (July–August 1997): 6.

57. Update on Action Proposals; "1990 Voting Body," B 9–10; and "New Network to Increase NYSNA's Legislative Clout," *Report* 24 (August 1993): 9.

58. Martha L. Orr to Board of Directors, Memo, 10 January 1989, NYSNA Archives; " [76th Convention]," B 1–30.

59. *New York State Nurses Association Annual Report 1992–1993* (Guilderland, N.Y.: NYSNA, 1993): [7]; and "NYSNA-PAC Charts Successes in 1994 Campaign," *Report* 26 (June 1995): 12.

60. "On the Front Lines of Health Care," *Report* 22 (October–November 1991): 7; "New York State Nurses Association 77th Convention" (Rochester, N.Y., 1992, stenotype transcript), 28; *Annual Report 1992–1993,* [8]; and "81st Annual Convention," 120.

61. "New York State Nurses Association Annual Meeting" (Saratoga Springs, N.Y., 1993, transcript), 21.

62. Board Minutes, 5–6 June 1986; "1990 Voting Body," B 15; and "Alcohol & Drug Problems: They Harm Patients, Nurses, and the Profession," *Report* 22 (March 1991): 5.

63. "NYSNA to Launch Expanded Peer Assistance Program," *Report* 23 (October–November 1992): 1–2; "NYSNA Names Regional Peer Assistance Consultant," *Report* 26 (June 1995): 3; and "Expanded Peer Assistance Program Poised for Action," *Report* 25 (January–February 1994): 3.

64. *Annual Report 1998–1999,* 10; and "NYSNA Lobbying Wins Funding for SPAN Program," *Report* 29 (October–November 1998): 9.

65. "A Plan to Restructure NYSNA Dues," *Report* 22 (August 1991): 8–9.

66. "First Fellows Complete Leadership Program," *Report* 22 (September 1991): 12; "They're Jolly Good Fellows . . . And You Could Be Too!" *Report* 23 (August 1992): 16; and "81st Annual Convention," 116–17.

67. "*Report* Wins Two National Awards," *Report* 23 (August 1992): 6.

68. "77th Convention," 109; "New Year Brings New Mandate for Infection Control Education," *Report* 25 (January–February 1994): 13; and *Annual Report 1996–1997,* 10.

69. Barbara Joyce, "From the President," *Report* 30 (October–November 1999): 2.

FEATURES

MARTHA L. ORR

1. "70th Convention," A 32.

2. "Martha Orr New NYSNA Executive Director; Appointment Effective December 1, 1984," *Report* 15 (September-October 1984): 1; and Report of the Executive Director to the Voting Body, 15 October 1999, NYSNA Archives.

A NEW HEADQUARTERS

1. New York State Nurses Association Strategic Plan, 1992–1997 (Guilderland, N.Y., 1992, mimeographed); and "NYSNA Outgrows Current Headquarters," *Report* 23 (July 1992): 3.

2. "New Headquarters Dedicated in Latham," *Report* 26 (October–November 1995): 1.

3. Ibid.

4. Report of the Executive Director to the Voting Body, 20 October 1995, NYSNA Archives.

EXCERPTS

1. "Membership Divided on Issue," *Report* 18 (September–October 1987): 1.

2. "1990 Voting Body Business Sessions" (Lake Placid, N.Y., 1990, stenotype transcript), C 102.

3. "Mandating Nurse-Patient Ratios," *Report* 24 (March 1993): 1.

4. "Nurses March on Washington to Protest Use of Unlicensed Workers," *Report* 26 (April–May 1995): 1.

5. "[Seventy-sixth Convention]," 22.

6. "Nurses Testify About Crisis in RN Staffing," *Report* 26 (June 1995): 4.

7. "The Aftermath: Solidarity, Confidence and Pride," *Report* 20 (July 1989): 6.

8. "Should Our Association Be for RNs Only?" *Report* 18 (July–August 1987): 1.

9. "[Seventy-sixth Convention]," 22.

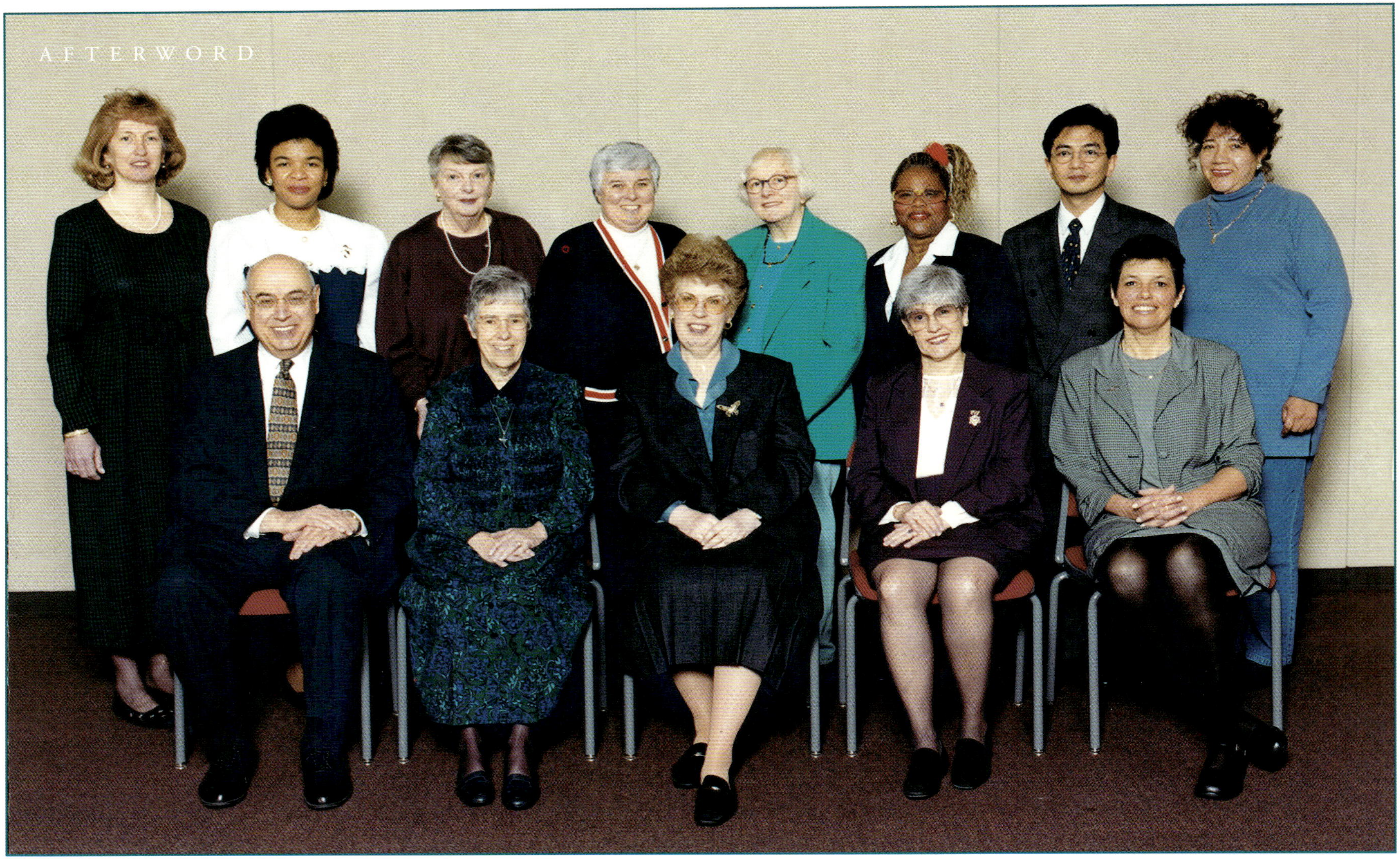

This NYSNA Board of Directors guided the association into the twenty-first century. Shown here is the board which took office in October 1999: standing from left to right are Joanne Billott, Lorna Samuels, Dorothy Williams, Sr. Theresa Graf, Nancy Sweeney, Joan Cumberbatch, Edmund Pajarillo, and Josephine Bolus. Sitting are President-elect Robert Piemonte, Vice President Sr. Mary Finnick, President Phyllis Collins, Treasurer Elizabeth Mahoney, and Secretary Ann Converso. *Photograph by Timothy Raab.*

A GLIMPSE INTO THE FUTURE

As we look to the future let us not focus on pessimism and hopelessness but rather on opportunity and challenge. Accordingly, while we celebrate our past let us profit from it and use it to build our preferred future. We have learned through a study of our heritage that change is an ongoing reality and that dilemmas and issues — nursing shortages, levels of educational preparation, equitable salaries, and questions of professional prestige — are cyclical.

Responding proactively to the trends in the health-care arena will be a significant force as nursing moves into the future. Simultaneously, we will continue to affirm the social contract that exists between the nursing profession and society. The unique position of nursing in the context of the health-care disciplines will be enhanced by advances in science and technology. As Americans continue to be more health conscious, have greater access to health care, and participate in their health-care decisions, the need for professional nursing interventions will escalate. Nurses will advocate for the individual's inalienable right to recognize and understand those options. When nurses educate clients, the locus of decision making control rightfully will remain with those individuals or their designated others. Nurses will provide care along the health to illness continuum throughout the life span and in all settings.[1]

In the past, the nursing profession has generally been regarded as a prestigious calling. This will not change as the future unfolds. A popular contemporary talk show host based in New York has provided priceless nationwide visibility for nurses. He has shared with his vast audience his perceptions of the extraordinary service and care delivered by registered nurses who were responsible for his well-being during his recent hospitalization for cardiac bypass surgery. During this celebrity's first show following this surgery, he featured two RNs (a staff nurse and a nurse practitioner) together with four colleagues (physicians) and thanked them publicly. His flattering and articulate comments describing his view of the importance of the registered nurses' interventions in his personal situation were accurate and cogent. This positive projection of the care received will do much to promote nursing as a competitive career at a time when professional opportunities for each generation become more exciting and diverse. Public testimony, such as this by national figures, will further enhance the current popular trust that the public feels toward nurses.

The volatility of the health-care delivery system and reform at local, state, and national levels will reinforce two constants — the need for flexibility and the management of change. Nurses will need to be visible and vigilant to *ensure their* input into decisions which will affect the quality of care. At the present time there is much media attention to medical errors and health-care quality. Nurses know that these problems often result from systems errors which have a ripple effect. They also know that such regrettable occurrences may be caused by inappropriate staffing, unsafe equipment, and poor communication. Technology will afford nurses new opportunities. It will simultaneously demand additional competencies in a high technology environment. Computers will be the primary source for contemporaneous information as printed materials become increasingly obsolete.

We have a professional responsibility to recruit and retain the brightest and the best from multi-cultural backgrounds into the profession. We are obliged to prepare RNs for their unique function in the health-care delivery system. We will need to continuously evaluate the means by which we educate nursing students to meet the multiplicity of competing demands in the changing workplace, characterized by the present demand for non-institution based services in home and community settings. With the expansion of nursing knowledge and responsibility, the demand that more nurses be prepared at the graduate level will become clear and unequivocal. At the same time, master's degree prepared nurses will facilitate the scientific investigation of clinical nursing problems and provide leadership in integrating appropriate findings into the clinical practice domain.

We have clear evidence that nurses have the tenacity to keep up with demands for better performance as well as assume leadership roles in health care, the profession, and the association. We will build on the strong foundation of our centennial leaders and NYSNA's mission of public protection and advancement of the profession as we begin to document a bicentennial history. I have every confidence that tomorrow's nurses can manage the challenges of the next century. The profession is in good hands. Unquestionably, we will *Honor our Past and Build our Future* with a cadré of confident, talented leaders who are visionary lifetime career professionals empowered for the changing health-care system.

PHYLLIS COLLINS, EdD, RN, CS-FNP
President 2000–2001

CHAPTER NOTE

1. Taken from NYSNA's statement of philosophy.

APPENDIXES

APPENDIX 1
CHARTER MEMBERS

All nurses who joined the association and signed the membership list before the date of incorporation in February 1902, were "charter members," or "founders." By law, these individuals had a lifetime vote in NYSNA matters.

Miss Annie Damer, New York
Miss Julie E. Bailey, Rochester
Miss Martha O'Neill, Brooklyn
Miss E. C. Sandford, Rochester
Miss Eunice A. Hentig, Rochester
Miss Ida R. Palmer, Rochester
Miss Annie R. Young, New York
Miss Emma J. Keating, Buffalo
Miss Anna L. Alline, New York
Miss Christina Hall, Jamestown
Miss Marian Detweiler, Jamestown
Miss E. A. Underhill, Rochester
Miss E. M. Burns, New York
Miss Lillie L. Waterman, Brooklyn
Miss E. H. Hall, Brooklyn
Miss Nellie W. Lee, New York
Miss Sylveen Nye, Buffalo
Miss L. L. Dock, New York
Miss M. Isabel Merritt, Cherry Valley
Miss Eva Allerton, Rochester
Miss Sophie F. Palmer, Rochester
Miss Mary E. Thornton, New York
Miss Anna J. Smith, New York
Miss Hermione D. Stone, New York
Miss Nancy E. Cadmus, Utica
Miss Frances Black, New York
Miss H. A. Staley, Schenectady
Mrs. M. L. Smith, Sandy Hill
Mrs. M. J. Martin, Albany
Mrs. Juliette Lee, Greenwich
Miss Jane G. Roberts, Utica
Miss Gertrude B. Cleveland (Mrs. W. S. Emberson), New Rochelle
Miss Jean Campbell, New York
Miss Laura Haltern, New York
Miss Tillie Both, New York
Miss Isabel Gahn, Buffalo
Miss Anna Davids, Richmond Hill
Miss Nellie S. Couzens, Yonkers
Mr. James J. Coakley, New York
Miss May Gifford, Troy
Miss Sara Burton, Troy
Mrs. May Curtis, Rochester
Miss Mary Brooks, Rochester
Miss Margaret A. Soule, Quaker City
Miss Marie A. Mowatt, New York
Miss Louise Bower, New York
Miss E. Robertson, New York
Miss A. H. Schwartz, Gloversville
Miss Lillian Best (Mrs. John P. Sisson), Gloversville
Miss L. M. Root, Gloversville
Miss Margaret M. Wallace, Auburn
Miss Emily I. MacDonnell, Auburn
Miss Richards, Brooklyn
Miss A. B. McDonald, Brooklyn
Miss Annie Rhodes, New York
Miss M. E. Cameron, New York
Miss Jennie Stillson, New York
Miss Ida M. Cooper, Rochester
Miss Mary H. Crocker, New York
Miss Georgiana Ramsden, New York
Miss Florence E. McDermott, Utica
Miss Bessie Hadley (Mrs. Simon), Utica
Miss H. C. Snell, Brooklyn
Mrs. Marian D. Lingenfelter, Amsterdam
Miss Belle Gardner, Amsterdam
Miss Irene B. Yocum, New York
Miss B. A. S. Taylor, New York
Miss Anna C. Maxwell, New York
Miss Mary Lord, Albany
Miss Mary E. Melville, New York
Miss Alice M. Myers, Brooklyn
Miss Anna M. Hooker, New York
Mr. John M. Hallock, New York
Miss Cathryn Ryan, New York
Miss Ellen Enright, New York
Miss A. W. E. O'Brien, New York
Miss Susan West, New York
Miss Mary A. Samuels, New York
Miss Annie Goodrich, New York
Miss Grace L. Gable, New York
Miss Eva M Gardner, Syracuse
Miss Harriet M. Webber, New York
Miss Bertha C. Cooper, New York
Miss Florence Y. Morange, Tenafly
Miss Mary Bohling, New York
Miss Isabel Burrows, Brooklyn
Miss J. Florence Moore, Brooklyn
Miss Anna M. Charlton, New York
Miss Ann D. Van Kirk, New York
Miss Jessie C. Sleet, New York
Miss Freda E. Wagner, New York
Miss Mary A. Miner, New York
Mrs. E. E. Green, New York
Miss Harriet Livermore, New York
Mrs. C. C. Brown, New York
Miss M. M. Brown, New York
Miss F. A. Stone, New York
Mr. L. Bissell Sanford, New York
Miss L. E. Anderson, New York
Miss Lora Hyde, New York
Miss Frances M. Traphagen, New York
Miss Laura T. Richardson, New York
Miss Mary E. Graf, New York
Miss Helen Sutherland, New York
Mrs. Ada S. Willard, New York
Miss Ida E. Berlet, New York
Miss E. J. Barnard, New York
Miss Isabel L. Evans, New York
Miss Martha C. Drew, New York
Miss C. K. A. McMartin, New York
Miss Agnes Handley, New York
Miss Edith Hooper, New York
Miss Clara L. Arend,Port Richmond
Miss Nellie G. Heck, Brooklyn

Appendix 2

District Nurses Associations

The District Nurses Associations with their original geographic boundaries and year of acceptance into NYSNA are listed below.

1919

District 1
Niagara, Orleans, Erie, Genesee, Wyoming, Chautauqua, and Cattaraugus Counties

District 2
Monroe, Livingston, Alleghany, Wayne, and Ontario Counties

District 3
Yates, Seneca, Steuben, Schuyler, and Chemung Counties

District 4
Cayuga, Cortland, Onondaga, and Oswego Counties

District 7
Madison, Oneida, Herkimer, and Ostego Counties

District 8
Essex, Hamilton, Clinton, and Franklin Counties

District 9
Albany, Rensselaer, Saratoga, Washington, Schoharie, Delaware, Columbia, and Warren Counties

(1919 continued)

District 10
Schenectady, Fulton, and Montgomery Counties

District 1
New York, Richmond, Bronx, and Westchester Counties

District 14
Kings, Queens, Suffolk, and Nassau Counties

1920

District 5
Tioga, Broome, Chenango, and Tompkins Counties

District 6
Jefferson, St. Lawrence, and Lewis Counties

District 11
Greene, Ulster, Sullivan, Orange, and Rockland Counties

District 12
Columbia*, Dutchess, and Putnam Counties

1937

District 15
Chenango and Ostego Counties

1942

District 16
Westchester County

1947

District 17
Rockland County

1955

District 18
Orange and Sullivan Counties

1988

District 19
Suffolk County

*Columbia County was moved from District 9 to District 12 in 1920.

Membership of Selected NYSNA Committees

". . . those who devote time and energy in fulfilling the responsibilities of committee work are the unsung heroes of our membership. Literally they are the backbone of our Association . . . It is at the committee level where much of the initial planning, the thinking through of a problem is done so that finally recommendations may be presented to the Board of Directors for decision and a final course of action decided upon . . . A committee member may be unsung or even misunderstood, but a member of a committee is never to be underestimated—responsible committee members are the basis of our future progress." ("Proceedings, 53rd Meeting of The New York State Nurses Association" [Rochester, N.Y., 1965, stenotype transcript], 8.)

The following is a small sampling of some of the committees, chairpersons, and committee members from NYSNA's first one hundred years.

1901
First Elected Officers
President, Sylveen Nye
Vice-President, Isabel Merritt
Second Vice-President,
Annie R. Young
Secretary, Elizabeth Sandford
Treasurer, Mary E. Thornton

1902
Executive Committee
Miss Garden
Miss Rhodes
Miss Van Kirk

1902
Committee Chairpersons
Revision of By-Laws
Miss I. R. Palmer
Legislation, Miss Allerton
Press and Publication,
Miss S. F. Palmer
Finances, Mr. L. Bissell Sanford
Credentials, Miss Maxwell

1910
Legislative Commitee
Mary D. Burrill
Sophia F. Palmer
Marion T. Brockway
Annie W. Goodrich
Amy M. Hilliard
Lina Lightbourn
Bella J. Fraser

1918–19
Legislative Committee
Miss Margaret Anderson
Mrs. Julia Kline
Miss Mabel Chase
Miss Margaret O'Farrall
Mrs. Anne L. Hansen
Miss Nellie Davis
Miss Lena Kranz
Miss Alice S. Gilman

1925
Committee on
Professional Ethics
Miss Elizabeth C. Burgess, chairperson

1927
Common Activities Committee
(NYSNA Representatives)
Miss Louise R. Sherwood
Miss Lily Strange
Miss Alta Dines
Mrs. Mae Woughter Strack

1933–34
Committee Chairpersons
Service, Miss Alta E. Dines
Legislative, Miss Geneva Hoilen
Men Nurses, Mr. Herbert Nash
Program and Arrangements,
Mrs. Anne L. Hansen
Public Information,
Miss Emma L. Collins
Nurse Practice Act,
Miss Marion Sheahan

1938–39
Registry Committee
Leah Blaisdell
H. Lenore Bradley
Ella G. Casey
Emma L. Collins
Stella M. Hawkins
Alice E. Snyder
Mrs. Genevieve M. Clifford

1943
Service Committee
Alta E. Dines
Blanche F. Mann
Mrs. Margaret Hogg
Arvilla E. Everingham
Mattie Washburn
Mrs. Tessa M. Klein

1946
Nursing Information Committee
Dorothy K. Anker
Frances R. Ball
Marjorie E. Connor
Mary Volweider
Emily L. Creevey

1949–50
Committee on Employment
Conditions for Nurses
Mary Perrone
Ruth M. Brooks
Dorothy E. Clark
Arlene Shaw
Mildred Gent
Mary V. Barrett

1951–52
Committee on
Counselling and Placement
Victoria Frederick
Mrs. Margaret Gile
Mrs. Helen Strong
William Wilkins
Carl E. Tremer
Mrs. Cecelia Abrahamer

1965–67
Committee on
Professional Nursing Practice
Florence Shumway
Celia Heffron
Cynthia Kinsella
Mary Jane Venger
Mildred Smith
Margaret Rogers
Maude B. Miller
Mildred Schmidt
(consultant)
Eleanor Gochanauer
(constultant)
Beatrice Latremore

1967–69
Committee on Education
Enda Scanlon
Olga Andruskiw
June Simpson
Sister Marie Michael
Eleanor C. Lambertsen
(consultant)
Esther M. Thompson
(consultant)
Sister Victoria
Margaret Tyson

1969–71
Special Committee to
Study the Nurse Practice Act
(NYSNA Representatives)
Mrs. Edith Benoit
Doris T. Geiss
Elizabeth Runkle
Sister Kathleen Nolan
Mary Wemett
Eleanor Lambertsen
(consultant)
Laura L. Simms

1980–81
First Human Rights
Committee
Thetis Group
Dorothy Hickey
William Santiago
Kathleen Sward
Juanita Hunter

1981–82
First Awards Committee
Elaine E. Beletz
Iris Brice
Ellen M. Burns
Ann M. Gothler
William F. Greiner
Kathleen M. Nokes

1986–87
Task Force to Establish
a Delegate Assembly
Dorla Alleyne
Elissa DeLorenzo
Patricia Gates
Diane Mackie
Barbara May
Elizabeth McLaughlin
Venolia O'Connor

1992
NYSNA Representatives to
First PAC Board
Connie Vance
Janice Viola
Harriet Brathwaite
Mary Eileen Callan
Barbara May
Marva Wade

Appendix 4
New York State Nurses Association Presidents*

1901–1902
Sylveen Nye

1902–1903
M. Isabel Merritt

1903–1904
Annie Rhodes

1904–1906
Annie Damer RN

1906–1907
Anna Davids RN

1907–1909
Mary D. Burrill RN

1909–1913
M. Louise Twiss RN

1913–1915
Beatrice Van H. Stevenson RN

1915–1916
Maud M. Jack RN

1917–192
Elizabeth Golding RN

1920–1922
Alice S. Gilman RN

1922–1925
Anne L. Hansen RN

1925–1927
Louise R. Sherwood RN

1927–1930
Genevieve M. Clifford RN

1930–1934
Elizabeth Greener RN

1934
Marie Swanson RN

1934–1939
Ethel G. Prince RN

1939–1943
Ruth G. Hall RN

1943–1947
Clare M. Casey RN, MA

1947–1951
Mabel Detmold RN

1951–1955
Mary E. Delehanty RN

1955–1959
Esther M. Thompson RN, MA

1959–1961
Lucille E. Notter RN, EdD

1961–1965
Cora E. Pike RN, MA

1965–1969
Katherine M. Disosway RN, MA

1969–1973
Evelyn M. Peck RN, MA

1973–1974
Laura L. Simms RN, EdD

1974–1975
Janet P. Mance RN, MS

1975–1976
Louise Pan RN, MS

1976–1977
Virginia L. Barker RN, EdD

1977
Grace Dowling RN, EdD

1978–1979
Paul T. Hageman RN, PhD

1979–1981
Elaine E. Beletz RN, EdD

1981–1983
Susan J. Fraley RN, MS

1983–1985
Cecilia F. Mulvey RN, PhD

1985–1987
Ellen M. Burns RN, MSN

1987–1989
Juanita Hunter RN, EdD

1989–1991
Madeline Naegle RN, PhD

1991–1993
Nettie Birnbach RN, EdD

1993–1995
Mary Eileen Callan RN, MS

1995–1997
Marva Wade RN

1997–1999
Barbara Joyce RN, PhD

1999–2001
Phyllis Collins RN, EdD

*Some credentials may be incomplete due to unavailability of the information.

Appendix 5
Executive Secretaries and Executive Directors*

1926–1927
Mae L. Woughter RN

1927–1929
Caroline Garnsey RN

1929–1944
Emily J. Hicks RN

1945–1948
Elizabeth Hall RN

1949–1963
Katherine E. Rehder RN

1963–1969
Marion M. Klappmeier RN

1969–1979
Veronica M. Driscoll RN, EdD

1979–1984
Cathryne A. Welch RN, EdD

1984–
Martha L. Orr RN, MN

*Some credentials may be incomplete due to unavailability of the information.

Appendix 6
Honorary Recognition Recipients

1971
Senator Thomas Laverne
Assemblyman Joseph Pisani

1972
Robert H. Jones III

1978
Ruth W. Harper
Laura L. Simms

1979
Marion Sheahan Bailey
Veronica M. Driscoll

1980
Sally Ann Donihee
Lucille E. Notter

1981
Iris Brice
Ellen Wulff

1982
Eleanor E. Lambertsen
Jerrold Nadler

1983
Mildred L. Green
Mildred L. Montag

1984
Ida O. Benderson
Evelyn M. Peck

1985
Catherine Leach

1986
Leota P. Brown
Cathryne A. Welch

1987
Elaine E. Beletz

1988
Kathleen Hoover

1989
Ada Patton

1990
Carrie B. Lenburg
Thelma Schorr

1991
Maggie Jacobs
Rita Reis Wieczorek

1992
Sylvia M. Barker
Robert Piemonte

1993
Ruth Watson Lubic

1994
James Tallon, Jr.
M. Elizabeth Carnegie

1995
Loretta C. Ford
Cecilia F. Mulvey

1996
Jane Fielding

1997
Erline P. McGriff

1998
Claire Murray

1999
Dorothy E. Ramsey

Selected Bibliography

Hundreds of primary and secondary sources were used in the preparartion of this history. These primary source materials included meeting proceedings and transcripts, minutes, association publications, annual reports, and correspondence. In the early years of the association, the *American Journal of Nursing* contained many editorial comments on meetings, official association reports, and articles by and about New York nurses and association activities. Additional information came from the national nursing journals, newpaper articles, general historical works, and nursing history publications. Readers interested in undertaking additional research are diretced to the footnotes, which contain full bibliographic information on all primary and secondary source materials, and to the slected works listed below.

Ashley, Jo Ann. *Hospitals, Paternalism, and the Role of the Nurse.* New York: Teachers College Press, 1976.

Baer, Ellen D. *Editor's Notes.* New York: National League for Nursing, 1990.

Bullough, Vern L., Olga M. Church, and Alice P. Stein, eds. *American Nursing: A Biographical Dictionary.* Vol. 1. New York: Garland Publishing, 1988.

Carter, Elizabeth and Jane Fielding, eds. *Professionalization of Nursing in New York State: Oral History Interviews with Six Leaders Who Helped to Advance the Mission of NYSNA.* Guilderland, N.Y.: NYSNA, 1988.

Dock, Lavinia L. *A History of Nursing.* Vol. 3. New York: G.P. Putnam's Sons, 1912.

Donahue, M. Patricia. *Nursing, The Finest Art: An Illustrated History.* St. Louis, Mo.: Mosby-Year Book, 1996.

Driscoll, Veronica M. *Legitimizing the Profession of Nursing: The Distinct Mission of The New York State Nurses Association.* Guilderland, N.Y.: Foundation of NYSNA, 1976.

Fitzpatrick, M. Louise, ed. *Prologue to Professionalism: A History of Nursing.* Bowie, Md.: Brady Communications, 1983.

Flanagan, Lyndia. *One Strong Voice.* Kansas City: American Nurses' Association, 1976.

Kalisch, Philip A. and Beatrice J. Kalisch. *The Advance of American Nursing.* 3rd ed. Philadelphia: J. B. Lippincott, 1995.

Melosh, Barbara. *The Physician's Hand.* Philadelphia: Temple University Press, 1982.

Roberts, Mary M. *American Nursing: History and Interpretation.* New York: MacMillan Company. 1954.

Stapleton, Darwin H. and Cathryne A. Welch, eds. *Critical Issues in American Nursing in the Twentieth Century: Perspectives and Case Studies.* Guilderland, N.Y.: Foundation of NYSNA, 1994.

Tomes, Nancy. "The Silent Battle — Nurse Registration in New York State, 1903 to 1920." In *Nursing History–New Perspectives, New Possibilities,* edited by Ellen C. Lagemann, 107–132. New York: Teachers College Press, 1983.

INDEX

T

U

V

W

Y

Z

PUBLISHING

First printing, 2000
Q Publishing LLC
Franklin, Virginia
757-569-0929

To purchase copies of this book, contact Organization Services at NYSNA, 11 Cornell Road, Latham, NY 12110. Telephone 518-782-9400.

Library of Congress Cataloging-in-Publication Data
Pavri, Julie M.
Honoring our past, building our future : a history of the New York State Nurses Association / by Julie M. Pavri.
p. cm.
Includes bibliographical references and index.
ISBN 0-9665228-5-0 (alk. paper)
1. New York State Nurses Association. 2. Nursing—New York. (State)—Societies—History. I. New York State Nurses Association. II. Title

RT5.N5 P386 2000
610.73'06'0747—dc21

00-030590

Printed in Iceland
Elizabeth B. Bobbitt, Creative Director

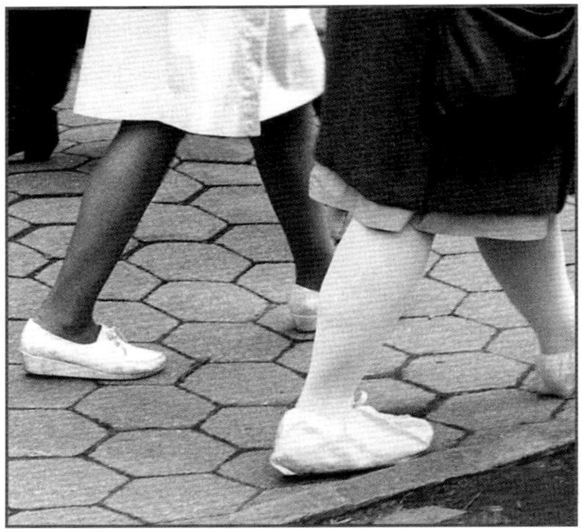

THESE FEET WERE MADE FOR WALKING . . .

Nurses pounded the pavements for better patient care and fair treatment as employees.

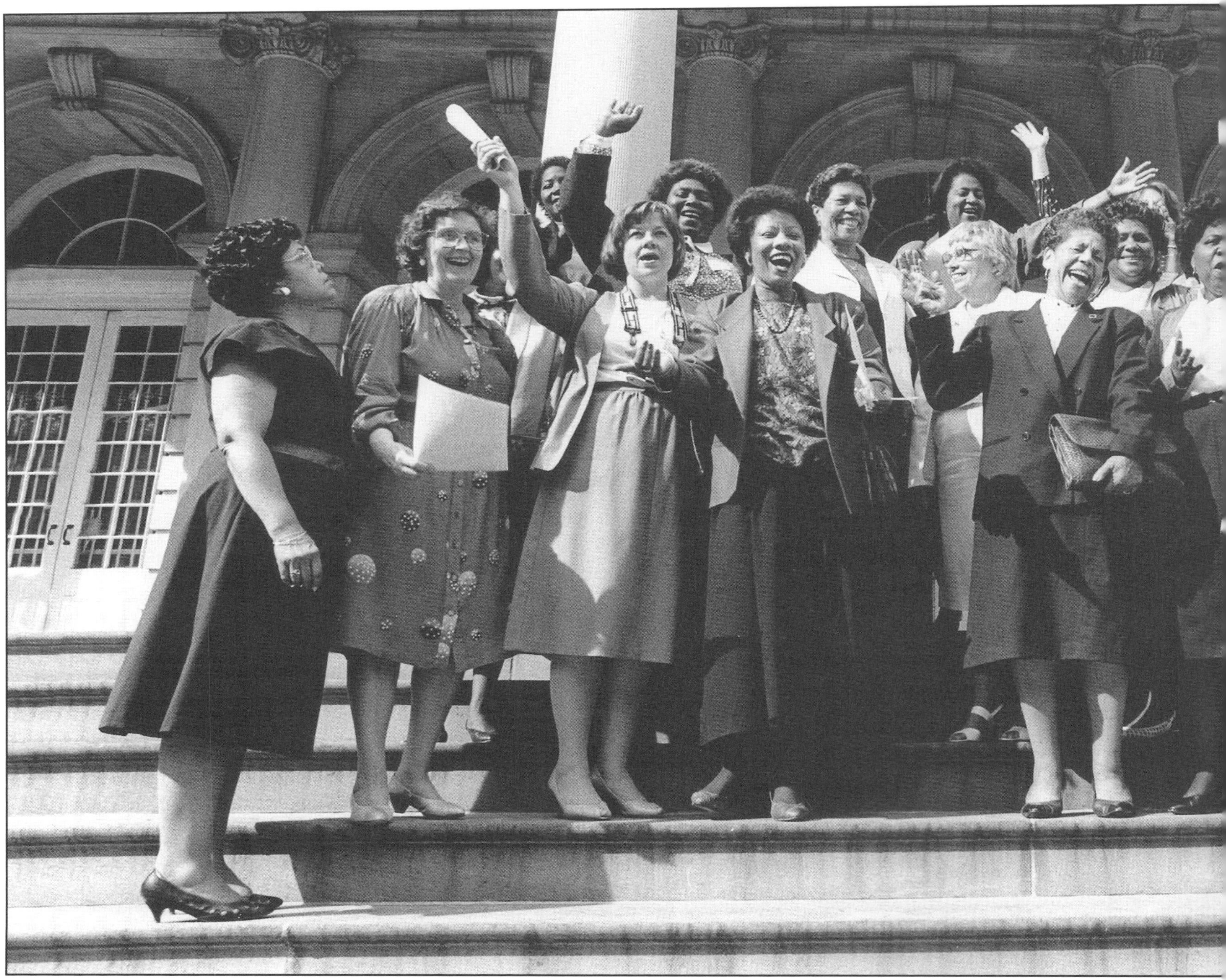